REAL FOOD KETO

Applying Nutritional Therapy to Your Low-Carb, High-Fat Diet

International Bestselling Author
Jimmy Moore
& Christine Moore, NTP
Recipes by **Maria Emmerich**

VICTORY BELT PUBLISHING

LAS VEGAS

Published by Victory Belt Publishing Inc.

ISBN-13: 978-1-628603-16-3

Cover Design, Interior Design & Illustrations by Justin-Aaron Velasco

Printed in Canada

TC 0118

CONTENTS

FOREWORD

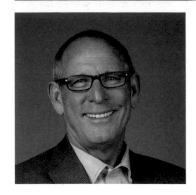

We are currently in the midst of a healthcare crisis of almost unimaginable proportions! To some degree, almost everyone is acutely aware of the crisis in the ways it affects us collectively as a society and the ways it touches our lives individually. However, from a societal perspective, we don't talk about healthcare, which is a problem. Oh, we talk about sickness care and how we individually and collectively pay for it, but that's not the only issue. The much deeper and more profound question is, "Why are so many people so sick?" Or maybe an even better way to put it is, "Why aren't people healthy?" As Jimmy and Christine Moore point out in this book, *Real Food Keto*, health is not just the absence of disease or infirmity; it's "a dynamic state of complete physical, mental, spiritual, and social well-being." More and more of us have diagnosable health problems, but the bigger problem is that very few people are actually living a healthy life!

I've developed a concept that I like to call the Hallway of Life and the Nightmare of Yet. The Hallway of Life is a continuum that goes from absolute, perfect health to death. You're reading this book about improving your diet and health, so you very likely know that you're not at a state of perfect health. (By the way, you're not alone; no one is in that state of perfection.) We all exist somewhere in this hallway, and we're all heading in one direction or the other—toward perfect health or sickness and death.

Along this hallway are markers that help us gauge where we are. The first marker for most of us is a symptom (or symptoms, in some cases). Many of us believe that if we don't have symptoms, then we're healthy. That's not exactly true. The human body is extremely adaptable, and long before we have symptoms, we have wandered away from perfect health. The mistaken assumption is that having a few symptoms—such as headaches, fatigue, minor allergies, heartburn, or poor sleep—are just part of life, and we need to put up with it. Maybe we take an over-the-counter medication to relieve the symptom, or, if we're more holistically minded, maybe we use a medicinal herb. There's nothing wrong with that, right? Wrong!

Every symptom you have is your body's way of telling you that you're doing something wrong, and you need to change whatever it is in your environment that's causing the occurrence of the symptom—be it your diet or your lifestyle. Taking aspirin might make your headache go away in the short term, but it won't address the reason you have a headache. Taking an antacid might make your heartburn go away temporarily, but it will not address why you have heartburn. When you cover up these symptoms without ever addressing the cause, they almost always get worse and worse. Your symptoms will likely become more worrisome or acute until you go to see a medical doctor. And that brings us to the next marker in our Hallway of Life—the diagnosis. In its most fundamental terms, medicine is the diagnosis and treatment of disease.

Within each of us is a fear that we'll eventually get "It"—some horrible disease that will ruin our lives. For some of us, it's heart disease; for others, it's cancer. More and more, we're learning to fear dementia as many of us are diagnosed at younger and younger ages with Alzheimer's or other forms of cognitive decline. When we seek medical care, it's important to realize that many doctors are not trained to make you healthy (although there are now some notable exceptions who are doing things differently). They're trained to diagnose and treat disease.

The good news is that doctors are very good at coming up with a diagnosis. They can tell you if you have "It" already, and that's a good thing because they have a lot of tools to keep "It" from killing you. For example, if you have heart disease, doctors can do open-heart surgery, put in stents, or give you powerful drugs to keep you from dying. If you have cancer, doctors can give you chemotherapeutic agents, radiation, or surgery. These are all good things because life is sacred, and I appreciate that modern medicine can save my life and the lives of the people I love. But what modern medicine can't do is make you healthy again. That's just not what most doctors are trained to do. If you get Alzheimer's disease, good luck; at this point, they can do next to nothing to help you with it.

So that's what we all need to understand: You don't go to the doctor to *get healthy*. You go to find out if you have "It" happening already. If you do have "It," you'd better pray that you have good insurance because having "It" in the United States of America is very expensive, and sometimes the cure is as bad as the disease. Which brings me to the second part of my concept: the Nightmare of Yet! What is the "It" that you fear? And, do you have "It" yet?

But there is good news. Wherever you are in the Hallway of Life, you get to choose which direction you're headed. In our culture, we've been taught to believe that life is a journey that brings us from a healthy place to a place where we develop symptoms, get sick, receive a diagnosis, and undergo treatment to keep us alive. In this book, Jimmy and Christine Moore show you that you can turn around and go the other way from most points in the Hallway! You can be healthier tomorrow than you are today, and you can be healthier next year than you are this year. Jimmy and Christine are living proof of that truth!

One important concept that Jimmy and Christine discuss is epigenetics. Although genes change very slowly, the way genes are expressed through these mechanisms (or epigenetics) can change very rapidly. And once changes happen, they can be passed down and exaggerated from generation to generation. So, when we don't take care of ourselves, we're also affecting the health of our unborn children and the generations that follow. Dr. Francis Pottenger, Jr. demonstrated this phenomenon in his famous cat studies (which Jimmy and Christine explain in *Real Food Keto*). A significant part of our current health crisis is the result of diets that have relied heavily on highly processed foods that we have been eating for several generations. From an epigenetics point of view, we have collectively dug ourselves into a deep hole with the unconscionable amount of sugar and highly processed carbohydrates we feed our children, and it's time to start digging our way out!

Modern societies have strayed away from healthy food choices for a long time now, but things have worsened in the last fifty years or so since we collectively started on the low-fat, high-carbohydrate diet that is considered to be "normal." It's simply not! In fact, this low-fat, high-carb way of eating is what I consider the ultimate fad diet, and it needs to stop.

Thankfully, things are starting to change. A real food movement is afoot. People like Jimmy and Christine Moore are leading the way as they shepherd us back to the whole foods that will restore our health, the health of our children, and the health of the planet itself.

I hope you embrace the wisdom in *Real Food Keto* whether you're doing it for a therapeutic intervention to restore your health or as a permanent lifestyle change. Either way, your body will thank you, and you will leave behind a legacy of health and vibrancy for generations to come.

Thank you, Jimmy and Christine, for this wonderful guide to living the *Real Food Keto* life!

Gray Graham, BA, NTP
Founder of the Nutritional Therapy Association (NTA)

INTRODUCTION

Perhaps you picked up this book because you're sick and tired of being sick and tired all the time, and you're searching for a solution to your health and weight problems. This book is for you. Or maybe you're already making a lifestyle change that has sent you down the path of including more real, whole foods in your diet, and you want inspiration as you trudge forward one step at a time on this journey. This book is also for you. And it's possible that seeing the term *keto* in the title of this book appealed to you because you've heard so much about how this incredibly healthy low-carb, moderate-protein, high-fat diet plan is helping millions upon millions of people get their lives back. That's right; this book is for you as well.

We called this book *Real Food Keto* for a reason: We believe that a well-formulated and highly effective ketogenic diet is one that needs to be customized to the individual and should include fresh foods that taste delicious, nourish the body, and heal you from the inside out. The goal of any health-promoting nutritional approach should be to optimize your health by tweaking it to your situation. We don't all start on the pathway to healthy living at the same point; therefore, we should never compare our journey with the people we see around us or online. Sure, it's human nature to make comparisons, but it would be like comparing a high school basketball player to Lebron James—they're not even close to being at the same level in their experience. If this concept about not comparing yourself to others is the only thing you take from this book, then it's a valuable lesson that will serve you well in the years to come.

Is this uplifting and encouraging message already resonating with you in some way? If so, then that's great, and we're happy to hear it! Keep reading for even more inspiration and education as you travel along this road to a healthier life. But perhaps you're still kind of skeptical about all this "real food and keto" talk and need a lot more convincing before you dive headfirst into it. Maybe you're wondering who exactly is behind this book and why you should believe anything we're sharing. That's fair, and we're happy to address your concern.

Our names are Christine and Jimmy Moore, and we live in Spartanburg, South Carolina. Christine is a Nutritional Therapy Practitioner (NTP) and health podcaster. Jimmy is an international bestselling health-book author (*Keto Clarity, The Ketogenic Cookbook, The Keto Cure, The Complete Guide to Fasting*) and top nutritional health podcaster (*The Livin' La Vida Low-Carb Show, Keto Talk with Jimmy Moore & Dr. Will Cole, The KetoHacking MD Podcast, Nutritional Pearls Podcast*). Everybody has heard Jimmy's inspiring story of weight loss and health gain that happened back in 2004 and launched his name into the health space, but not many people have heard about Christine's health struggles, which had very little to do with needing to lose weight and much more to do with other health issues. Let us formally introduce you to Christine so you know where she's coming from in this book and how her experience has influenced what she's sharing with you.

CHRISTINE'S STORY

I almost didn't make it in this world; I was born prematurely after only six months of gestation. I weighed just two and a half pounds. The doctors had to use oxygen therapy to help keep me alive, and back then they weren't as knowledgeable about the physical dangers of overexposing a baby to oxygen as we are today. As a result, the blood vessels in my left eye tore the retina, and now I'm completely blind in that eye except when bright lights are shining in it. The same damage started to happen in my right eye. The doctors weren't aware that the oxygen they were using was causing damage to my eyes. The damage had been done, though, and my prospects for a normal life with the ability to see well were bleak. (In fact, when Jimmy asked my dad for his permission to marry me, my dad told Jimmy that the doctors had said I'd be completely blind by the age of thirty-five.)

I was born on November 11, and the doctors had planned for me to be in the hospital until the new year. However, against their better medical judgment, they gave my parents a gift by letting them take me home on Christmas Eve. I was fragile but alive. My parents had no idea their newborn baby had come into this world with health issues.

My eyesight problems didn't become apparent to my parents until I was about two years old; that's when they realized I wasn't focusing on objects like I was supposed to. They received the devastating news that I was blind in my left eye and had significant vision damage in my right eye. Because of the physical challenges I was going to face, my parents kick-started my education

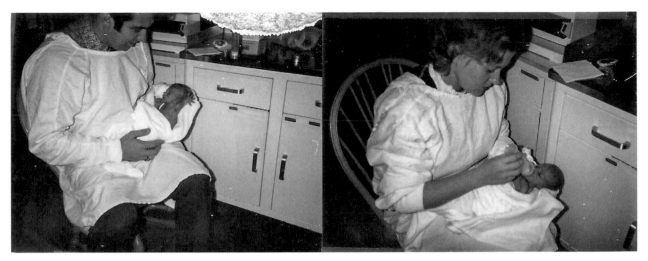

November 29, 1972

when I was three by enrolling me in pre-kindergarten classes for special-needs kids. My mom and dad had the great foresight to do this for me, and it helped me keep up with the rest of the kids in class when I got to elementary school. My parents sacrificed much time and money to give me as many advantages as possible, and I'll forever be grateful to them for what they did. This book truly is a miracle and never would have happened without John and Elizabeth Woodward. I thank God for them daily for loving me despite the challenge I presented them. They taught me at an early age that I was just like all the other kids and to always believe in myself. Thanks to them, I did, and I still do.

While my mom got me interested in singing, playing piano, drawing, and other extracurricular activities to distract me from my visual impairment (and the really thick Coke-bottle glasses that other kids made fun of me for wearing), I started to notice various health issues rearing their ugly heads. I was often sick throughout my childhood, and I was in and out of the hospital far too many times to count with pneumonia and other respiratory issues. I was probably put on ten different rounds of antibiotics before I was a teenager. Of course, no one realized that the antibiotics were significantly damaging my gut health, and they would eventually negatively impact my health even more when I became an adult.

When I was eleven years old, my parents took me to the doctor because I was complaining of low back pain. The doctor ordered a battery of tests and found only a slight curvature of the spine, but the pain I was experiencing in my back quickly spread to joints all over my body. Never in a million years was it on my mom and dad's radar screen that what we were eating could possibly be related to my back pain. No one made a connection between our diets and what happened to our health, so nothing changed, and my pain persisted. I took aspirin daily to manage the discomfort. Nobody needs to be taking medications every single day at that age! However, it's what I had to do because mainstream medicine didn't have another answer for me.

By the time I turned sixteen, my back pain was worsening each time I had my monthly menstrual cycle. When my parents took me back to the doctor, yet again there were no answers for us; the doctor stated that there was nothing wrong with me. My periods were often very irregular and extremely painful. Over time, I learned to deal with the pain and resigned myself to the idea that this was just my lot in life. If I had known then what I know now, life would have been so much better for me. (I hope that reading my story is showing you that you're never too far gone to make changes in your health. Keep reading and you'll see what I mean.)

Through all the pain I endured, I never had a problem with being overweight. In fact, I had the exact opposite problem—I was severely underweight for the first twenty-one years of my life. We never made the connection between my diet and the health issues I was having because they didn't manifest as excess weight. If anything rebuts the adage that what you weigh determines whether you're healthy, then this is it. I was certainly very thin, but I was *not* healthy. Jimmy and I address this topic again later in the book because it's shocking how many people think their weight determines their state of health, and it's just not true.

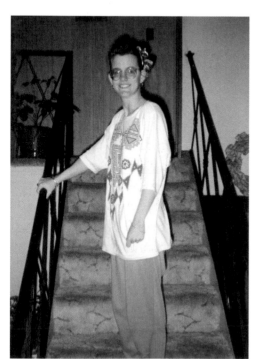

I graduated high school in 1991 and was salutatorian of my class. I decided to pursue an associate degree in elementary education at the local community college, and while I was taking classes there, I met a man named Jimmy Moore. He was working on his master's degree and started attending my church. We both loved to sing and were in the church choir together. Little did I know that Jimmy was interested in me, but he was hesitant about asking me out because he thought I was way too old for him. I was stick thin (about 90 pounds at the time) and wore really thick glasses and a hairstyle that made me look older than I was. He told one of the choir members that he thought I was thirty-five years old. I was only twenty-one! When he found this out, the boy couldn't ask me out fast enough.

Jimmy was already a very large man at six-foot-three and 330 pounds. So where did this future ketogenic diet leader take me on our first date? McDonald's, of course. We both ordered a Big Mac, super-size fries, and a large Coke, and it was the first of many fast-food meals that we would share over the years. Once again, we were oblivious to what these "foods" were doing to our bodies. (We now call them "foodlike disease agents" because none of them can be even remotely considered real food, even if Mickey D's brags about having "fresh beef" in its burgers.) When we married on August 5, 1995, the difference in our weights was nearly 250 pounds. We were far from being the happy, real food–eating keto couple that people know us as today. We had many more years and lots more health problems to work through first.

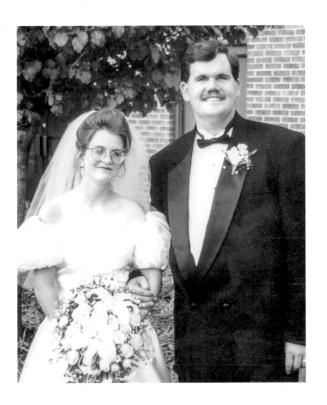

In our first two years of marriage, I was under a great deal of stress from the financial difficulties many young couples face; I also didn't realize that I had a very poor diet. For example, I would regularly consume fast food from Chick-fil-a and McDonald's, pasta, rice, M&Ms, Skittles, and Dr. Pepper. Keep in mind that I was still very underweight, and I thought my low weight gave me license to eat anything and everything I wanted because it wouldn't make me pack on the pounds as it had with Jimmy. Little did I know that eating whatever crappy food I wanted was doing significant damage to my health.

The signs of damage continued to pop up, though. For example, I had a series of urinary tract infections in the first year of our marriage that required me to be on a round of very strong antibiotics for three months straight! If I had known then what I know now about having a healthy gut microbiome, I never would have allowed myself to do that because, in the long run, it certainly didn't help my overall health. (Later in the book, Jimmy and I talk at great length about healing the gut.) And this was only the beginning of my ever-growing laundry list of health woes that seemed to be getting worse and worse as the years went by.

Eventually, I started having anxiety attacks and struggling with bouts of depression, which required me to take antidepressants like Zoloft and Paxil. Both my mom and my sister Jennifer took these medications, so I just thought it was a genetic thing that we all had to do to function. It never dawned on me at the time that I didn't have a pharmaceutical drug deficiency; I had a nutrient deficiency, and my body was screaming at me to correct it. My crappy diet was catching up to me, but I was still oblivious to the connection between my nutrition and my health. We've all been in this position at some point in lives, right?

In 2002, the day before my thirtieth birthday, I started noticing what felt like sunburn in the middle of my back, and I discovered I had a rash in that area. I also had a feeling of being run-down, like I was coming down with a cold. So, the next day, on my birthday, I went to see my family doctor. He looked at my back and first thought I might have had an allergic reaction to a new detergent. I informed him that I hadn't changed anything and that I didn't feel well aside from having the rash. He finally concluded that I had come down with shingles. He was pretty shocked because shingles normally manifests in older people. However, because of my crappy diet and the amount of stress I was under, my immune system was weakened to the point that shingles had developed. What a wonderful birthday present for me . . . not!

In 2004, after receiving a book from my mom for Christmas called *Dr. Atkins' New Diet Revolution,* Jimmy went on the low-carb Atkins diet to deal with his morbid obesity and health issues. He was doing so well—losing 100 pounds in the first 100 days—that he wanted to get more exercise. One of our favorite activities was volleyball, which Jimmy loved playing because, as a tall man, he could spike and block from the front row. One particular evening, we were playing a friendly game at our church when someone spiked the ball down hard directly on my right eye, which is the only eye I could actually see out of! It scared the bejeebies out of all of us, but I thought I was okay. About a week later, though, I started seeing flashes of light and black spots in my vision, which the doctor said were signs that my retina was becoming detached in that good eye. I was thirty-one years old and feared I was going to become permanently blind in both eyes, just as my dad had warned Jimmy might happen by the time I was thirty-five.

I went to see the retina specialist, and he confirmed that my retina was starting to detach. They did emergency laser surgery, and while they were in there looking around, they discovered a cataract had developed in my left eye (the one I'd never been able to see out of). Because the cataract could cause issues down the road, the eye doctor also did surgery to remove it. Later that same year, I had yet another eye surgery to correct the weak muscles that caused me to have a lazy eye. Because I had dealt with vision issues from birth, I never imagined my eyesight had anything to do with what I was eating. Later in this book, we discuss the role blood sugar imbalances play in leading to a whole host of problems, including eye issues.

So, with all this "stuff" going on with my health, you probably think I ironically had a dog named Lucky, right? Well, unfortunately, my problems were far from over.

In 2006, my gallbladder started causing me so much pain that I had to have it removed. I have since learned that eating a low-fat diet for many years contributes to the bile becoming thick and sludgy so that it can't pass through the bile ducts, which can lead to gallstones and inflammation of the gallbladder. It makes me rethink and regret every decision I ever made about eschewing fat in my diet because I thought a low-fat diet was making me healthier. It did precisely the opposite, making my health worse—much worse. Fat-phobia has directly contributed to so many of the health problems people are dealing with today. We talk about the role of healthy fats, which include saturated fats, later in the book.

During this time, my doctor ran an endoscopy as he tried to determine whether it was indeed my gallbladder that was causing the pain. The endoscopy revealed that I had tiny ulcers all over my stomach, which came as a big surprise to me because I wasn't experiencing any pain from them. The doctor put me on a proton pump inhibitor (Nexium is an example). Little did I know that I wasn't suffering from a stomach acid surplus but a stomach acid deficiency. Jimmy and I cover the importance of stomach acid in Chapter 10. Although I still seem to have a little trouble with my stomach, I'm working on healing those issues through vitamin and mineral supplementation.

Then in 2007, I found out that I had a severe case of endometriosis, an autoimmune disease that creates abnormal tissue growth along the outside of the uterine lining. It's extremely painful and can contribute to infertility. The reproductive endocrinologist who found the endometriosis finally gave me some answers to the nagging pain I was having. He performed surgery to remove it, and Jimmy and I were hopeful that this would solve our problem with conceiving.

The very next year, we went through an in vitro fertilization/intracytoplasmic sperm injection (IVF/ICSI) cycle that failed to produce a baby despite the many daily hormone injections I was giving myself. The lack of success nearly caused us to give up on having kids forever, but we weren't willing to surrender just yet. By this time, I had watched Jimmy successfully lose more than 100 pounds on a low-carb, high-fat diet and completely change his health, and I decided I wanted to try this low-carb thing, too. Unfortunately, despite Jimmy's enthusiasm for livin' la vida low-carb (as he called it), I wasn't that serious about it yet, so I was only sorta, kinda eating low-carbish. I now know that you can't eat low-carb and high-fat (commonly known as keto, short for the ketogenic diet) and expect results without fully committing yourself to it. It's a lifestyle change that you need to implement fully, or you might as well not even bother. Once again, I didn't see the undeniable connection between all my health issues and the nutrition I had been led to believe was "healthy."

In 2009, I was thirty-six, and I had been dealing with nagging joint pain since my childhood. I went to see a rheumatologist about it, and the doctor told me nothing was wrong with me. Because the autoimmune condition known as rheumatoid arthritis runs on my mother's side of the family over at least three generations, I was concerned I might be developing it, too. Interestingly, my doctor ordered a test that I'd never had before—25-hydroxy vitamin D—which measures the level of vitamin D in the blood. I had no idea how important the results of this test would become in my health journey. The so-called "normal" range for vitamin D is 20 to 50 ng/mL,[1] but a better functional medicine range for optimal health is closer to 40 to 60 ng/mL.

Imagine my surprise when I learned that my vitamin D level was a measly 9 ng/mL! NINE! My rheumatologist said it was probably the lowest level he'd ever seen, and he speculated that it might be a contributing factor in my many health issues. We go into more detail about vitamin D in Chapter 9, but suffice it to say that I was in desperate need of raising that level to get it closer to normal. Jimmy had already interviewed a few vitamin D experts for his podcast who recommended high-dose vitamin D3 gel caps along with regular sun exposure.

So I started taking 10,000 IU of vitamin D3 daily and noticed that something pretty remarkable started happening—the chronic joint pain I'd learned to deal with suddenly started to subside. I also no longer needed those antidepressant and anxiety medications that I had taken for about a decade. I just stopped taking them and never went back on them again! Is it possible that I went through years and years of taking these powerful prescription drugs when all I was dealing with was a vitamin D deficiency? Yep. I was finally waking up to the realization of just how important nutritional optimization was in my health.

Soon after, I went to see my primary care physician for a physical, and he conducted a standard lipid panel, which includes LDL, HDL, triglycerides, and total cholesterol. When the results came back, my triglycerides (the truly bad fat in the blood that is much worse than LDL will ever be) came in at a whopping 298. The standard lab test says to keep this number below 150, but we now know that the functional healthy range is actually below 100 and optimally under 70. (If you're interested in learning more, Jimmy wrote an excellent book about this subject called *Cholesterol Clarity*.) As soon as I showed Jimmy my results, he said, "You know how to fix that," insinuating that I needed to start eating a low-carb diet immediately to bring that number down. That meant giving up my beloved Dr. Pepper, Skittles, and M&Ms. Boo-hoo! However, I knew my health was at stake, and I was determined to turn things around. Simply cutting these sugary, empty-calorie foods out of my diet for six weeks helped me drop my triglycerides to 135, which is an example of how profoundly and swiftly change can happen in your biomarkers when you stop feeding your body "carbage" and start embracing whole foods. That's the very essence of what we aim to teach you in *Real Food Keto*.

Just as I was coming to terms with my years (decades!) of proverbially sticking my fingers in my ears about how the foods I was eating were affecting my health, a medical doctor friend of Jimmy's told us about an alternative-medicine physician who did intravenous chelation therapy to remove heavy metals from the body. When I visited this physician, and he tested me, my results included off-the-charts levels of cadmium, thallium, and tungsten. I had figured out another key piece of my health puzzle with very little help from mainstream medicine.

As I was talking to the chelation doctor about how these heavy metals had built up in my body, he explained that the high-carbohydrate diet I'd eaten most of my life spiked my blood sugar levels so much that my body couldn't effectively detoxify the metals from my body. (We discuss detoxification at great length in Chapter 13.) I went on several rounds of intravenous chelation therapy over the course of a week to help address the chronic joint pain I'd dealt with for so long. My body was healing from years upon years of needless damage, and that motivated me to become a lot more engaged and purposeful in my food and lifestyle choices. I was becoming passionate about nutrition and health the way Jimmy had just a few years prior.

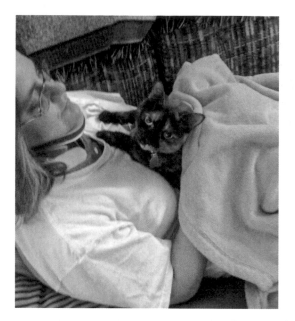

Beginning in 2009, I had the first of what would be not one, not two, but *three* surgeries on my neck. (Yes, I had a pain in the neck, and it wasn't Jimmy this time!) The first surgery addressed a herniated disc with a spinal fusion of the C4/5 vertebrae. For the second surgery, the doctor had to go in through the back of my neck to shave down a bone spur that was pressing against a nerve and causing me pain. I later learned through my training as a Nutritional Therapy Practitioner that the bone spur was probably due to vitamin K2 deficiency. My blood calcium levels were completely normal according to lab test results, but it's K2 that tells the calcium where to go in the body. (We share more about this in Chapter 9.) My third surgery was for another spinal fusion—this time of the C5/6 vertebrae. The spinal fusions probably could have been prevented had I made better nutrition choices earlier in life and achieved an adequate micronutrient intake. Again, this underscores just how important it is to have proper nutrition from an early age.

In 2011, Jimmy and I tried one more time to have children through embryo adoption, which meant I experienced lots of long needles full of progesterone being pushed into my hips on a daily basis, and I became pregnant with twins. Because I was feeding myself and two babies, I really got serious about my diet and lifestyle. I became more purposeful about eating low-carb, high-fat, and ketogenic. All the research we had seen at that point for fertility and pregnancy showed massive benefits to combining keto with nutrient-dense foods like liver. (Jimmy actually cut cow liver into pill shapes and then froze them to help me get more vitamins A, C, and E, zinc, selenium, copper, chromium, iron, and this funny-sounding nutrient called molybdenum!)

Two months after getting the happiest news of our lives (we'd been trying to get pregnant for sixteen years at that point), we lost the babies. We were devastated because we had gone from the highest of happy highs to the lowest of lowly lows in an instant. The realization that having children of our own probably wasn't going to happen brought Jimmy and me closer together. (If one more person told us to "just adopt" after this traumatic experience, I think I would have screamed.) We have come to terms with being a childless couple, but that doesn't alleviate the frustration I feel from the complications that went back to all the untreated childhood health issues that nobody helped me figure out. It wasn't my parents' fault. They didn't know because no one told them. How many other people are dealing with these sorts of issues and thinking they're just a normal part of life?

Shortly after losing my twin babies, another key element in this gigantic health puzzle became clear to me. Through his podcast, Jimmy had heard about a genetic test called methylenetetrahydrofolate reductase, or MTHFR, which can be run by practically any doctor if you ask for the test by name. I asked to have the test conducted, and the specific gene mutation I have is the C677T, which I inherited from both my mother and my father (which is known as heterozygous gene mutation). Because of this mutation, my body can't turn folic acid into folate. (Anyone who discovers they have this MTHFR gene mutation can supplement with methylated folate, which provides the much-needed micronutrient folate for various functions of the body.) The lack of adequate folate combined with the crappy carbage-laden, generally low-fat diet that I'd followed for most of my life is probably one of the major contributors to why we couldn't have kids, which is something that underscores the critical role of dietary fat in making the body function as God intended. We get deeper into this subject later in the book.

I was three months into going keto when I had an appointment with my ophthalmologist for my annual checkup. Because I had been born prematurely and doctors had given me excess oxygen, which seemingly had caused permanent eye damage, my vision had gotten progressively worse and worse with every single yearly checkup. Each new prescription required brand-new glasses that cost more than $1,000. Yikes!

At this ophthalmologist appointment, I was bracing for another eye-popping bill, but, to my amazement, something happened for the first time in my life—my prescription went the other direction! In other words, my eyesight got *better*. What the what?! When I told my parents, who had spent a fortune buying me glasses over the years, they were amazed. How in the world could a simple dietary change make such a miraculously profound impact? Here's the best part: Since that appointment, I've been wearing the same prescription for seven years and counting. If that's not an endorsement for embracing healthy nutrition, then I don't know what is!

As I continued on keto, almost all my remaining joint pain went away. I still have bad days when a change in weather is coming, but it's nothing like it was just a few years ago. I began to notice that I had increased energy, and my head felt clearer than it had in years. My anxiety attacks diminished significantly, and over time they disappeared. I don't suffer from them anymore. Thank God!

In 2015, I was diagnosed with an autoimmune disease known as Hashimoto's thyroiditis. I had been noticing the telltale signs of this disease for more than a decade before I even started keto—hair loss, sensitivity to cold, tiredness, and weight gain—and I was getting frustrated because my primary care physician was running lab tests for only TSH, T3, and T4. I knew from Jimmy's work that there were more relevant markers that a full thyroid panel could check, including reverse T3, free T4, free T3, calcitonin, thyroglobulin, and thyroid antibodies. My doctor, like most mainstream medical professionals, ran only the TSH test and said that everything was normal. However, I could tell that everything was *not* fine, and even though I asked, my doctor never bothered to run all the other numbers for me. This disconnect between educated patients and old-guard physicians is one of the great travesties of the American healthcare system.

Jimmy suggested that we run the full panel ourselves and have some of his doctor friends help us interpret the results. So we went to an online lab test company (we used PrivateMDLabs.com) and ordered the test, paying out of pocket. When the results came in, we noticed the thyroid peroxidase antibodies were double what they should have been, which indicated very clearly that I had Hashimoto's. When I took these test results to my doctor and asked him if he would put me on Armour Thyroid, which is made from desiccated pig thyroid to mimic human thyroid hormone, he agreed to let me try it. I'm still taking this hormone pill to this day. Interestingly, my thyroid antibodies have slowly come down since I've been following a ketogenic diet. BAM!

Because I already had one autoimmune disease, I was prone to others. One of the other autoimmune issues that I had to deal with was the endometriosis for which I'd had surgery in 2007 before I went strict keto. It simply wasn't getting better. In fact, it came back with a vengeance, causing abdominal pain like never before. When I went to see a doctor about it in 2016, he said that if we were no longer pursuing having children, then I should have a complete hysterectomy to remove the endometriosis. When he got in there to do the surgery, he realized I had one of the worse cases of endometriosis he'd ever seen. As difficult as it was to decide to have the hysterectomy, in hindsight I'm so glad that I did. No amount of change in my diet or increase in my consumption of nutrient-dense food could have helped me come back from this condition.

Of course, the hysterectomy opened a whole new can of worms in my health because it surgically put me into menopause and exposed me to all the fun stuff that comes with it. Six days after the surgery, I was having more than twenty-five hot flashes a day. Jimmy would play the Chipettes' version of Katy Perry's "Hot N Cold" on his phone (he made it his ringtone, too!) to make me laugh whenever I had a hot flash. As we discuss later in this book, the adrenal glands help control hot flashes with estrogen production. When the ovaries are removed and can no longer produce estrogen, you have to replace that estrogen with proper amounts of exogenous sources (similar to what a type 1 diabetic has to do in injecting insulin because the pancreas can no longer make it). I use an estrogen patch twice weekly because my adrenal glands are still trying to heal. They're still worn out from the poor nutritional habits I had when I was younger, so the glands can't produce adequate amounts of estrogen to help prevent the hot flashes. Take it from me: You might think you can get away with bad food choices when you're young, but it eventually catches up to you. As Baptist preacher Robert G. Lee said in a famous sermon, "Pay Day Someday."

As if having Hashimoto's and endometriosis wasn't bad enough, when I was forty I won the trifecta of autoimmune disease by developing psoriasis on the back of my scalp. The elevated inflammation in my body from the endometriosis probably triggered these itchy, burning scalp attacks, and they were particularly profound when I ate dairy. After my hysterectomy removed the endometriosis and the inflammation ostensibly came down, I quickly noticed that the psoriasis outbreaks stopped for the most part. I've had only one issue with psoriasis since my hysterectomy, and that was after I had consumed a very large amount of dairy. Nowadays, I can have small amounts of full-fat dairy without any trouble.

With all that I've gone through with my health and coming out the other side many years older, wiser, and healed, I knew I wanted to do something to help others on their journeys to optimizing their health. For many years, Jimmy has been afforded opportunities with his online health podcasting, social media presence, and bestselling books to live that dream. In late 2016, he helped open a door for me to follow him into the wonderful world of inspiring and educating others in the health community when he discovered an organization called the Nutritional Therapy Association (NutritionalTherapy.com) and its Nutritional Therapy Practitioner (NTP) and Nutritional Therapy Consultant (NTC) programs. I had long desired to go back to school and add to my associate degree, even though it had been twenty-plus years since I had been in any formal educational setting. Although it lasts only nine months, this course is one of the most intensive, comprehensive nutritional health programs I've ever seen. I thought I knew a lot about nutrition from listening to Jimmy blabber on about it for years, but now I say words and even he doesn't know what they mean. Prostaglandin. Duodenum. Cholecystokinin. Oh, my!

Another reason I wanted to pursue this Nutritional Therapy education was to continue to learn ways to heal my body through natural means and leave behind all the questions left unanswered by mainstream medicine. I was so proud to graduate in November 2017. I was excited about the prospect of passing on this great knowledge to help other people like me who are needlessly hurting because of inadequate information regarding how to fix their diet and their health. I wish I had known about the concepts we share in this book earlier in my life so I wouldn't have had to deal with so many health issues when I was younger. We all did the best we could with what we knew at the time. Now we know better, and we can help the next generation be better than us. The knowledge I now have is what drives me to promote both real food and keto for the people who need it (which is most people).

Now, Jimmy and I both do our part to promote healthy living to anyone who needs to hear about it. Because we don't have any kids of our own, we have four fur babies (cats) and twenty-nine feather babies (backyard chickens) to keep us company. We get close to two dozen organic eggs daily from those free-range chickens. We even have a garden in our front and back yards and a greenhouse in our backyard for fresh, organic vegetables and herbs anytime we want them. If you want to try to incorporate more real, whole foods into your diet, the best way to do it is to grow your own food and take care of animals that produce nutrient-rich foods. Part of following the ketogenic lifestyle is understanding the importance of food quality and knowing the source of your food. Once you eat an egg from your own chickens, you'll never buy another egg from the grocery store.

As a result of the information I learned while becoming an NTP, I jumped into the world of health podcasting that Jimmy has been participating in for more than a decade. Together, we created a podcast called *The Nutritional Pearls Podcast* (NutritionalPearlsPodcast.com). We knew that a large segment of the population, including people who think they're living a healthy lifestyle, needed to hear some clinical pearls of wisdom about nutrition that just weren't being shared elsewhere. I'm honored to see clients over Skype and in person to assist them in implementing the diet and lifestyle changes that will make them better than they are now. *Real Food Keto* is our way of putting this information into your hands so that you can benefit from this life-changing message.

DIVING INTO
REAL FOOD KETO

What you're about to read, in our eyes, will revolutionize your eating habits and health. You should throw out the window everything you thought you knew about diet and the impact that it has on your body. Hardly anyone thinks deeply about digestion, the importance of eating the right kinds of fat and what healthy fats are, ways to get proper mineral balance, the critical nature of hydration, and the controversial yet important subject of detoxification, which sadly has been hijacked by fruit juicing and other such nonsense. In this book, we set you straight on all these subjects and more, looking at them all through the prism of eating a low-carb, moderate-protein, high-fat, ketogenic diet.

You think you might already know a lot about nutrition. Well, buckle your seatbelt, folks, because you're about to embark on a wild and crazy ride. It's real food, it's keto, and it's time to get started!

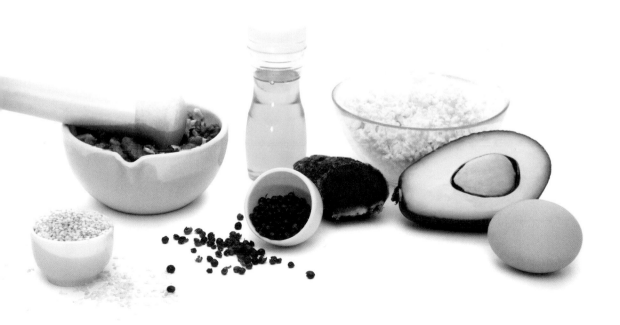

part 1
WHAT'S THE POINT?

Why do we need a book about eating real food? Come on, what's the point? Food is food, isn't it? It should be hard to go wrong. Well, stick around, and you'll see just how messed up our food system has become. It's a far cry from the traditional foods of just a few generations back that served people well and kept their health and weight in check. Furthermore, because of the metabolic damage brought on by what we have long thought of as food (but really isn't), a diet that can heal and restore our bodies—like a low-carb, moderate-protein, high-fat, ketogenic diet—may be just what the doctor ordered.

What you're about to read is perhaps some of the most revolutionary information you've ever encountered about nutrition and health. Think you're ready for it? If so, come on in and make yourself comfortable. This could be a bumpy ride.

CHAPTER 1

Why *Real Food* Keto?

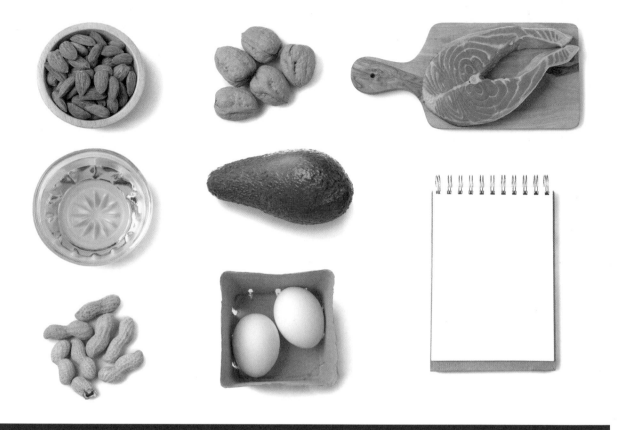

We speculate that there are three very different groups of people who are reading this book, and each group has varying reasons for doing so. Maybe you're already following the ketogenic diet, but you want to incorporate more real, whole foods into your eating plan. We're glad you're here. Or perhaps you picked up this book because you're already into real food, but you don't know anything about the ketogenic diet, and you want to learn more. Splendid! Or maybe this is the very first book on nutrition you've ever read, and you need to find out more about both the ketogenic diet *and* real food. Excellent! *Real Food Keto* speaks to all three groups with a unified message to bring you quality nutritional health knowledge no matter where you're coming from.

If you're in the first group of people who already eat keto, perhaps you've read one or more of Jimmy's best-selling books on the subject—*Keto Clarity, The Ketogenic Cookbook,* and *The Keto Cure,* for example—and you've already embraced this healthy low-carb, high-fat lifestyle. That's fabulous! Here's the sobering reality, though: Not all ketogenic dieters consume real, whole foods as part of their eating plan (although many do). They go keto and obsess about reducing their carbohydrate intake and raising their fat intake without paying any serious attention to the quality of the food they put in their mouths. Conventional mayonnaise made with soybean oil (which describes most of the products on store shelves) is a prime example of a low-carb, high-fat food that ketogenic dieters are encouraged to eat but that's less than ideal for a healthy diet. In Chapter 4, we explain why the fats you eat matter when you're eating keto, and later in the book we give you good resources for purchasing or making better alternatives to beloved foods like mayo.

One of the major goals of this book is to teach people who already eat keto about the incredible value of adding micronutrient-rich real foods to their routine. We honestly believe that this could be one of the biggest missing links in addressing some of the health challenges you still might be facing. The eating habits we describe in this book match how we try to eat most of the time, and we've seen great benefits from shifting from low-carb junk-food products to better-quality foods such as bone broth, grass-fed beef, and homemade sauerkraut. This ever-so-slight shift in our nutrition has paid big dividends for our health. It's not about being 100 percent perfect; it's about embracing real food in day-to-day life to see the best possible health results from your keto approach. Adopting a real food approach could be a game-changer for many people.

The second group includes those people who already embrace real food and have thought that making that decision alone would give them the desired results in their weight and health. Although eliminating processed junk food and fast food from your diet can and will certainly help improve your health, many people who only switch to real food without making other changes don't necessarily see the results they expected. Many people do see dramatic changes in their health simply by eating more whole foods, but this doesn't necessarily happen for everybody. And there's a perfectly good reason.

Our bodies are very adaptive to whatever we choose to feed them, and they attempt to cull whatever nutrients they can to run the way they're intended to. However, if you don't feed your body well and instead choose to consume highly refined, processed foods and fast food on a regular basis—which is typical of many people these days—the result is metabolic damage and a condition called *insulin resistance,* which is something on which we want to shine a bright light. When you have insulin resistance, your body's natural ability to handle the foods you eat is impaired. Insulin resistance develops over many years and decades of eating poorly, and you can't magically heal it simply by choosing real foods again. For some people, the damage is so great that consuming even certain nutrient-rich and higher-carb real foods starts to become a problem.

A sweet potato is the perfect example of a real food that might not be good for someone to eat because of their level of insulin resistance. Yes, you can grow a sweet potato in the ground, and it's definitely considered a real food. However, for someone with years of poor diet under their belt who now has a damaged metabolism that has led to insulin resistance, even this so-called healthy sweet potato can cause blood sugar and insulin levels to rise—and that means it's no longer a food that's health promoting. Having an elevated glucose response after eating a sweet potato means that your carbohydrate tolerance is much lower than normal, and you need to restrict carbohydrates based on your tolerance level.

The lesson in all this is that we're not all just a bunch of lemmings with identical nutritional needs. We have this incredible thing that you might never have heard talked about within mainstream nutritional health circles: *bioindividuality.* Every person has a unique metabolism, and how your body reacts to the food you eat now is based on past diet and lifestyle choices. Bioindividuality is the reason nutrition can be so incredibly complex for some people to understand; they just want to be told what to eat. Sadly, it's just not that simple.

Your unique circumstance requires you to customize your nutrition plan to *you.* That's where a Nutritional Therapy Practitioner (NTP) like Christine can step in to help you figure out what you should be eating to set you on a path to healing. There's no such thing as a one-size-fits-all approach to diet. That's why comparing what you eat with what someone else eats and getting jealous about it is as silly as becoming green-eyed over someone with a size six foot when you wear a size ten. There's nothing you can do about it, and you both have to find the shoe that's right for you. The same goes for your diet.

Finally, the third group reading this book includes people who don't know anything about eating real food or keto. Many people—including us—have found their way out of the depths of ignorance about the significant role nutrition plays in health. Lots of people are talking about the locavore movement and eating farm to table, communities are experiencing an astronomical rise in the popularity of farmers markets, and the number-one most searched diet term is *ketogenic or keto.* You might be realizing that something desperately needs to change to prevent your health from rapidly declining in the coming years. That decline isn't an inevitable fate, and we're so glad you chose our book as your foray into the wonderful world of nutritional health. Stick around, because we'll teach you the specifics about how and why you should combine the two awesome concepts of eating real food and eating a ketogenic diet into one fantastic way to optimize your weight and health. It's never too late to make the best possible you, no matter where you start.

WHY REAL FOOD?

The greatest challenge we face in trying to communicate what real food is to the general public is that most people have a skewed view of what food actually is. Some people think what they are feeding their families *is* real food. What else would it be, right? After all, how can manufacturers call all those products in grocery stores *food* if they're not actually food? Well, our definition of *real food,* which is at the heart of what we share throughout this book, isn't what many modern-day humans are feeding themselves. Many of the foods that people eat every single day have been in our food supply for only a little more than a half century. Jimmy likes to call these foods "crappy carbage"; another accurate description is "foodlike disease agents." Some of them make claims about their health benefits, such as cereals that are promoted as having heart-healthy benefits, but the truth of the matter is these items are very likely making your health worse over the long run, one bite at a time.

You know what we're talking about.

Highly processed and refined sugary foods like cakes, doughnuts, pies, candy, milk chocolate, and soda, as well as grain-based and starchy foods such as chips, white bread, crackers, pasta, and bagels, are simply not real food. We're sure this isn't groundbreaking news to many of you. But perhaps this is a major newsflash for some who have been eating this way without a care in the world about what these foods are doing to your body. You might need a moment to grieve and lament all those years you wasted on a bad diet. Go ahead; take your time. We'll be here when you get back.

Jimmy was there at one point in his life, drinking sixteen cans of soda a day, eating whole boxes of snack cakes in one sitting, going to fast-food restaurants daily, and worse. He'll be the first to tell you he simply *did not care* what he was eating. He never considered the ramifications of what all those "foodlike disease agents" were doing to his body. Had he been awakened to the value of good nutrition that comes from consuming real food, perhaps he could have warded off the obesity and insulin resistance that nearly took his life at an early age. You see, as difficult as it might seem to embrace real food and leave behind all those products you think you can't live without, the reality is that you're just putting yourself one step closer to destroyed health and possibly

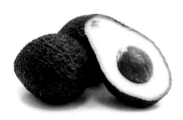

premature death. It's a sobering thought, but it's one you have to come to terms with if you're serious about reclaiming your health.

When you're ready to learn more about what real food actually is, it might blow your mind to discover how much of what you know about the foods you eat is just a big façade. We've been purposely deceived and manipulated through highly suggestive and aggressive marketing tactics to buy what the food manufacturers want us to buy. (We tell you how in just a moment.) If you walk into any supermarket these days, what you find, particularly in the middle aisles, is anything but real food. Sure, a few real, whole foods—like brown rice, steel-cut oats (not instant oats), olive oil, and coconut oil—are in those center sections, but most of what's there is pure, unadulterated junk. It's not real food. Not even close.

Yet this is the kind of stuff that dominates our food choices and ends up in the grocery carts of the American public. (This is less of a problem in other Westernized countries, like Australia and South Africa, where people put a higher priority on real food, but the United States definitely isn't the only nutritional wasteland.) The most disgusting aspect of this flawed food system is the deliberately deceptive role that food manufacturers are playing. Those companies pretend that their products are real food by making grandiose claims about what will happen in your health if you eat them. The result is that people obediently gobble up those products and come back for more. The greatest travesty is how this is happening right under our noses, and so few of us even realize it.

Here are the facts: The boxed and bagged foods in the center aisles are junk food pure and simple, no matter what the marketing slogan on the packaging states. And most of these so-called food products are made for just pennies on the dollar, which makes them incredibly lucrative to the bottom line of major food manufacturers. There's certainly nothing wrong with a business making money, but that business has a duty to be transparent with its customers about the truth about its products. However, major food manufacturers have no desire to tell the truth, the whole truth, and nothing but the truth when marketing their products. What's the upside of doing that when you know what you're selling is junk?

Only ten companies own the major food brands that people around the world are buying for their families. TEN! This juggernaut of food domination by some of the most highly recognized food and beverage brands—including PepsiCo, General Mills, Kellogg's, Associated British Foods, Mondelez, Mars, Danone, Unilever, Coca-Cola, and Nestle[1]—is the biggest reason why the concept of real food has had such a difficult time gaining traction among average consumers. People are bombarded by multibillion-dollar advertising campaigns that urge them to buy more and more of this junk all day, every day. From television and

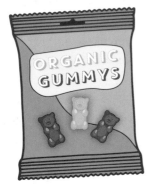

radio commercials, magazine ads, and billboards to banner and pop-up ads across every nook and cranny of the Internet, there's just no hiding from the messages the companies want you to hear about their food products.

The unintended consequences of the food industry's pursuit of greater and greater profits has been a swift and steady rise in obesity rates and the development of major health epidemics, including type 2 diabetes, heart disease, Alzheimer's disease (which we now know is related to blood sugar and insulin levels and is being referred to as type 3 diabetes), and cancer. Big Food (or, more accurately, Not Real Food) can no longer turn a blind eye to the elephant in the room. The food manufacturing industry is threatened to the very core by the prospect of people getting their food from any other source, and real food is its target. But here's the truth—real food is the *answer* to all these health woes. Is this really so difficult to understand?

Now that the general public is beginning to open its eyes to the manipulative marketing games that food companies are playing, manufacturers have upped their game and taken it one step further to cater to consumers who are becoming savvier about their food-purchasing habits. Companies now market foods as "healthy" by slapping various hip marketing terms right on the packaging. Following are some examples of buzzwords you might see on packaging:

- Made with healthy whole grains
- Low-fat
- Sugar-free
- No sugar added
- Organic
- GMO-free
- All-natural

Our favorite gimmick is when a company puts the American Heart Association's "heart health" symbol on the package.

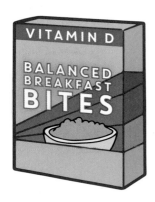

We saw organic gummy bears at the store and just shook our heads in disgust at all the moms who would buy this product thinking it's a better option for their kids. Even breakfast cereals have a bogus health claim plastered across the top of the packaging stating that it's a "good source of vitamin D." The truth is, it's not a good source of vitamin D because one serving provides only 188 IU, whereas a relatively small amount of sun exposure gives you the recommended amount of vitamin D.[2]

The manufacturers' health claims are only meant to sucker people into buying fake processed food products under the auspices of reaping health benefits when, in truth, the exact opposite will happen.

There are so many mixed messages about healthy foods and products that people get whiplash trying to keep up. Whole grains are a perfect example. Just walk down the bread or cereal aisle of your local grocery store to see many claims such as "a good source of whole grains," "rich in whole grains," or "21 whole grains and seeds." Because the general public has heard that whole grains are healthy, and dietitians and other so-called health experts have reinforced that notion, people obediently buy these foods, oblivious to their effect on blood glucose and insulin levels. People neglect to consider the other ingredients in these products, including various forms of sugar, fake fats, and additives. The products are often fortified with vitamins and minerals to replace the nutrients that have been stripped away during processing. If something has to be fortified to put back nutrients that processing removed, can you still call it a real, whole food? We don't think so.

The reality is that there are very few truly whole-grain foods on the market that aren't highly processed. Those barley breads, seven-grain bagels, multigrain crackers, and whole-grain cereals you enjoy eating and think are doing something good for your health have likely gone through heavy processing, just like junk food does, that makes them less than ideal for consumption. The truth of the matter is that genuine whole grains are incredibly difficult to find, and even then they need to be properly prepared, which most people don't have the time or the know-how to do. Proper preparation includes soaking and sprouting the grains to remove toxins and make them more digestible. Who's gonna take the time to do that? Consequently, the ruse about grains being healthy continues because people aren't privy to the truth. Are you getting angry about this yet?

Highly processed vegetable oils that you commonly see in clear, plastic containers on supermarket shelves are another problematic food that people who eat a standard American diet consume under the pretense that they're healthy. These oils have the word *vegetable* in their names, so they have to be good for you, right? We're gonna pull out our inner Brooklynites and say fuhgeddaboudit! These oils don't come from vegetables at all. They're from seeds, and they go through significant processing, including deodorizing, bleaching, and a chemical extraction process that would make your stomach turn. This process involves high heat, which makes these oils very unstable. Just do an Internet search for "How Canola Oil Is Made" and watch the shocking video.

What you'll realize is that these "healthy" vegetable oils do a lot more harm than good. If you walk down the grocery store aisle and look at all the corn oil, canola oil, soybean oil, cooking spray, and other such products, you'll see they all have the American Heart Association's heart symbol on them because they're low in saturated fat and cholesterol. But frankly, most of these vegetable oils are so highly inflammatory that they aren't healthy for anyone to consume because of the way they've been processed. Later in the book, we share more about why these are the last fats you want to be eating if you're embracing the *Real Food Keto* concepts, and we explain why saturated fat isn't the great enemy to your health that you've been led to believe. We explain how to look for better versions of these oils that have been cold-pressed and packaged in dark bottles to maintain their stability. (These versions are okay to consume.)

With the popularity of the real food movement growing—thanks to the promotion of such nutritional concepts as Whole30, Paleo, primal, and keto—we hope the monopoly the food industry has had on what people are eating is finally starting to lose its grip and that major food companies are beginning to feel the pinch in their bottom line. The best way to slap back at the degradation they have brought into our food supply is to start supporting local farmers, farmers markets, and natural food stores. Additionally, you could grow a home garden, get backyard chickens, and start making sauces and condiments at home (which taste better, anyway). We do all these things now, and we can tell you there's peace of mind in knowing where your food comes from.

Now that you're beginning to realize what real food is, you can start cleaning up your diet and benefiting from all that it has to offer you. But focusing on real food isn't the only thing that improves your health. There's also the popular diet that so many people are trying with great success—keto!

WHY KETO?

Since the publication of Jimmy's book *Keto Clarity* in 2014, we've seen a steady rise in the popularity of the ketogenic way of eating. Blogs, social media pages, podcasts, and books galore have been created for people to share information, inspiration, and tons of recipes about the ketogenic diet, and for good reason—it's worked incredibly well to heal the many diseases of civilization that plague us today. Yes, it's the antithesis of what mainstream health experts tell us is healthy: reduce your carbohydrate consumption rather than eating more whole grains, legumes, and starchy vegetables and increase your fat consumption, especially saturated fat, instead of avoiding dietary fat like the plague. However, the sensational results people have with this nutritional health plan are impossible to ignore.

Keto is a diet low in carbohydrates (determined by your tolerance level) and moderate in protein (to your threshold for blood sugar control) with the remainder of your nutrition coming from dietary fats—namely saturated fats, monounsaturated fats, the right kinds of omega-6 fats, and omega-3 fats. So a keto breakfast plate might feature two eggs, two slices of bacon, half an avocado, a slice of cheddar cheese, and a dollop of full-fat sour cream. (Okay, now we're hungry!) You could even throw in some leafy green and nonstarchy veggies to make an omelet. And if you're already inspired to start incorporating the real food element, add a scoop of sauerkraut for some healthy probiotics to start your day on the right foot. This isn't rocket science, people! It's the very essence of *Real Food Keto*.

Keep carbs low

Eat more fat

Test ketones often

Overdoing protein is bad

Let us say one thing very clearly, so you don't misunderstand us: A one-size-fits-all keto diet doesn't exist. People like to have macronutrient ratios to follow to make eating keto a math equation. Don't do that! Instead, you need to tinker and test with varying levels of macronutrients to find what works for you. (Remember, it's all about that bioindividuality we discussed earlier.) Your keto diet might look different from what your friends, family, and coworkers eat on their keto diets, and that's okay. The important thing is that you maintain the low-carb, moderate-protein, high-fat diet that's right for you, and the result is that you should be producing the by-products of fat metabolism known as *ketones*. Health professionals have unfairly maligned these molecules, but more and more people are coming around to the idea that ketones are not at all harmful and instead are helpful in getting you to your health goals.

What's so special about nutritional ketosis? When you make the shift from being primarily a sugar burner to being primarily a fat burner, which can happen in as little as a few days to upward of two months, your body rewards you with lower inflammation, insulin, and blood sugar, all of which are signs of robust metabolic health. Although not everyone needs to eat a very low-carb, high-fat diet to get these effects, some people, like the insulin-resistant population, do. Arizona-based family physician Adam Nally, DO, notes in his book with Jimmy, *The Keto Cure,* that 80 to 85 percent of his patients have some level of insulin resistance that requires them to be in ketosis most of the time. This isn't to say that everyone needs to adopt a ketogenic lifestyle or pursue nutritional ketosis—but there's certainly no harm in trying it, especially when you add the real food element. This could be the one-two punch you've been looking for in your pursuit of optimal health!

How exactly do you know whether you're in a state of ketosis? Excellent question. (Fair warning: We're about to get super nerdy on you!) You can measure three different ketone bodies:

- **Acetoacetate** in the *urine*
- **Beta-hydroxybutyrate** in the *blood*
- **Acetone** in the *breath*

Let's take a look at the pros and cons of testing one over the others.

ACETOACETATE

You easily can test the ketones in the urine with an inexpensive product called Ketostix, which you can find at your local drugstore. The testing strip turns pink to purple to indicate that ketones are spilling over into the urine. However, the challenge with acetoacetate is that it begins to be converted to the more usable form of ketones found in the blood, called beta-hydroxybutyrate, which is why some (but not all) people see their urine ketones disappear once they become keto-adapted. And when the urine ketones disappear, people tend to freak out about what they're doing wrong. Consequently, urine testing is recommended only during the first two weeks of going keto; after that, you should switch to blood or breath testing.

BETA-HYDROXYBUTYRATE

If you're looking for accuracy on how well you're doing in your pursuit of ketosis, then testing for beta-hydroxybutyrate in your blood is hands down the best way to do it. Blood ketone testing is considered the gold standard. The major downside is the need to prick your finger to determine ketosis. If you prick the side of your finger with the lancet (instead of the pad of your finger), it doesn't hurt as much.

You can test blood ketones with a device that's like a glucometer. The one we use now is the moderately priced Keto-Mojo ketone meter from BestKetoneTest.com. In 2012 and 2013, Jimmy was testing daily for nutritional ketosis as part of an N=1 experiment (which means the study includes just one participant), and he was spending more than $5 per strip for the only blood ketone testing that was available at the time. Because more people are pursuing nutritional ketosis now, the prices have come way down, to closer to $1 per strip.

ACETONE

High levels of acetone in your breath is a clear indication of fat-burning and being in a state of ketosis. You can test breath ketones using a variety of meters that measure for acetone in the breath in different ways. The Ketonix (ketonix.co) is a moderately priced, USB-powered device that you blow into so you can evaluate how the color changes; it also offers a more sophisticated number system that can be graphed on your computer. You can test thousands of times using this device.

The LEVL (levlnow.com) is a higher-priced breath ketone testing device that's relatively new to the market. It offers a high-tech way to measure for acetone, with a numerical result that indicates the level of acetone in your breath. To ensure accuracy, the LEVL requires that you calibrate it and change the sensor monthly. The sleek accompanying app that tracks your readings keeps a visual graph of your progress. Although breath ketones don't necessarily correlate with blood ketones, many people like to test the breath as an alternative to pricking a finger.

BENEFITS OF NUTRITIONAL KETOSIS

Now that you know how you can start burning ketones and how to test for them, you might be wondering about the benefits of doing so. Well, we could spend the rest of this book sharing in great detail all of the incredible positive health effects of pursuing nutritional ketosis, but here are just a few to get you started:

No hunger	Fewer acne breakouts
Normal blood sugar	Feelings of happiness
Deeper sleep	Improved insulin sensitivity
Robust energy	Lower triglycerides
Calmness	Higher HDL ("good") cholesterol
Lower blood pressure	Induction of spontaneous fasting
Mental clarity	Slowing of aging
Lower inflammation	Being in control of food
Improved immunity	Real fat loss (not just weight loss)
Better memory	

If you want to dig deep into the ins and outs of ketosis, then definitely read Jimmy's books *Keto Clarity* and *The Keto Cure* for all the science you could ever want to know about low-carb, high-fat living. What we share in *Real Food Keto* is how to merge the worlds of eating real food through the prism of a ketogenic lifestyle. The real food element needs keto as much as keto needs real food. The two go hand in hand to optimize your health.

Before we get into the various areas of a healthy lifestyle, such as digestion, hydration, mineral balance, and endocrine function, we have to get to the essence of what *Real Food Keto* is all about. If you don't get this basic information about nutrition down from the start, then everything else we share in this book will likely be meaningless. You may need to read Chapter 2 a few times to soak it all in, but it will be worth the effort.

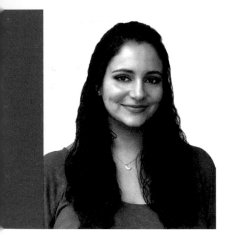

LAUREN ARONSTAM, NTP www.bodyandsoulsustenance.com

The ketogenic diet has helped not only me heal from fungus, mold toxicity, and HPA axis dysfunction but several of my clients as well. I've seen a number of people with chronic blood sugar and mood issues, pathogenic infections, autoimmune conditions, and thyroid and adrenal dysfunction whose health and quality of life have substantially improved by adopting this diet. On the other side of the spectrum, I've also worked with endurance runners who've used it to improve their performance during training and high-stakes races, as well as top-level executives who've wanted more mental clarity and energy for their high-stress jobs. It is overall a highly healing and customizable diet that can fit almost anyone's needs.

REAL FOOD KETO TAKEAWAYS FROM CHAPTER 1

- If you already eat keto, try adding in the real food element for nutrient density.

- If you already eat real food and still struggle with weight or other health issues, start eating low-carb and high-fat to enhance the benefits.

- Insulin resistance makes it more difficult for your body to handle carbohydrates—even carbohydrates from real food.

- Bioindividuality means that the same diet and lifestyle won't work for everybody.

- If you've never embraced real food or keto before, then merge the two for a perfect match in optimizing your health.

- Knowing what real food is can be challenging because of heavy marketing from Big Food. Health claims on the packaging of food products are about selling you, not helping you reach your health goals.

- Not everything you see available for consumption in a grocery store can be considered real food.

- Real food isn't the enemy in our health; it's the answer to it.

- Commercially available whole-grain food products are not the health panacea we have been led to believe they are.

- Vegetable oils are promoted as heart-healthy but are highly inflammatory to your body.

- The best ways to combat the fake food monopoly are by supporting farmers, buying from farmers markets and natural food stores, and growing your own garden and raising backyard chickens.

- Eating keto consists of lowering carbs, moderating protein, and eating healthy fats, including saturated fats, to satiety.

- Getting into nutritional ketosis isn't about macronutrient ratios or counting calories; tinker and test to find the proper amounts of carbohydrates, protein, and fat that are right for you.

- The only way to know how well you're doing in your pursuit of ketosis is to test for ketones in your urine, blood, or breath.

- The list of ketogenic health benefits is long.

CHAPTER 2

The Nuts and Bolts of *Real Food Keto*

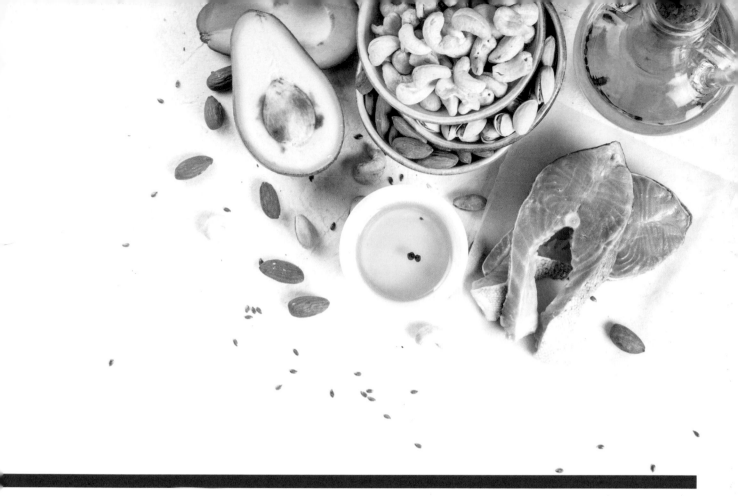

Before we get into some of the specifics about a healthy diet and lifestyle and how to make sure our bodies are functioning at their best, we want to cover some basic information that's the nuts and bolts of what we share in *Real Food Keto.* Our goal in this chapter is to lay the groundwork for the rest of the information in this book.

Here's just a glimpse of what we have for you in this chapter:

- Identifying what health, nutrition, and nourishment are

- Listing the essential nutrients that your body needs to function well

- Recapping the major benefits that you receive from these nutrients

The last thing we want to do is overwhelm you with gobs of information until you become cross-eyed. Instead, we give you information in chunks so that you can properly digest it (without the need for digestive enzymes). So hold on tight; here comes some of the most important information about nutritional health that you've likely ever seen. After you finish this chapter, you'll know more about nutrition and its role in your health than most doctors and other medical professionals.

DEFINING *HEALTH, NUTRITION,* AND *NOURISHMENT*

Let's start by defining the term *health*. According to the World Health Assembly, *health* means "a dynamic state of complete physical, mental, spiritual, and social well-being and not merely the absence of disease or infirmity."[1]

That's a very highbrow definition of health, so how about we create an acronym that makes it much easier to understand? This HEALTH acronym should help you remember the major concepts involved in it.

Holistically healed and optimized

Exercise the body and mind

Absence of disease or sickness

Loving yourself and others

Trusting God or a higher power

Handling day-to-day stressors

Ahhh, now that makes more sense, right?

As you can see, health is not just about what we put in our mouths to give us nutrition. It encompasses every aspect of our lives, including how we feel, what gives us purpose in life, and our interactions with other people—this is real life, and how we handle it can either positively or negatively affect our overall health. What you'll find is that some of these lifestyle issues are more important to health than even the food we eat. That's surprising to hear, but it's the reality in many cases.

You could have the cleanest, most whole food–based, low-carb, high-fat diet in the entire world and stick to it faithfully day by day by day and not see the results you're looking for in your health if you allow stress from mental, spiritual, or social issues in your life to creep in. Maybe that's you right now, and you can't for the life of you figure out why you can't drop those last few pounds or bring some health marker back into line with the stellar diet and exercise program you're following. You're not alone. Many people ignore the role of something called *epigenetics* that can have a profound impact on how your genes are expressed based on your lifestyle choices.

The primary instigators of epigenetic expression include a poor diet; toxins from household cleaners and beauty products; stress from life circumstances such as financial problems, death of a loved one, or marital issues; thyroid dysfunction; adrenal fatigue; prescription and non-prescription medications; compromised gut health, blood sugar imbalances, vitamin and mineral deficiencies, and stored toxins in the body, including heavy metals, food additives, and more.[2] All these criteria can uniquely affect your ability to lose stored body fat and attain the ever-elusive health you so desperately desire. We address many of these topics in much greater detail later in the book.

Now that you understand what *health* means, let's shift our attention to defining what *nutrition* is. It seems pretty easy to understand at first blush, but let's see what the Merriam-Webster online dictionary has to say about it. *Nutrition* means "the act or process of nourishing or being nourished; specifically: the sum of the processes by which an animal or plant takes in and utilizes food substances. Foods that are necessary for human nutrition."[3]

Well, isn't that fancy? Most people probably need a dictionary to help them interpret what that definition means. How about we make things a whole lot simpler for you and give you the established definition of *nutrition* from the Nutritional Therapy Association (NTA):

"A science focused on the interactions between living organisms and their food. It includes the study of the biological processes used by the body to break down, absorb, and utilize the nutrients contained in food."

The NTA goes even deeper in its explanation by defining that nutrients are chemical substances contained in food and are necessary to sustain life. They provide energy (calories), contribute to the body's structure, and regulate and assist in body processes.

The greatest challenge for those of us who are attempting to add more nutrition to our diets by ensuring proper nutrient intake is that we don't eat nutrients—we eat *food,* and the majority of people have no idea which vitamins and minerals are in the foods they eat. Maybe you've heard that you can get potassium from a banana or vitamin C from an orange, but your knowledge might not go much deeper than that. The serious lack of knowledge and understanding of the nutrient content of real foods is an obstacle in attempting to attain optimal nutritional health that we hope to resolve with this book. Later, in Part 3, we share exactly which vitamins and minerals you get from the various foods you consume.

When you think about the word *nourishment,* what's the first thing that pops into your head? It's food, right? Consuming healthy real, whole foods can and will nourish your body. But true nourishment goes so much deeper than that. *Nourish* derives from the Latin word *nutrire,* which literally means "to feed, cherish." Other good definitions that make the point about nourishment going so much deeper than just our diet include the following:

- Provide with the materials necessary for growth, health, and good condition

- Keeping (a feeling or belief) in one's mind, typically for a long time

- To strengthen, build up, or promote

- To support or encourage (an idea, feeling, etc.)[4]

As you can see, nourishment encompasses the mind, body, and spirit in one cohesive package. Keep that in mind as you implement the tenets of *Real Food Keto* into your life. Both eating real food and keto are important, but genuine, holistic nourishment is critical to your goal of being healthy.

ESSENTIAL NUTRIENTS

Now that we've given you a foundation for understanding health, nutrition, and nourishment, we're going to get very practical and explain what nutrients are. Honestly, it's very simple. There are various essential nutrients that you need to sustain life. They're called *essential* because your body can't make them endogenously (meaning from within), and if you don't consume them exogenously (meaning from outside sources), you will die. The essential nutrients are water, fatty acids (dietary fat), amino acids (proteins), most vitamins, and minerals. That's it!

Did you notice anything conspicuous missing from that illustrious list of essential nutrients? Oh yeah, that's right—where are the essential carbohydrates? We have essential fatty acids. We also have essential amino acids. The definition also includes vitamins, minerals, and water. But there's just no such thing as an essential carbohydrate acid. It simply doesn't exist, no matter how many mainstream dietitians, nutritionists, doctors, and other health experts claim that you need them. It's why people who eat a ketogenic diet do more than just survive; they thrive, even with minimal carbohydrate intake.

The major mainstream objection to low-carb/keto diets boils down to the glucose-dependent functions of the body, especially in the brain. Dietitians often tell their clients that they need to eat a minimum of 130 grams of carbohydrates a day for their brains to function properly. What they fail to acknowledge, though, is that your body is very efficient at creating all the glucose it needs from the proteins you consume (a process known as *gluconeogenesis*), as well as the proteins that are floating around in your body. These are the materials your body can use to create adequate glucose for the various functions that require it.

However, we're not saying that we should be eating zero carbs and gnawing on a grass-fed beef steak all day long. A carnivorous diet might sound appealing to some people, but it's probably not ideal. You can still get incredible nutrients from nonstarchy and leafy green vegetable carbohydrates as part of your *Real Food Keto* approach, which adds some variety, texture, and flavor to your healthy plate of food. The point is these carbs aren't *essential*. Got it? Good. (We go much deeper into the metabolic pathway of how all this works in Chapter 11, which is about blood sugar.)

The following is a list of all the essential nutrients that the body needs to function properly:

ESSENTIAL NUTRIENTS

Water	Fats	Amino Acids	Vitamins	Minerals
	Linoleic acid	Isoleucine	A	Calcium
	Alpha-linolenic acid	Leucine	B1 (thiamine)	Phosphorous
		Lysine	B2 (riboflavin)	Potassium
		Methionine	B3 (niacin)	Sulfur
		Phenylalanine	B5 (pantothenic acid)	Sodium
		Threonine	B6 (pyridoxine)	Chloride
		Tryptophan	B7 (biotin)	Magnesium
		Valine	B9 (folate/folic acid)	Silicon
		Histidine*	B12 (cobalamin)	Iron
		Arginine*	C	Boron
			D	Zinc
			E	Vanadium
			K	Selenium
				Manganese
				Iodine
				Molybdenum
				Chromium
				Lithium*
				Rubidium*
				Germanium*

*Essential for children

Rest assured, we explain how you can get adequate amounts of these nutrients into your diet. This is fun, right? Like putting together the pieces of a puzzle. Let's keep learning.

THREE MAJOR CLASSES OF NUTRIENTS

The nutrients your body needs and uses fall into three major classes:

- Water
- Macronutrients (fat, protein, carbohydrate)
- Micronutrients (vitamins, minerals)

Let's start with water. Good old H_2O. Did you know your body is 60 percent water? SIXTY PERCENT! Boy, that's a whole lotta water. So it's probably not surprising that water is a critical nutrient that you cannot live without. We give much greater detail of all the ins and outs of getting adequate amounts of water in Chapter 7.

Next up are macronutrients, which make up about 35 percent of your body. Proteins account for 18 percent, fats weigh in at 15 percent, and carbohydrates are responsible for a mere 2 percent. Isn't it interesting how mainstream nutritional health experts want us to be eating upward of 65 percent of our diet as carbohydrates, yet our bodies are only 2 percent carbs? If you're still teetering on whether this ketogenic thing is for you, that statistic alone should make you rethink eating a high-carb diet, even if the carbs come from mostly real foods.

Finally, the micronutrients, which include both minerals and vitamins, fill up the remaining 4 percent and 1 percent of the body, respectively. Later we explain how even slight deficiencies in these micronutrients can have a profoundly negative effect on your total health. Don't worry; we also explain how to help prevent and shore up any deficiencies you might have.

Now let's look at the specific benefits of all these nutrients.

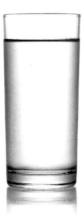

BENEFITS OF WATER, PROTEIN, FAT, CARBOHYDRATES, VITAMINS, AND MINERALS

It's one thing for us to talk generally about the three major classes of nutrients, but you're probably wondering what actual benefits you get from each one. We start your education by scratching the surface of each nutrient to introduce you to them, and in later chapters, we give much more information about them.

WATER

As the most prominent nutrient in the body, water serves some tremendous purposes that you shouldn't overlook. It helps shuttle oxygen and other nutrients into the cells. The result of insufficient hydration is an inefficiency in taking these nutrients into the cells. Adequate hydration is needed for electrolytes to work properly. When you don't drink enough water, you might experience muscle cramps, headaches, heart palpitations, constipation, and fatigue. Betcha didn't know that, did ya?

NOTE FROM CHRISTINE

Another critical benefit of water is maintaining a safe body temperature. I know from personal experience the importance of this one. We have a garden, and I enjoy getting out there in the heat of the day to pull weeds and harvest the crops. On far too many occasions, Jimmy has come outside to see me gasping for air and looking flushed because I wasn't drinking enough water and had become overheated. I get so busy working that I forget to hydrate myself properly, and thankfully I have a husband who helps me stay on top of that. See, even those of us who know better aren't perfect!

Finally, water plays a key role in flushing the body of toxins. Many people neglect to hydrate themselves properly because they don't want to pee so much. If you're in that boat, every time you urinate or defecate, remind yourself that you're ridding your body of toxins that cause harm. Additionally, when you skimp on water consumption, you can get constipated, which is no fun at all. So drink up! Er, drink water, that is.

PROTEIN

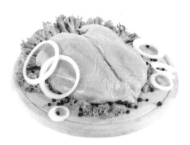

You've probably heard that proteins are the building blocks of the body, and it's true. Without protein, growing the tissue of every single aspect of your body would be impossible. Your organs, your skin, and even your bones need protein to develop properly and regenerate. Additionally, proteins help the enzymes in your body complete all the biochemical processes that make it work. Simply put, your body won't correctly function if you don't eat adequate amounts of protein. Proteins even do their work all the way down at the cellular level, aiding in every single aspect of the inner workings of the body by helping to maintain the cell's shape and developing connective tissue. One specialized protein that helps deliver oxygen throughout the body are the red blood cells, and proper protein levels are necessary for this critical part of life. No red blood cell production and you're dead. So do you think it's pretty important? You betcha!

FATS

Fat is perhaps the most vilified of the macronutrients, and that irrational fear has led us to be so scared of eating fat that we've now put ourselves in danger of being deficient. Proper fat intake is critical, especially when you're on a ketogenic diet, because it becomes your primary fuel source, replacing the carbohydrates you consumed when you were mostly a sugar burner. Fat provides a long-lasting source of energy, so you don't get hungry as quickly between meals. The reason it works so well for satiety is that it helps slow the absorption of the carbohydrates and proteins you eat, blunting the blood sugar and insulin effects. If you need to snack between meals, then you didn't have enough fat in your previous meal.

The cell membrane is made primarily of fat, so adequate dietary fat intake is required for proper cell membrane health. And here's a reason why you should never, ever eat a low-fat diet again—without fat in your diet, you can't absorb the fat-soluble vitamins A, D, E, and K. If you don't get sufficient fat intake, then these valuable vitamins are excreted from the body without having benefited you. It would be like winning a brand-new Rolls-Royce and never being allowed to drive it. As we explain in Chapter 9, each of these fat-soluble vitamins is a vital part of a healthy lifestyle.

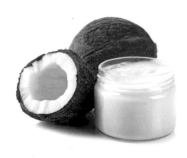

Ask any professional chef how to infuse flavor into a dish, and the answer is hands-down to add butter, coconut oil, lard, or some other real food fat source. One of the most freeing aspects of eating keto, for example, is that focusing on consuming fat blunts the cravings and desire for sugary foods. No kidding. So many people think they could never live without sugar and starch in their diet, but fat is the great equalizer that makes the transition easier. You might already know this is true because you've tasted something like low-fat cheese. It's gross! Often in products like fat-free yogurt, the manufacturer has added a ton of sugar to make it palatable without the fat. Without that added sugar, nonfat yogurt would taste nasty. We love the full-fat versions of our favorite ketogenic foods because they taste so good and are actually good for us, too.

CARBOHYDRATES

Even though this book is partly about a low-carb, high-fat, ketogenic diet, there are some compelling reasons why you might want to consider adding certain carbohydrates to your diet beyond having variety in your meal choices. The primary sources of these healthy real food, keto-friendly carbs are nonstarchy and leafy green vegetables. Although these carbohydrates aren't essential in your diet, there's reason to add them to your meals because they do the following:

- Provide fuel for the brain
- Supply a quick source of energy for muscles
- Help regulate protein and fat metabolism
- Provide fiber, which helps feed the microbiome in the gut and helps with regular elimination of waste
- Fight infections
- Promote tissue growth, including bones and skin
- Lubricate joints

That's not a bad list of reasons to eat more healthy carbohydrates, right?

It should be obvious that, because of our bioindividuality, we each should have a different level of carbohydrate intake. Because we're focusing on a ketogenic diet in this book, the recommended carb intake is certainly low for everyone relative to the standard American diet. But if you're an athlete or very active, then perhaps you can eat more carbohydrates than someone who's less active. Like we've said before, you have to tinker and test and find what works for you. Determining your carbohydrate tolerance level isn't an exact science, so keep working on it if you still struggle with what the right amount is supposed to be for your body. Testing your blood sugar after eating carbs is the perfect way to see what effect it has on your biochemistry.

If you want to test to see how you react to a real food, such as a sweet potato, follow these steps:

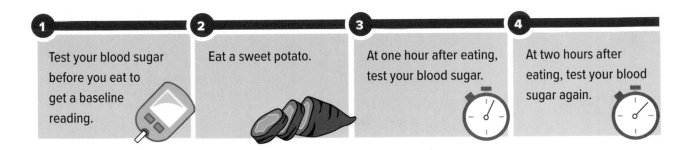

1	2	3	4
Test your blood sugar before you eat to get a baseline reading.	Eat a sweet potato.	At one hour after eating, test your blood sugar.	At two hours after eating, test your blood sugar again.

At one hour, your blood glucose should not have risen more than 20 points. At two hours, your blood glucose should be back down to baseline. So, if your baseline blood sugar number (before eating the sweet potato) is 90 mg/dL and two hours after eating the sweet potato your number is 92 mg/dL, your body has a perfect response. You probably can have a sweet potato now and again. However, if you started at 90 mg/dL and one hour later your blood sugar is 139 mg/dL, and two hours later it's 106 mg/dL, then you probably can't handle many carbohydrates. You must remain vigilant about testing your response to carbohydrates. Otherwise, you're playing a guessing game about how your body reacts to them.

VITAMINS

We all know about the importance of proper vitamin intake because most of us grew up taking Flintstones multivitamins and other supplements along with the foods we ate. Many of the metabolic processes that our bodies perform require an adequate amount of vitamins to run efficiently. Additionally, vitamins play a critical role in supporting tissue growth, aiding in digestion, helping the body eliminate waste, and boosting your immune system to keep you strong and healthy. Many chronic diseases that people develop are a direct result of an inadequate amount of vitamins and can easily be remedied by shoring up these deficiencies. We get into much greater detail about vitamins in Chapter 9.

MINERALS

Minerals are the kissing cousin to vitamins. When they're at proper levels, minerals facilitate many enzyme reactions, and they're responsible for the ability of the muscles to contract and relax. Some minerals are used to tightly regulate the pH balance (ranging from 7.35 to 7.45) in our blood. Without certain minerals, the nutrients we consume can't transfer across the cell membrane. Minerals like electrolytes (primarily sodium, potassium, magnesium, calcium, and chloride) play an important role in maintaining proper nerve communication and conduction, which is so important when you're eating keto; we'll explain more in Chapter 8, which is all about minerals.

We know we've given you a whole lot of information in just a few pages, but rest assured, we explain all these things in much greater detail later in the book. In Chapter 3, we pay homage to the pioneers who paved the way for teaching us about proper nutrition and offer a bit of history about how society moved away from real food principles to put us in a position where we now need to fine-tune our habits to move toward ketogenic nutrition as a means for healing.

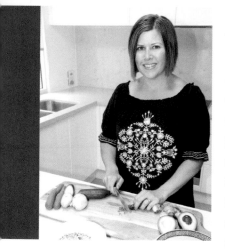

LEAH WILLIAMSON, NTP

www.nourishingconversations.com

I work with clients to choose nutrient-dense, real foods to better utilize the healthful fats they're eating in their ketogenic diet. Good food does not need to be complicated, and I am all about getting delicious, nutrient-dense food on the table as quickly and easily as possible to nourish yourself and your family. I have a 55-year-old client who is a registered nurse. She has rheumatoid arthritis and is prediabetic. She had attempted keto herself but had not managed to lose weight, struggled to get into ketosis, was constantly stiff and sore, and had bowel urgency each time she ate. At her initial consultation, she had issues with digestion in terms of her liver and gallbladder and was not digesting her fats. She also had blood sugar dysregulation and was overworking her adrenals. I worked with her on a five-week nutrient-dense, real food ketogenic protocol with additional real food nutrients to better digest the fats she was eating. I had her emulsify her fats for better digestion and remove any potential foods that were causing inflammation in the body. She lost approximately 44 pounds, her bowel movements were regular, and she had more energy and no muscle stiffness.

REAL FOOD KETO
TAKEAWAYS FROM CHAPTER 2

- Health is about much more than what you eat.
- Epigenetics can have a profound effect on how your genes are expressed based on lifestyle choices.
- Proper nutrition incorporates all the necessary nutrients to give your body the nourishment it needs.
- There are essential proteins and fats, but there is no such thing as an essential carbohydrate.
- Water, macronutrients, and micronutrients are the three major classes of nutrients.
- The benefits of water, protein, fat, carbohydrates, vitamins, and minerals are immense.

CHAPTER 3

Reviving and Thriving on *Real Food Keto*

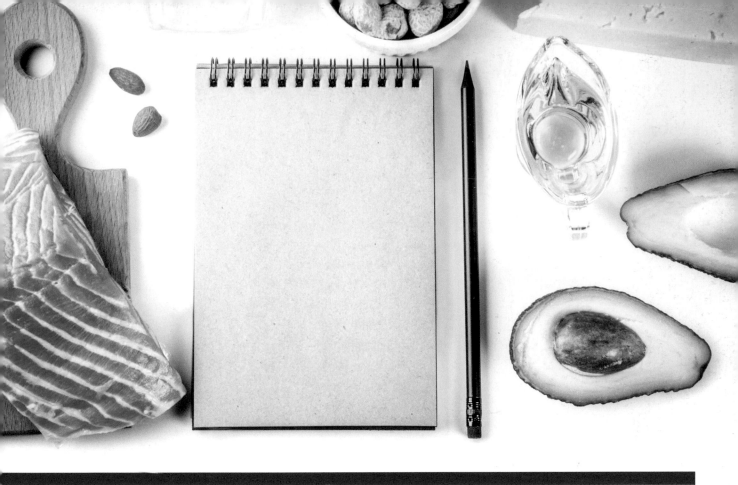

As you can already see from what we've shared so far in this book, much of the conventional wisdom about nutrition and its relationship to our health is far different from what we're teaching you in *Real Food Keto.* It's very sad that all the misinformation shared with the public about what people should eat and how to be healthy has veered so far from the previously taught tenets of reviving and thriving in our nutritional health.

Two major pillars of nutrition wisdom who we're paying homage to in this chapter are Dr. Weston A. Price and Dr. Francis Pottenger, Jr. You need to be abundantly aware of the foundation these two men laid so that you have a clearer understanding of how we have gone so terribly wrong with how we eat today.

TWO MAJOR PIONEERS IN NUTRITION

At the turn of the twentieth century, the world of nutrition was turned on its head by the forward thinking of two incredible men who researched how shifting the way humans were eating to a more traditional diet would affect health. Without the work of these forefathers, we would still be wandering in the wilderness, trying to figure out the inner workings of nutrition and health. If you've never heard of Dr. Weston A. Price and Dr. Francis Pottenger, Jr., we hope that after you've read this chapter you'll understand their historical importance.

DR. WESTON A. PRICE (1870–1948)

What is fascinating about the work of Dr. Weston A. Price (widely considered the "Isaac Newton of nutrition") is that he wasn't a medical doctor or nutrition researcher when he started traveling the world in the early 1930s to observe various traditional cultures and their diets. He was a dentist, and his primary concern was to see what effect eating a traditional, real, whole foods–based diet free from processed foods had on oral health. Dr. Price's findings were seminal work, and it's possible that even he had no idea how profound it was going to be.

Among his many observations, Dr. Price noticed that although groups of people in different areas of the world ate a wide array of diets, nearly all the cultures that ate real food experienced robust health. People in those cultures wouldn't have recognized the processed "convenience" foods that dominate the food supply in today's Western society. That's because nothing in those traditional diets was a refined or denatured food.

Interestingly, even though vegan and vegetarian diets are labeled as "healthy" in our modern world, every single one of the traditional cultures Dr. Price studied consumed animal products, including some that were raw. No kidding. These traditional diets were a whopping four times higher in calcium and other minerals, and they were an astronomical ten times higher in the important fat-soluble vitamins (A, D, E, and K) than the modern Western diet. This is a huge indication of nutrient density that gave people in these cultures their incredible health.

Additionally, the traditional diets that Dr. Price observed had a high enzyme content because of the fermented foods they included. In addition to the fermented foods in the diet of these traditional cultures, people also consumed

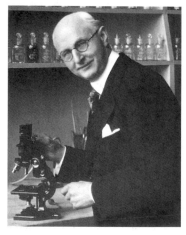

seeds, grains, legumes, and nuts that were soaked, sprouted, fermented, and/or naturally leavened. Far too many modern nutritional health experts are telling people to eat whole-grain foods without any caveat regarding the need for these foods to be properly prepared. Dr. Price noted that the lack of the type of processing that a lot of foods go through today and the preparation methods used by these traditional cultures were what made the foods healthy. Those traditional methods are far different than the processing used to make the whole wheat bread you can buy in the grocery store today.

Although a ketogenic diet doesn't contain grains, that doesn't necessarily mean that you shouldn't eat them. Some people can handle grains as long as they're properly prepared and haven't been refined. Most of us who have metabolic issues and autoimmune conditions that require us to eat keto, though, need to stay away from grains altogether.

If you're skittish about adding higher amounts of dietary fat into your *Real Food Keto* approach, you'll be pleased to learn that Dr. Price made a keen observation about the fat content of the traditional diets people were eating. It ranged from as low as 30 percent of caloric intake to as high as 80 percent! Now that's what you call a high-fat diet! Curiously, these fats were mostly saturated and monounsaturated fats, with a mere 4 percent coming from polyunsaturated fats. And yet dietitians and other nutrition gurus today tell us to make polyunsaturated fats the preponderance of what we consume as we eschew saturated fat.

Dr. Price went on to note that the traditional diets he studied were nearly identical in the amounts of omega-3 and omega-6 fatty acids they contained. The standard American diet has closer to a 30-to-1 omega-6 to omega-3 ratio because of the recommendation to consume high amounts of polyunsaturated-rich vegetable oils. In traditional cultures, this ratio was 1-to-1 because they omitted seed oils and regularly consumed fish and other omega-3-rich foods. People in these cultures were healthy, and we are not. When you compare these traditional diets to our diet, can you start to see the effect our diet is having on our health?

Another hot nutritional health topic is the fear of consuming salt. Just as we fear saturated fat nowadays, salt raises the eyebrows of uneducated consumers. But Dr. Price noted that traditional cultures had a diet that included copious amounts of unrefined salt. Remember, these cultures were virtually free from disease. It's irrational to cut down on your salt intake (unless you're in the minuscule 1 to 2 percent of the population that is truly salt-sensitive) for the sake of improving your health. Instead, use pink Himalayan salt or any colored sea salt and reap the benefits it brings. The colors of the salts indicate they're full of minerals that are beneficial for your body.

Another food Dr. Price observed these traditional cultures eating was bone broth. People consumed it with basically every meal and reaped the benefits in their health. They also had nose-to-tail diets, meaning they consumed every part of the animal, including the brain, heart, liver, and more. People—especially Americans, but really people from any modern-day Western society—can get squeamish when you start talking about eating any part of an animal other than the muscle meat. However, in traditional cultures, people gladly ate all parts of the animal, even without knowing they were getting tremendously rich nutrition for their bodies. It was an instinctive practice, and it's something we need to incorporate in our diets.

The most significant conclusion that Dr. Price made about nutrition from his many observations of traditional cultures around the world was that certain dietary laws are both inflexible and unchangeable. It all boiled down to these two key concepts:

- We must get fat-soluble vitamins from animal sources.
- Foods must be properly prepared and consumed in their whole forms to ensure that they provide optimal health benefits.

Interestingly, people in traditional cultures that have been introduced to the Western diet of processed foods have developed the same chronic health issues that plague us in Western society. This development underscores the importance of learning from our mistakes by returning to what worked in the past. Because of the metabolic damage poor dietary choices have brought on, a ketogenic approach can be an adjunct to a real food protocol for health and healing.

The single greatest disappointment for Dr. Price was the failure to find a single traditional culture based on a vegan diet that also experienced robust health. He noted that plant-based diets led to significant vitamin and mineral deficiencies because of the lack of key fat-soluble vitamins and complete proteins that come from animal products. Although we don't necessarily consume grains or legumes on a ketogenic diet, Dr. Price noted that the people in traditional cultures who consumed mostly grains and legumes were still healthier than people in our modern society. However, he also noticed that those who consumed grains and legumes had a higher incidence of cavities and abscesses as a direct result of phosphorus deficiency than those who ate mostly meat and fish. Meat is rich in phosphorus and helps develop proper bone and tooth health. This is why Dr. Price was far ahead of his time nearly a century ago when he promoted meat as a health food and warned people about vegan diets.

Dr. Price wrote a book that became an instant classic about his research. You can still find the book, *Nutrition and Physical Degeneration,* today.[1] In fact, this book was on Christine's required reading list when she was training to become a Nutritional Therapy Practitioner. We owe Dr. Price a huge debt of gratitude for his willingness to share such incredible insights into the power of food on our health.

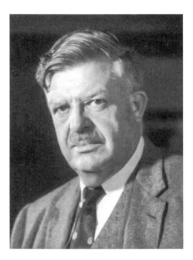

DR. FRANCIS M. POTTENGER, JR. (1901–1967)

Following in the footsteps of Dr. Weston A. Price was a physician named Francis M. Pottenger, Jr. who successfully implemented many of the same principles that Dr. Price had found. Dr. Pottenger used the dietary principles to treat patients who had respiratory diseases such as tuberculosis, asthma, and emphysema, as well as all kinds of allergies. Beginning in 1932, Dr. Pottenger began a ten-year study of what would become a total of 900 cats (a sample set of first-generation cats and their offspring). Dr. Pottenger studied two groups:

- The diet for Group 1 was two-thirds raw meat, one-third raw milk, and cod liver oil as a supplement.
- The diet for Group 2 was two-thirds cooked meat, one-third raw milk, and cod liver oil as a supplement.

All the cats had the same daily routine, and Dr. Pottenger kept a chart with notes for each cat. By the end of the study, a total of 600 cats, which included both the first-generation cats and their offspring, had recorded health histories. One thing became obvious to Dr. Pottenger as he pored over the results of his comprehensive feline study: The raw meat diet resulted in better overall health than the cooked meat diet, not just for the first-generation cats but also for the later generations. The results for the raw meat diet group were the following:

- The size of the kittens born to this group and their skeletal development were uniform.
- They maintained a regular, broad face.
- They exhibited good dental health.
- Their tissue tone was healthy.
- There were few signs of shedding.
- They had resistance to infections, parasites, and fleas.
- Their temperament was good, and they were easy to handle.

- The mother cats had fewer miscarriages and an average litter size of five kittens.
- The mother could nurse her kittens without difficulty.

What about the cats that ate the cooked meat? What happened to them? Well, it was much different, and some outcomes have parallels that are eerily similar to what we see as a result of the severe processing of the foods in the human diet in modern society. The results for the cooked-meat-diet group were the following:

- The kittens born to this group were of different sizes.
- Their bones were not as strong and subject to osteoporosis.
- There were signs of heart disease, kidney disease, nearsightedness, and many types of infections.
- There was an increased amount of inflammation in the cats' bodies.
- The female cats showed greater signs of irritability and were dangerous to handle.

One of the most interesting discoveries about the cooked-meat study group was that when Dr. Pottenger returned the cats to a raw meat diet, it took a total of four generations before their offspring fully returned to an optimal state of health. FOUR GENERATIONS! He did a follow-up Milk Study to examine the use of raw milk versus cooked milk, and the results were nearly identical to the raw meat versus cooked meat study. The results of this study for the raw-milk-diet group were the following:

- They maintained good overall health.
- Their fur was shiny and healthy.
- They had no signs of allergies.

Meanwhile, the results of the Milk Study for the pasteurized-milk-diet group were the following:

- They had difficulty in reproduction.
- Their kittens had more respiratory issues.

Dr. Pottenger decided to shake things up even more by adding another intriguing element to his study. What would happen if he introduced evaporated milk to the mix? Here were the results:

- The cats had more fat deposits.
- They showed more signs of extreme irritability compared with the other groups.

In the end, the cats that were fed raw meat, raw milk, and cod liver oil were the ones that maintained optimal health throughout their lives and in the generations that followed. Although Dr. Pottenger conducted his research on cats, he said the lessons he learned from his studies were applicable to humans as well. The cooked meat, pasteurized milk, and evaporated milk the cats consumed mimic the effects of the processed foods that dominate our diets today. Conversely, the raw meat and raw milk diet with cod liver oil equates to the real food diet we share with you in this book. Dr. Pottenger did yeoman's work dealing with all the cats to help us come to this conclusion, and, like Dr. Price, he deserves our appreciation for helping us understand why real food nutrition is the path to health that lasts for generations.[2]

A TIMELINE: TRADITIONAL DIET TO THE MODERN DIET

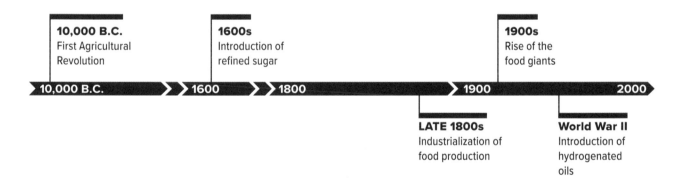

10,000 B.C.
First Agricultural Revolution

1600s
Introduction of refined sugar

1900s
Rise of the food giants

10,000 B.C. 1600 1800 1900 2000

LATE 1800s
Industrialization of food production

World War II
Introduction of hydrogenated oils

After completing all this phenomenal research, you'd think that Dr. Price and Dr. Pottenger would have made a compelling argument for the use of a traditional diet full of real, whole foods with minimal carbohydrates. But that didn't happen. So how did we go from understanding the importance of real food to seemingly no awareness of the effects of processed foods on our health? Let's take a look.

Human beings started out as hunter-gatherers, which means if they wanted to eat, they had to hunt wild game or gather vegetation to consume. Then, about 12,000 years ago, the Agricultural Revolution took place, and people started growing and saving food to consume later. In the 1600s, refined sugar came on the scene and was popular among the most affluent members of society. These people started replacing fat and protein in their diets with sugar. By the 1800s, the Industrial Revolution had started, and companies began automated production of foods. It was at this point in history when traditional food preparation and cooking techniques started to fall by the wayside, and Big Food stepped in to offer convenience.

As more and more people began working in factories in the 1900s, they had less available free time for growing a garden, raising animals, and fermenting foods, so they turned to food manufacturers to do the work. The 1900s is also when hydrogenated oils were developed, but they didn't really take off in sales until after World War II. The process of hydrogenation gave us the ability to preserve and store foods for long periods of time. Ultimately, we turned over responsibility for feeding our families to companies whose only goal was to make money off of our desire for convenience—and that was perhaps the biggest mistake we've ever made. We opened Pandora's Box, and now all these years later we're still fighting to shut it.

The production of man-made chemicals took off in the early twentieth century. Since World War II, more than 75,000 man-made chemicals have been introduced into people's lives through household items, pest-control products, health and beauty products, and, yes, even the food supply. Food companies love these chemicals because they help the companies make more money, but the unintended consequence is that the chemicals are slowly destroying the health of the consumers.

17 WAYS TO OPTIMIZE YOUR DIET AND LIFESTYLE— RIGHT NOW!

With all this seemingly impossible-to-overcome gloom and doom in our food supply today, you might be wondering, "How exactly am I supposed to live a healthy lifestyle?" It takes a little forethought, but there are specific things you can do right away in your diet and lifestyle to turn this tide.

1. **Try to eat as many different foods as possible.** If you eat the same foods over and over again (called *monoeating*), then you can develop food sensitivities that can make even healthy foods harmful to you. Jimmy developed an allergy to eggs in 2017; he showed sensitivity to both the yolks and the whites that was five times higher than normal. He needed to abstain from consuming eggs for several months before slowly adding them back to his diet. Now he doesn't eat them every day—which is hard because we have backyard chickens!

2. **Try to include more raw vegetables in your daily diet.** Cooking vegetables can leach the nutrients out of them, making them less healthy than they are in their raw state. However, consuming raw vegetables might be hard on you if you have gut health problems. (We help you determine whether you have gut problems later in the book.) For people with Crohn's disease, IBS, and leaky gut, for example, raw foods tend to be harder on the digestive system. In this case, cooking vegetables is probably a good idea. Pull out your slow cooker to help you cook these foods low and slow. When you've cooked your vegetables in the slow cooker, you can drink the broth to get even more nutrients that might have leached from the vegetables into the cooking liquid.

3. **Purchase your food from local sources such as farmers markets or directly from the farmer.** Buying local gives you a personal connection to your food, where it comes from, how it's raised and treated, and more. You might also consider growing a garden, installing a greenhouse to grow crops year-round (something we added in 2018), and even having backyard chickens if your local ordinance allows it. The point is to get reacquainted with where your food comes from. If you ask most kids these days where food comes from, they'll say "a grocery store." That's just wrong!

4. **Eat seasonally.** Our bodies were never meant to eat certain foods year-round. Although grocery stores stock strawberries throughout the year, the truth is they're in season locally for only a few months, and not at all during the winter. However, because of modern shipping practices, you can find the red, juicy goodness of strawberries tempting you in January because they were grown in some far-flung place where they're in season. It's difficult to resist foods you love when they're out of season locally, but when you understand the purpose of eating seasonally, you know that it's better for you to eat only in-season foods. As difficult as it is, we don't usually consume strawberries in the winter anymore, although we love them.

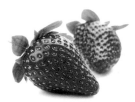

5. **Avoid refined sugars and hydrogenated oils.** Avoiding refined sugars and hydrogenated oils is next to impossible if you're still eating foods that come in a box or can because processed sugars, grains, and oils are the lifeblood of the mainstream food supply. Removing yourself as a consumer of these products will improve your health and send a message to food manufacturers that we're not buying what they're selling anymore.

6. **Don't purchase foods that are labeled low-fat.** This guideline is a difficult one for people to understand because anti-fat propaganda has been shoved down our throats for decades. If you struggle with the idea that low-fat manufactured foods are bad, we have some news that might help you better understand why they're unhealthy: When fat is cut out of foods, that fat has to be replaced with something else—which usually means more sugar, toxic additives, and other fillers that your body doesn't need. The fat might be gone, but lots of other unhealthy stuff is added, and you don't want to consume that stuff.

7. **Switch to raw dairy.** The milk we've been consuming over the past few decades is pasteurized and homogenized as a means of making it safer to drink. Also, when fat-phobia set in, the fat was stripped out for skim and low-fat milk. If you're fortunate enough to live somewhere where you can get raw milk and dairy (as we can here in South Carolina), then choose the raw options. There is so much nutrition in unprocessed forms of dairy that you'll taste the difference and reap the benefits in your health.

8. **Switch from man-made salt to sea salt.** We've all purchased the blue-and-white canister of table salt thinking we were getting real salt. Nope. Real salt is from natural sources that contain large quantities of minerals—quantities so large that the salt isn't the white color you've always known. Our favorite sea salt is pink Himalayan salt.

9. **Add fermented foods to your diet.** Consuming a small portion of fermented or cultured food with each of your meals will improve your gut health tremendously. These foods help support digestion, strengthen metabolism, help balance blood sugar levels, and boost immunity. Some examples of what you can consume include kombucha (fermented tea), kefir (fermented milk), sauerkraut (fermented cabbage), pickles (fermented cucumbers), kimchi (a Korean dish using fermented vegetables, spices, and seasonings), raw milk (especially goat's and sheep's milk), full-fat raw cheeses (especially goat's and sheep's cheese), and full-fat plain yogurt. If you prefer to eat mostly plant-based foods, consider tempeh (fermented soybeans), miso (fermented soybean, barley, or brown rice with koji, which is a fungus), and natto (a Japanese dish made from fermented soybeans). We include several resources for making or purchasing fermented foods in the Recipes and Resources sections of the book.

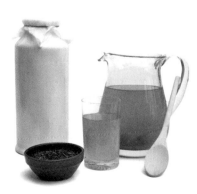

If you have gut health issues, please add fermented foods to your meals slowly. Too much of them can cause issues like gas and bloating.

10. **If you're going to eat grains, nuts, and seeds, prepare them properly.** Although we don't recommend consuming grains on a ketogenic diet, nuts and seeds are most certainly a part of the menu. Make sure you understand soaking, sprouting, fermenting, and other preparation tactics for nuts and seeds. The Weston A. Price Foundation website has an awesome video on this topic; search for "Proper Preparation of Grains and Legumes."[3]

11. **Get adequate sleep.** No, it's not something in your diet, but it's a critical element in your pursuit of optimal health. Because we're all bioindividual, the amount of sleep we need can vary between seven and nine hours of sleep each night. Some people need more and others less. But, as with food, quality matters over quantity. It's critical that you advance through the four stages of sleep. Blue light exposure is the biggest culprit in preventing a good night's sleep; it prevents our bodies from being able to produce proper amounts of melatonin and disrupts the body's natural circadian rhythm.

    Here are two tips that we've found help us immensely: First, limit exposure to blue light at night by wearing blue blocker glasses and using the Night Shift mode on devices, which turns the screen orange. Second, put red light bulbs in lamps to cut the blue light emitted from your lighting fixtures. How do these practices help you? They allow your body to heal, repair, and detoxify from the stresses of the day. Just one poor night of sleep can throw your entire health goal off kilter. It raises blood sugar higher than normal, which then makes you hungry and creates cravings for all that carbage that Big Food wants you to eat.

12. **Implement a fun exercise routine.** Again, this is not diet-related, but it's important to a healthy lifestyle. Most people abhor exercise because they have visions of agony, pain, and lots of sweat in a gym with a beefy trainer who barks orders. Who wants that? You need to find a way to move your body that's also fun for you. For example, we've found a much better way that doesn't seem like exercise to us. Movement specialist Darryl Edwards has a concept called Primal Play (www.primalplay.com). The key element in Darryl's philosophy is to make exercise fun and constantly change things up, just like we did when were kids.[4] When we were kids, we never viewed playing as exercise. We just played, and our bodies were rewarded with lower inflammation, lower insulin, improved oxygen delivery throughout the body, better mood, a lower risk of cardiovascular disease, and so much more. It's good to get a mixture of strength training and aerobic exercise each week. If the Primal Play method doesn't appeal to you, then try hiking, biking, playing tennis, or anything that gets you moving. The important thing is that you move.

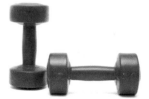

13. **Avoid using the microwave.** Microwaving food is convenient, but it alters the food, leading to an increased risk of digestive disorders.[5, 6] Also, the chemical alterations that happen in the microwaving process can disturb your lymphatic system, which directly impacts your body's ability to detoxify and inhibits the transport of your hormones to where your body needs them. That's not good. Also, using the microwave on a regular basis is potentially carcinogenic. EEEEK!

14. **Avoid using Teflon and aluminum cookware.** Whether you realize it or not, elements of your cooking vessels can be transferred to your food, so you consume and absorb them. So, when a Teflon skillet starts to chip, you're *eating* those flakes of Teflon. And that chemical is *no bueno* in the body. Also, cooking food regularly on aluminum increases heavy metals in the body, which can lead to all sorts of health problems down the road.

15. **Express gratitude for your food daily.** It seems so simple to be thankful for the blessing that you have food to eat, but how many people actually do it? When you take time to express gratitude, your body goes into a parasympathetic state, which helps you better use the food as intended. Being grateful in general leads to new relationships, improved physical health, stabilized psychological health, enhanced empathy, reduced aggression, improved sleep, greater self-esteem, and optimal mental health.[7]

16. **Find easy-to-grab, real food keto options.** We all live busy lives, and it's convenient to have foods when you're on the go in your car, traveling on a plane, or just going about living life. There are some amazing companies selling some outstanding on-the-go foods made with high-quality whole-food ingredients for those times when a meal just isn't an option. Some of our favorites include Drop an F Bomb nut butter packets, PaleoValley grass-fed meat sticks, pili nuts, and Adapt bars. We have a thorough list of some stellar companies doing things the right way in the back of the book. Meanwhile, please avoid products that have a mile-long list of questionable ingredients, even if those products claim to be healthy. Even so-called "healthy" products include funky-monkey ingredients like soy lecithin, maltitol (which can cause gastric distress and blood sugar spikes), soluble corn fiber, oat fiber, chocolate-flavored coating (what's that supposed to mean?), partially defatted peanut flour, nonfat dry milk, peanuts, and more. You'll save yourself a lot of frustration in your pursuit of optimal health if you simply keep these ingredients out of your diet.

Many low-carb and keto product manufacturers use something called "net carbs" as a means to get you to buy what they're selling under the guise that they're lower in carbohydrates than they actually are. Net carbs are the total carbohydrates in a food minus the fiber and sugar alcohols. Dr. Michael Eades, the low-carb diet author of the best-selling book *Protein Power,* created net carbs as a way for people watching their carbohydrate intake to have a little more flexibility in their diet because the fiber in food is absorbed at a much slower rate than other nutrients. Unfortunately, food companies took this concept and ran with it, putting "net carbs," "net effective carbs," and other similar phrases on packaging to fool customers on low-carb diets into getting more carbs than they bargained for. Don't fall for the net carb scam. The only intellectually honest way to know your carbohydrate tolerance level is to count total carbohydrates. Period.

17. **The changes you make are about progress, not perfection.** It would be easy for us to pretend like we've got this whole diet and health thing nailed down and that everything is hunky-dory every single day. Yeah, right! That ain't real life, and the reality is, we're not always perfect. Far too many people refuse to try to make the kinds of changes we're sharing in *Real Food Keto* because they're afraid of what friends and family might say about them in person or online. The Internet, in particular, seems to bring out the very worst in people, especially complete strangers, when you're sharing your health journey.

We've seen this firsthand since Jimmy has become more of a public figure. Think of some of the vilest, most vicious language you can imagine, and he's been called that and worse in the comments on social media and YouTube; some insults even come directly to his email inbox. The expectation that he should look a certain way if he's supposed to represent what health is has resulted in a daily barrage of hate-filled insults and not-so-subtle innuendo that he needs to stop talking about diet and health. Most of the time, these people are anonymous and would probably never say any of these things to Jimmy's face, especially when they see his six-foot-three-inch-tall body. (He could probably body slam most of these people!) Christine hasn't been immune to it, either; she's been called fat, four eyes, and much worse. We've been online long enough to realize that this abuse comes with the territory, but we're human beings with feelings and hurts that are affected by this constant onslaught of ugliness.

The reality is that the people making comments about our weight don't know our journey, and they assume that being thin means being healthy. That's the biggest lie we've ever been told. (Christine's story in the Introduction is a perfect illustration of someone who is thin but was not healthy.) The truth is that managing weight is more difficult when you have an autoimmune condition like Hashimoto's thyroiditis as Christine does or insulin resistance as Jimmy does. Christine also had a total hysterectomy in 2016 to deal with another painful autoimmune disease she was dealing with—endometriosis—that led to all sorts of hormonal changes that she's still getting used to. Through these challenges, both of us have remained highly engaged in our health, seeking to make it the best we can and helping others along the way.

It's tempting to judge people based on looks, but let us encourage you to look deeper at the people you encounter and extend a hand of compassion and love to counter the insults and hatred that have pervaded our culture. It's through this that you learn a lot more about these people who you think are unhealthy and realize how incredibly healthy they really are. Your fellow human beings deserve respect, forgiveness, and the benefit of the doubt when you don't know anything more about them than what you see on the outside. The contributions that these lovely people have to offer this world are priceless, and we should never squelch the voices of those who have something to share.

In the end, this is *your* journey to better health and no one else's. Find what works for you and then do that confidently with nary a thought or concern with what others think. The only person you are ultimately accountable for is yourself. All the rest is just chatter. Perfectionism will eat you from the inside out because it induces stress and robs you of the enjoyment of creating a meal and then consuming it for nourishment. Think of it this way: trying to be perfect makes you imperfect because of the inflammation it brings on. In fact, we know that hanging on to "hurt causes toxicity, malabsorption, and genetic dysregulation,"[8] and that isn't a good thing, ever.

As you can see, these are a few small changes you can make right away to start your *Real Food Keto* journey to success in your health. Don't overthink it or stress about it. That's not good for you, anyway. Take it all in stride and take baby steps in the right direction at your own pace. Your progress on this journey is about so much more than just your weight. The primary goal is not necessarily weight loss. Instead, your focus should be the many health gains you will see when you eat this way, and you'll realize the nirvana of being right where you want to be in your health. That's what we hope to help you achieve with this book.

Now that you get the point of what we're communicating, it's time for us to get down to business and share more about the *Real Food Keto* diet and how you're going to want to eat. Everything we've shared up to now has laid the foundation of what's coming in Part 2, where we discuss the various macronutrients that make up your diet. If you're still unsure about what exactly you'll be eating, then pay attention to the next few chapters, where we sort it all out for you.

REAL FOOD KETO TAKEAWAYS FROM CHAPTER 3

- We need to honor the great contributions of Dr. Weston A. Price and Dr. Francis Pottenger, Jr.

- When we allowed industrialized food into our lives, traditional food preparation went away.

- The advancements in chemical development introduced a means for preserving food longer (hydrogenation), but that development resulted in a cost to our health.

- There are a multitude of things you can do right away to optimize your diet and lifestyle.

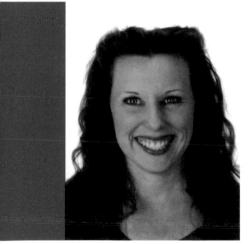

KATRINA FOE, NTP, CPT-PMA

www.PersonalizedPilates.com/nutritionaltherapy

In my practice I have found that people on a ketogenic diet are looking for health benefits—weight loss, improving thyroid issues, heart disease/cancer/Alzheimer's prevention, diabetes management, etc. With nutritional therapy, I've been able to help by testing exactly what will support their bodies best to maximize and accelerate those health benefits. It is not about diagnosing or symptom-chasing but about personalizing the ketogenic diet for a specific client. I also integrate my Pilates background with the keto diet and nutritional therapy to create a customized plan to bring balance to their muscular system, which greatly improves their movement mechanics and therefore enhances their body's performance both in everyday life and athletic endeavors.

I adopted a ketogenic diet in order to finish my natural cancer therapy and found that it miraculously resolved my manic depression, which I had suffered for over 25 years. However, there were still other lingering issues that I have used nutritional therapy to fine-tune by being able to test what exact foods/supplements best support my body at a particular time. I have been surprised many times that what I thought would be the best choice of a treatment (herb, glandular, mineral, vitamin, etc.) would not be at all what my body wanted. It's profound to be able to ensure that the time and energy spent on treatment will be effective!

part 2
THE MACROS (AKA THE DIET)

In Part 1, we gave an overview of why we've chosen to merge the worlds of real food and a ketogenic diet into one cohesive concept. Now that you understand more about the basics of what nutrition is and how we've come to where we are today, it's time to dig deeper into the various nutrients—especially the essential ones—that make up a healthy diet. When you better understand why what you eat matters, you can take that knowledge and progress to the next level of properly forming a healthy meal on a plate. It's time to get our hands dirty and go into much greater detail about the three main macronutrients as we discuss fats, proteins, and carbohydrates. We even throw water into this section because it's widely considered the fourth macronutrient. It's time to get down to business and look at the various macronutrients and how they apply to your pursuit of a healthy lifestyle.

CHAPTER 4

Fat Is Where It's At

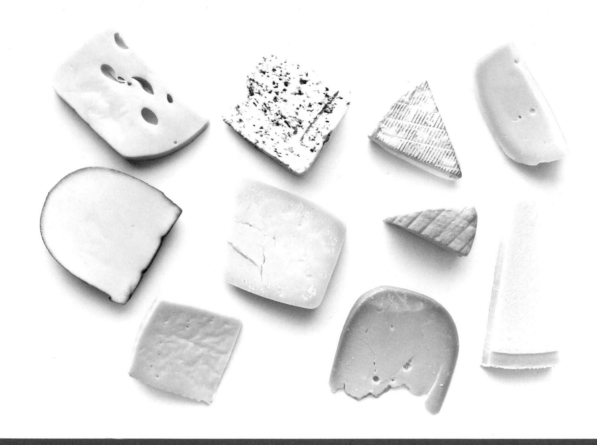

Among the macronutrients is one that's considered the most controversial—fat! For decades, well-meaning health professionals have told us that dietary fat is the single greatest enemy in the pursuit of weight loss and optimal health. They make this claim almost entirely based on the fact that fat is so rich in calories that you can cut the amount you eat to reduce your total caloric intake, and they say that single change will help you lose weight, which, in turn, will improve your health. Sounds logical, right? But many experts don't stop there. They claim that consuming fat—especially the evilest of all fats, known as saturated fat—will clog your arteries, give you a heart attack, and quite possibly kill you! Why on earth would you ever want to consume fat under these auspices?!

The truth of the matter is that fat isn't an enemy in your health when it comes from real food sources and is the primary macronutrient in your meals as part of a healthy low-carb, high-fat, ketogenic nutritional approach. The reality about obesity and heart disease is that these health conditions have much less to do with the fat and calories you consume and more to do with the processed carbohydrates and sugars that dominate what we eat collectively as a society (as well as a deficiency in healthy fats). We have a lot to say on this subject, and it's the foundation for your success in implementing the tenets of *Real Food Keto* into your life.

As we already discussed, the availability of crappy carbage and rancid vegetable oils that oxidize your cells should make it crystal clear why people are overweight and obese and why chronic disease is still rising at an alarming rate. The causes have less to do with the foods consumed than with the inflammation those foods bring on. You see, there's no disease without inflammation. The things that we know raise inflammation the most are what Jimmy calls "the twin villains": carbohydrates, especially processed ones, and vegetable oils. There also are certain disease states—including sleep apnea, arthritis, ulcerative colitis, autoimmune diseases like Hashimoto's thyroiditis, infectious diseases like HIV, periodontal disease, hyperlipidemia, and type 2 diabetes—that are brought on by these poor dietary choices and can exacerbate the inflammatory pathways.[1]

So how exactly did we get to this point of vilifying what we know is an essential macronutrient in a healthy diet, especially when we're in pursuit of nutritional ketosis? And if what we are doing now and have been doing for decades—telling people to lower their fat intake—has been working, then why in the world have the rates of obesity, heart disease, and type 2 diabetes risen to all-time highs, with no sign of the sharp upward trend stopping?

It's time for a little history lesson. Be prepared to be shocked by the dubious beginnings of how this low-fat mantra became such an integral part of the fabric of our culture.

THE GENESIS OF FAT-PHOBIA

Ask people whether consuming dietary fat is healthy or unhealthy, and it's very probable that the overwhelming response will be that it's harmful. But have you ever stopped to wonder why we as a society believe that fat is a bad thing to consume?

It all started about sixty years ago when an American scientist named Ancel Keys began looking at the connection between saturated fat, cholesterol, and heart disease and developed what would become known in research circles as the Diet-Heart Hypothesis. It was only a hypothesis, a theory, a whim, yet Keys took it and ran with it—even though he had to pull some underhanded shenanigans to substantiate it.

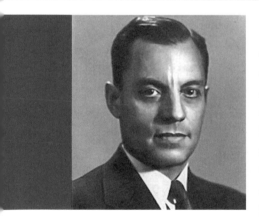

DR. ANCEL KEYS

As he started compiling data from countries around the world on saturated fat and cholesterol intake and the corresponding rates of cardiovascular disease, Ancel Keys became more and more convinced of the truth of his hypothesis and sought to spread it in the medical research community. At first, others laughed at him, scoffing at the idea that the high-fat foods people were commonly eating could cause harm to their heart health. But then, in 1958, Keys published his famous Seven Countries Study, which concluded that in the countries where saturated fat and cholesterol consumption was the highest, including Japan, Italy, Great Britain, Australia, Canada, and the United States, there was a correlating rise in heart disease rates.

Keys received accolades for his innovation, and this newfound health discovery landed him on the front cover of *Time* magazine in 1961. The American Heart Association and many other prominent health groups lined up to embrace the idea of cutting fat, especially saturated fat, for improving cardiovascular and overall health. There was only one problem—Keys didn't share all the data in his study. That's right; he lied by omission. In a court of law, this would be considered not telling "the whole truth."

Although the Seven Countries Study certainly looked like an open-and-shut case proving that saturated fat raised cholesterol levels, which led to heart disease, what most people didn't realize at the time was that Keys had data from sixteen *other* countries that didn't fit his theory. Populations like the Australian aboriginals consumed less saturated fat and had lower cholesterol rates but had higher rates of heart disease; people in countries like Switzerland consumed more saturated fat and had higher cholesterol levels but had lower rates of heart disease. The connection between fat, cholesterol, and heart disease simply was not there. But media darling Keys got exactly what he wanted—a big splash in the research world and in the public eye that would lead to a fundamental shift in the way America and Westernized society would eat for health. And he had plenty of help promoting this position as influential political leaders accepted the Diet-Heart Hypothesis and eventually would make low-fat eating the "law" of the nutritional land.

Meanwhile, behind the scenes, some dirty shenanigans went on to help promote the idea that saturated fat and cholesterol were our enemies, despite there being a lack of solid science to support this theory. People like British physiologist and nutritionist John Yudkin (whose seminal 1972 book *Pure, White, and Deadly* warned the world about sugar decades before we heeded his call[2]) were mounting evidence against sugar and its negative implications on health. The sugar industry knew it had to take drastic measures to protect itself—even if it meant crossing a line of ethics in research.

Because of documents published in the November 2016 issue of *JAMA Internal Medicine,* we now know that the sugar industry paid scientists in the 1960s to tell people that saturated fat was what caused heart disease instead of the true culprit—sugar.[3] Internal documents from the Sugar Research Foundation (now known as the Sugar Association) came to light and revealed that three Harvard scientists had received today's equivalent of $50,000 to publish a bogus paper hyping the negative effects of saturated fat on heart disease while ignoring the role of sugar. And it worked.

One of those Harvard scientists was a man named D. Mark Hegsted. Because of his willingness to accept hush money from sugar lobbyists and shine a bright light on fat as the culprit in heart disease and obesity, he received a position at the United States Department of Agriculture (USDA), where he was named the head of nutrition. In 1977, he continued to promote the fat-phobia message by helping to draft what would eventually become the very first government-sanctioned and -approved Dietary Guidelines for Americans in 1980. That's right; not only was the fear of fat that we still have to this day predicated on faulty data by Ancel Keys, but our fate of having fat-free everything in our food supply was sealed by the sugar industry throwing a small amount of money at researchers to make a stink about it. We're still paying the consequences of that bribery today.[4]

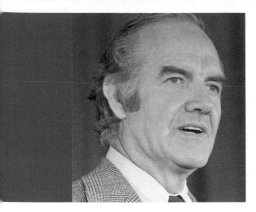

SENATOR GEORGE MCGOVERN

Senator George McGovern was so heavily influenced by the work of Ancel Keys that he looked for a way to push the idea of cutting fat on the American public. In 1977, he promoted what would become the first dietary goals for the United States as a means of combating heart disease. These guidelines instructed people to cut their fat and cholesterol intake, eat fewer processed grains and sugars, and consume more complex carbohydrates from fruits, vegetables, and whole-grain sources. In 1980, the USDA latched on to this idea and put the federal government's seal of approval on a low-fat, high-carb diet when it developed the Dietary Guidelines for Americans that were accompanied by the Food Pyramid[5] (which has morphed into today's MyPlate[6]). The USDA has updated these guidelines every five years, and not much has changed in nearly forty years.

Water
Minimum of 8 Servings

Milk, Yogurt &
Cheese Group
2–3 Servings

Vegetable Group
3–5 Servings

Fruit Group
2–4 Servings

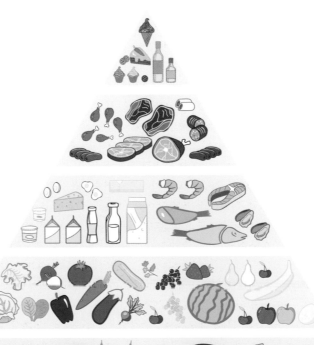

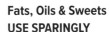

Fats, Oils & Sweets
USE SPARINGLY

Meat, Poultry, Fish,
Dry Beans, Eggs &
Nuts Group
2–3 Servings

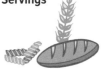

Bread, Cereal, Rice &
Pasta Group
6–11 Servings

Alcohol in Limited
Quantities

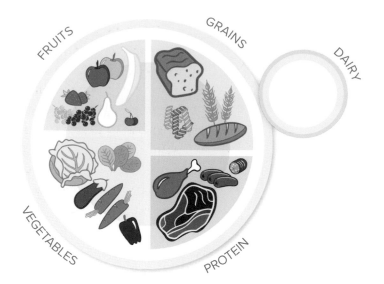

My Plate

Although incremental changes have taken place, the sad reality is that these guidelines still heavily promote a low-fat diet that was never, ever proven to be healthy for your heart or to help you shed a single pound.

In 2015, Nina Teicholz, author of the *New York Times* best-selling book *The Big Fat Surprise,*[7] created a 501(c)(3) nonprofit, nonpartisan educational organization called the Nutrition Coalition (nutritioncoalition.us), which is seeking to make major fundamental changes to the Dietary Guidelines for Americans by encouraging evidence-based nutrition instead of flawed science. Undoing the negative perception of fat in our culture seems like an impossible task right now, but at least some people are trying.

Telling people that consuming saturated fat is good for them is like telling people that Darth Vader is a good guy. But nobody would believe you because we so strongly associate Darth Vader with being a bad guy that people never really question it. The same can be said about fat, especially saturated fat. We have believed it to be harmful to our health for so long that it'll take a miracle or a major reversal by scientists, government leaders, and health organizations to turn the conversation around. Our intent in this book is to show that it's possible to eat a high-fat diet and thrive. Real food–based fats are not and never will be enemies in your health.

The push for a low-fat diet as a means for getting healthy has been a complete and utter disaster in America and in other countries that have adopted similar dietary policies. The unintended consequence of telling people to cut their fat intake is that they had to replace that fat with something else—and that something else was carbohydrates, especially processed ones! Consumption of carbohydrates skyrocketed because of the Food Pyramid recommendation that we eat six to eleven daily servings of bread, pasta, and other grain-based foods. (We get into the good and bad about carbohydrates in Chapter 6.)

Suffice it say that the low-fat diet has been a failed nutritional health experiment that was thrust on us by people who should have known better. Even with all the knowledge we now have about how saturated fat isn't as harmful as once thought, people still believe fat is bad, and shifting that mentality could take years or even decades. Family doctors are still recommending to their patients to cut their fat intake as a means of losing weight and improving health, and healthy lifestyle advocates on television and radio often still promote a low-fat diet. Something has got to wake us up from this sixty-year nightmare that Ancel Keys kicked off with his deceptive research and slick propaganda!

THE LEGACY OF THE LOW-FAT LIE

If you spend a little time reading about obesity rates and trends or take one look at the alarming rise in obesity shown in the graph below, then it's clear that encouraging people to cut fat and increase carbohydrate intake has led to people gaining weight at an alarming rate. There are similar trend lines in statistical analyses conducted on heart disease, type 2 diabetes, and other obesity-related disorders and diseases. Keep in mind that all these conditions get much worse as carbohydrate intake increases, not as dietary fat intake increases. Carbohydrates raise blood sugar and insulin levels, whereas fat is basically benign. So why do we vilify fat and give carbohydrates a free pass?

PREVALENCE OF OBESITY AMONG U.S. ADULTS AGES 20–74[8]

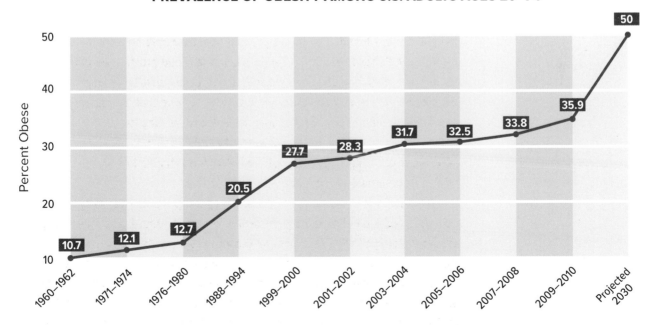

In a book like *Real Food Keto,* fat is most certainly where it's at for health and vitality like you've never experienced on any other diet. We can't tell you how many times we've dreaded attempting to lose weight and get healthy using the same old advice to cut fat and calories. The low-carb, moderate-protein, high-fat, ketogenic diet was a game-changer for both of us, and adding in the real food element is the key to the health you've always dreamed of.

Now that you know you want to eat high-fat, let's examine some reasons why you need more fat in your diet.

THE BENEFITS OF CONSUMING FAT

Now that you realize just how bamboozled we have been about dietary fat and that real food fats like butter, coconut oil, and lard are actually pretty good for you, you might be wondering specifically what's beneficial about consuming fat. Well, you've come to the right place. We're going to make your head explode with so many truth bombs about fat that you'll want to run to the kitchen to have a tablespoon of coconut oil right now! Ready? Let's go.

We could spend all day listing the many benefits of consuming fat, but here are thirteen (lucky you) compelling reasons why you need to start eating more real food fats right away:

1. **Fat is the perfect source of energy.** Many people think they get their energy solely from the carbohydrates they consume. Although carbs do provide energy when you're a sugar burner, you shift to being a fat burner when you eat a ketogenic diet with increased fat consumption. Because dietary fat has more than twice as many calories per gram (nine) than protein and carbs (four each), you get a powerful load of energy with less food intake. Have you ever noticed that when you eat a breakfast of just bacon and eggs, you don't get hungry for many hours afterward? That's the power-packed punch of energy that you get when you're fat-fueled! In fact, more and more athletes are tapping into using fat for energy because they've found it sustains their energy and helps them perform at their best.

2. **Fat provides better satiety (hunger control).** One of the biggest benefits of eating more fat is its unique ability to slow the absorption of the protein and carbohydrates you eat, which lessens the blood sugar and insulin response to those foods. The result is that you feel fuller, longer, which means you don't have to reach for something else to eat so soon after a meal. There's

no greater feeling of control over food than experiencing true satiation. If you have to eat again less than six hours after your last meal, then you clearly didn't consume enough fat in that meal.

3. **The brain health benefits of eating fat are spectacular.** Don't take this personally, but you're a fathead. That's right, more than 70 percent of your brain is fat, so it stands to reason that your brain would thrive and run quite efficiently on fat and ketones as compared with glucose. Without adequate amounts of real food fat in your diet, you'll notice you are crankier and have difficulty thinking clearly; perhaps you'll think you're having a nervous breakdown. Many people turn to the medical profession to give them prescription drugs to deal with the side effects of not consuming enough fat, but the reality is that they just need more butter in their diet! How many people suffer needlessly with brain health issues when all they needed was a little more fat? Far too many!

Christine saw big improvements in her mood and anxiety levels once she added more healthy fats to her diet. The increase in healthy fats allowed her to finally absorb fat-soluble vitamin D, which helped to stabilize her moods and lessen her anxiety and panic attacks. She was able to get off all the medications she had been taking for depression and anxiety once she started feeding her brain the nutrient it needed—fat.

4. **Fat makes your heart healthier.** What?! You read that right—eating dietary fat is *good* for your heart. Just as fat is the preferred fuel source for the brain, it's likewise what the heart uses to function well. Consuming real food–based good fats—including saturated fats like butter, coconut oil, and lard; omega-3 fats such as fish oil, grass-fed beef, pastured eggs, and walnuts; and omega-6 fats like pumpkin seeds, raw sunflower seeds, pine nuts, and pistachios—will energize your heart and keep it ticking as the good Lord intended. So much for artery clogging, right?

5. **Fat helps improve oxygen delivery to the cells.** If cells aren't getting adequate amounts of oxygen, then they experience an increase in inflammation, leading to chronic health issues and possibly even death. Other than that, you'll be okay. (Just kidding.) It's our cells that use fats (lipids) to produce adenosine triphosphate (ATP), which is the body's main source of energy. So, if you want to oxygenate your cells, then you'd better darn well eat more fat. That's an order!

6. **Fat allows the body to absorb the critical fat-soluble vitamins.** Chapter 9 explains that the four essential fat-soluble vitamins are A, D, E, and K. "Fat-soluble" means that the body requires fat to absorb and use them properly. If you don't have proper fat intake, then your body can't do anything with these vitamins, which would lead to significant negative consequences in your health. A vitamin A deficiency, for example, can lead to dry skin, an increase in susceptibility to infections, and even blindness. A vitamin D deficiency can cause poor bone structure because vitamin D helps the body use dietary calcium to strengthen bones. Additionally, a lack of adequate amounts of vitamin D increases arterial inflammation that leads to cardiovascular disease. A deficiency in vitamin E contributes to infertility and reproductive issues, fragile red blood cells, neurological issues, and mild anemia. Lastly, a vitamin K deficiency makes you susceptible to bruising easily, having heavy menstrual periods, and excessively bleeding from wounds. In the end, it doesn't matter how much vitamin A, D, E, or K you take; if you don't have enough fat in your diet to absorb them, your body can't use them. Can we get you pat of butter?

The wrong kinds of fat—including the polyunsaturated seed (vegetable) oils that are so commonly found in grocery store aisles—can easily oxidize cells throughout the body. This process of cellular oxidation causes serious damage to the cell membranes, cellular proteins, lipids, and DNA, which wreaks havoc on the entire body because of the development of dangerous free radicals. These free radicals steal electrons from other molecules, which can cause major damage in your body.

7. **Fat makes healthy cell membranes.** Most people are unaware that their cell membranes are composed of fat. Thus, it stands to reason that you want to consume adequate amounts of fat to keep your cells happy and healthy. If your cell membranes aren't getting adequate fat, then you won't be able to absorb all the nutrients your body needs to function effectively because fat is what helps transport nutrients across the cell membranes. In fact, the makeup of these cell membranes is the same as the makeup of the tissues of your heart and arteries. So, yet again, eating fat is shown to be beneficial to heart health when you give your cell membranes this key macronutrient that makes them work.

8. **Fat makes food taste good.** Professional chefs know how to get flavor into their dishes, and they will be the first to tell you that adding healthy fats is the secret to the flavor of a dish. Bacon and butter are incredibly tasty because they're chock full of the saturated fats your body craves. And when you restrict carbohydrate intake to your tolerance level, these fatty foods are incredibly good for you, too! We don't know about you, but we'd much rather have the fattier cut of steak, like the rib-eye, with some butter on top than a lean sirloin with steak sauce. There's just no comparison.

9. **Fat helps reduce inflammation in the body.** One of the primary ways fatty acids lower inflammation levels is that they're used to create prostaglandins (more on this in a moment), which control inflammatory pathways in the body. Getting the appropriate mix of fatty acids is crucial for managing inflammation levels. Inflammation is at the root of all the major chronic diseases of civilization, including heart disease and type 2 diabetes.

Fatty acid deficiency can cause our bodies not to use calcium properly; this is because K2, a fat-soluble vitamin, is needed to help transport calcium to the appropriate places in the body. The result of not getting enough dietary fat is that calcium deposits form in inappropriate places, like the coronary arteries. So, too much fat isn't the problem in the development of heart disease; it's the *lack of* adequate amounts of fat that is the real culprit!

10. **Fat is necessary for healthy immune function.** Consuming too much of any one type of fat can lead to an improper immune response, assisting in the formation of the antibodies that can lead to food allergies. Balancing your fat intake among saturated, monounsaturated, omega-6, and omega-3 fats can keep your immunity in tip-top shape. We discuss this balance later in this chapter.

11. **Fat aids the endocrine system in creating hormones.** Adequate fatty acid intake ensures that communication between the cells and hormones takes place. The fat-soluble hormones—the steroid hormones and thyroid hormones—especially need dietary fat to be produced in the proper quantities. Fat also is important for the three classes of what are called *eicosanoids:* thromboxanes, leukotrienes, and prostaglandins. That might seem like a bunch of gobbledygook right now, but don't worry; we explain what all this means in Chapter 12, which covers the endocrine system. Suffice it to say that eating fat is doing some great things in your body.

12. **Fat keeps the gallbladder and liver functioning properly.** Fat stimulates the gallbladder to produce bile and keeps that bile flowing smoothly without letting it get too thick. Bile has two primary functions—it helps break down fat, and it helps remove toxins from the body. Christine knows firsthand why adequate fat intake is so critical. Because she ate a low-fat diet throughout her twenties, she started having issues with her gallbladder that required its removal in 2006. Her body couldn't produce bile, and that prevented her liver from getting rid of toxins that were building up in her body. See how easy it would have been to prevent this had she simply not feared fat?

13. **Fat helps with detoxification.** Your body stores most toxins in your fat tissue as a means of protecting you from harm. So, when you start eating a low-carb, moderate-protein, high-fat diet that produces ketones, you begin to mobilize that stored body fat, which releases toxins into your body. However, as we said in reason 12, you also produce the bile necessary for removing these toxins from your body for good. Having a good balance of fats in your diet allows the toxins to be cleared from your body promptly because cell membranes are permeable, and permeable cell membranes allow nutrients and other substances to pass in and out of the cells with ease. Are you getting the idea of how everything is intricately interconnected?

THE PROBLEM WITH HAVING A FAT DEFICIENCY

Perhaps you're finally realizing the importance of fat as a macronutrient, and maybe you're starting to view it for the first time in your life as the healthy nutrient it has always been. Or maybe you're still quite skeptical and need some more convincing to start embracing fat. Fair enough; we get it. We've been where you are, and we eventually had an epiphany that woke us up from our fat-phobia nightmare. We have plenty more evidence to present, including the myriad problems that can occur as a direct result of a fatty acid deficiency.

Eating a low-fat, high-carb diet that follows the Dietary Guidelines for Americans or even the standard American diet (SAD), which includes lots of sugar and processed carbohydrates, can lead to gallbladder dysfunction (where bile becomes viscous) and the formation of painful gallstones. Unhealthy dietary fats contribute to these problems as well. If you're not producing proper amounts of bile from real food fats in your diet, then you can't and won't digest and absorb the nutrients that are critical to optimal health. Period. End of story.

Another key problem with having a fat deficiency is the inability to absorb and use the fat-soluble vitamins A, D, E, and K. You could supplement your diet with very high doses of these vitamins and still be unable to use them if you don't consume enough fat. The results of not absorbing fat-soluble vitamins are some serious health consequences down the road; we explain more about these in Chapter 9. Are you starting to get a little more convinced? Keep reading; there's more.

When you eat a low-fat diet, your body can't deal appropriately with inflammation. Getting a healthy balance of omega-3 fats and omega-6 fats (polyunsaturated fats), saturated fats, and monounsaturated fats—broken down as 10 percent polyunsaturated fats, 30 percent saturated fats, and 60 percent monounsaturated fats—calms the inflammatory pathways and vastly improves your health. There's a really geeky reason why this happens: Hormonelike substances, known as *prostaglandins,* are fatty acid compounds present in every single tissue in your body. They aren't secreted from a gland like most hormones are. Instead, they're made by a chemical reaction that occurs where they're needed most. (We're going super nerdy on you, but there's an invaluable point to knowing this.)

There are three types of prostaglandins you need to know about. Each one derives from a different fat in your diet:

- Prostaglandin 1 (PG1) comes from omega-6 fats (linoleic acid), and it's anti-inflammatory.

- Prostaglandin 2 (PG2) comes from saturated fat (arachidonic acid), and it's slightly inflammatory as a means of bringing about healing.

- Prostaglandin 3 (PG3) comes from omega-3 fats (alpha-linolenic acid), and it's anti-inflammatory.

Additionally, adequate prostaglandin production requires other things (cofactors), including proper digestion, optimal liver function, and the right amount of amino acids, vitamin B6, magnesium, and zinc. On top of this, prostaglandin formation can be inhibited when you consume trans fatty acids, aspirin, NSAIDs (pain medications like Aleve and Tylenol), alcohol, and steroids. While many NSAIDs lower inflammation and pain levels (which is the purpose of using them), they can block the conversion of arachidonic acid from saturated fat into PG2, which can prevent proper healing of inflammation from taking place. Plus, if the healthy inflammatory process of PG2 doesn't take place, then PG1 and PG3 can't do what they're supposed to do. See how one thing leads to another, and everything can quickly cascade downhill?

One of the reasons we're such staunch advocates for the ketogenic way of life is because it's not only anti-inflammatory (for the reasons stated earlier) but it's also highly effective at lowering insulin levels. When you don't eat enough fat, though, your insulin production can increase and prevent proper prostaglandin formation. When you have elevated insulin, PG1 is blocked, and your body can't properly deal with inflammation. The result is a state of chronic inflammation, particularly in the circulatory system, which manifests physically as hypertension (high blood pressure) because the inflammation reduces the space that your blood has to flow through your veins. It's a wicked process that you easily could prevent by eating more fat.

Do you ever experience depression, muscle aches, bone spurs, osteoporosis, cardiovascular health concerns, adrenal issues, allergies, or autoimmunity? These ailments could all be related to a fatty acid deficiency. One of the telltale signs that you have a deficiency is that your body can't absorb and use calcium correctly. This calcium can be deposited in other parts of your body, including your coronary arteries. The fat-soluble vitamin K2 is incredibly important for helping to put calcium where it's supposed to go. If you eat a low-fat diet, choose the wrong types of fats, or can't digest and absorb the fats you eat, then the K2 doesn't work.

THE THREE MAJOR KINDS OF FATS:
SATURATED, MONOUNSATURATED, AND POLYUNSATURATED

This section describes three major types of fats that should be included in your ketogenic lifestyle and lists sources of those fats so you know what to look for when you're grocery shopping. The three types of fats are saturated fats, monounsaturated fats, and polyunsaturated fats.

Keep in mind that if you're like Christine and you don't have a gallbladder, then you should stick with butter and coconut oil as your primary saturated fat sources because they don't require bile to break them down. Add in the other saturated, monounsaturated, and polyunsaturated fats slowly. Once your body learns to make enough bile to handle the increased dietary fat that comes with a ketogenic diet, then you can eat fat to satiety without any issues.

SATURATED FATS

Saturated fatty acids (SFAs) are highly stable. They have no double bonds between carbon atoms and are saturated with hydrogen molecules. These fats are typically solid at room temperature. Good sources include coconut oil, full-fat raw dairy, fatty cuts of meat (like rib-eye steak and pork belly), and lard. There are many more sources of saturated fats, including the following:

- Palm oil
- Butter
- Animal fats like lard, tallow, suet, duck fat, and goose fat
- Chocolate (unsweetened)
- Fish like sardines, menhaden, cod, herring, and salmon
- Cheese (full-fat), like goat cheese, cheddar, Colby, Cheshire, cream cheese, fontina, Monterey Jack, blue cheese, gjetost, Roquefort, Gruyère, Swiss, Romano, Brie, Parmesan, and feta
- Heavy cream (full-fat)
- Nuts like pili nuts, macadamia nuts, Brazil nuts, and cashews

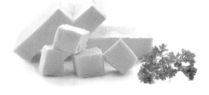

One type of fat that is extremely beneficial to your health on a ketogenic diet is medium-chain triglycerides, or MCTs. This saturated fat is a concentrated by-product of coconut oil or palm oil and is an excellent precursor to the formation of more ketones (fat-burning). Four types of MCTs are found in food, including caproic acid (C6), caprylic acid (C8), capric acid (C10), and lauric acid (C12). More than 75 percent of MCT oil is from C12, which the body metabolizes slowly. C8 makes up 12 percent, and C10 comprises 10 percent of MCTs; both of these provide rapid ketone conversion for a quick boost of energy. You can use MCT oil as a supplement (just go slowly; some people report gastrointestinal issues from consuming too much too fast), or you can drizzle it on top of a salad for a healthy fat boost. It's also popular in fatty coffee and smoothies.

MONOUNSATURATED FATS

Monounsaturated fats (MUFAs) are relatively stable. They have one double bond (thus *mono*) in the fatty acid chain, and the remainder are single bonds. These fats tend to be liquid at room temperature but start to solidify when chilled. A good example is olive oil. Use caution, though: A lot of the olive oils on grocery store shelves are mixed with various hydrogenated polyunsaturated fats (as much as 40 percent). So you need to make sure that the oil you choose is 100 percent olive oil and from the same source. Look at the label of an olive oil bottle in a store, and you'll sometimes find upward of twenty different countries of origin. Plus, a lot of companies add polyunsaturated oils to their olive oil to keep costs down. You have to be vigilant in reading the label on each bottle. We share an excellent source for olive oil in the Resources section on page 358.

The quality of these oils is very important. Make sure to choose cold-pressed and organic oils.

Here's a list of other healthy monounsaturated fats you can consume:

- Avocados
- Nuts and nut butters (unsweetened)
- Safflower oil (high oleic)
- Sunflower oil
- Sesame oil[10]

POLYUNSATURATED FATS

The quality of these oils is important. Read labels to make sure they are not hydrogenated.

Polyunsaturated fatty acids (PUFAs) are relatively unstable. They contain more than one double bond. These fats tend to be liquid at room temperature but start to solidify when chilled. The way these oils are processed is very important. Most of the ones you see on store shelves are hydrogenated (you might see a term like "partially hydrogenated," and this is a huge warning flag). Hydrogenated fats are the worst fats of all, and you want to stay away from them. Try to find oils that are cold-pressed and organic. Read labels. PUFAs are generally frowned upon by various health communities, but there are good ones that people following the *Real Food Keto* approach should be eating, which are listed here:

- Fish, such as salmon, mackerel, herring, albacore tuna, and trout
- Flax seeds and flax oil
- Safflower oil
- Sunflower seeds
- Walnuts[11]

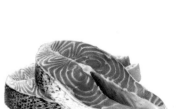

ESSENTIAL POLYUNSATURATED FATS:
LINOLEIC ACID AND ALPHA-LINOLENIC ACID

There are two essential polyunsaturated fatty acids, and you'll recall why they're essential—our bodies can't make them, so we have to get them from external sources. These oils are sensitive to heat and light, so you shouldn't cook with them, and you should purchase brands that come in dark bottles, which helps keep them stable. The first is linoleic acid (LA), which contains ample amounts of the healthy kind of omega-6 fat. Good examples include raw nuts and seeds. Be sure to avoid nuts and seeds that are roasted in highly unstable and inflammatory oils like soybean or cottonseed oil, which only adds more oxidative stress to your body. The second essential polyunsaturated fat is alpha-linolenic acid (ALA), which contains the healthy kind of omega-3 fat. A perfect source that we love using for its heart-health benefits is cod liver oil.

The ratio of omega-6 to omega-3 in the diet should be approximately 1:1, which mimics what Dr. Weston A. Price observed in the diets of people living in traditional cultures. (Read Chapter 3 for more information about Dr. Price's findings.)

Good Sources of Linoleic Acid/Omega-6 Fatty Acids:

- Eggs
- Nuts, including pine nuts, pistachios, Brazil nuts, and walnuts
- Poultry
- Seeds like pumpkin seeds, raw sunflower seeds, and sesame seeds
- Vegetable oils that are cold-pressed and organic[12]

Good Sources of Alpha-Linolenic Acid/Omega-3 Fatty Acids:

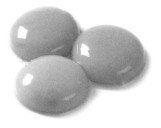

- Chia seeds
- Egg yolks
- Fish like mackerel, herring, salmon, whitefish, sardines, and anchovies
- Some green vegetables like Brussels sprouts, kale, spinach, and watercress
- Walnuts[13]

OMEGA-9 FATS

With all the attention paid to omega-3 and omega-6 fats, you shouldn't ignore the important role of omega-9 fatty acids. We don't hear as much about this omega fat because the body doesn't require as much of it as the others. Unlike omega-3 and omega-6 fats, which are essential because the body can't make them, omega-9 fats are nonessential because the body can make them from various foods that we consume. There are two omega-9 fatty acids—oleic acid and erucic acid. Oleic acid is the more common; it's in keto-friendly real food sources such as extra-virgin olive oil, almond oil, avocado oil, and macadamia nut oil. The primary benefit of omega-9 fat is how well it raises HDL ("good") cholesterol, which is good for your cardiovascular health.

WHY HYDROGENATED OILS AND FOODS ARE BAD FOR US

When we talk about good fats, we're referring to whole-food sources of saturated fats, monounsaturated fats, and polyunsaturated fats (including omega-3, omega-6, and omega-9 fatty acids, as described in the preceding section). So what exactly are considered bad fats? The ones you need to avoid at all costs are hydrogenated oils, partially hydrogenated oils, and trans fats. You might not know what hydrogenated oils are from their name, but you've probably consumed foods like margarine, shortening, and vegetable (seed) oils.

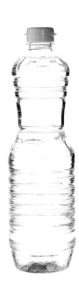

Food companies love to put oils through heavy processing to hydrogenate them because it helps make their products more shelf stable. The oils stay solid at room temperature to keep things like snack cakes moist for a very long time. Can you imagine what that hydrogenated oil is doing inside your body? You don't want to know. (But we're still going to tell you in a moment.) In a nutshell, our bodies simply don't recognize these oils as real foods—because they're not.

These hydrogenated oils are very bad news for your health. In fact, they can cause you to develop a fatty acid deficiency. How exactly do they do this? The hydrogenation process changes the makeup of the oil and causes your cell membranes to stiffen, which hinders the ability of nutrients and other substances to pass through. So these oils that were once natural and unprocessed become unnatural to the body as a result of hydrogenation. These oils also raise LDL (bad) cholesterol and lower HDL (good or protective) cholesterol, and they can even possibly lead to cancer and diabetes because of the inflammation they create in the body. Fully hydrogenated oils don't contain trans fatty acids like partially hydrogenated oils do because fully hydrogenated oils are saturated with hydrogen.

As bad as hydrogenated fats are, they have an evil cousin called trans fatty acids, which are commonly referred to as trans fats. Partially hydrogenated oils contain trans fatty acids. Packaged cakes, cookies, crackers, muffins, pies, and all sorts of other crappy carbage contain trans fats, and most people are oblivious to them. When an oil is partially hydrogenated, not all of the fat is saturated with hydrogen—hence the *partially hydrogenated* in the name. A small percentage of the unsaturated fats become trans fats, which have been shown to have very harmful effects on the body, including an increased risk of heart attack. They raise LDL cholesterol and lower HDL cholesterol. These oils also block the production of chemicals that combat inflammation and, ironically, actually *promote* inflammation (which is something real food–based fats don't do). Trans fats can cause the immune system to become overly active, and they're linked to an increased risk of developing heart disease and type 2 diabetes.[14]

This information makes you never want to touch another fast-food french fry or doughnut, right? Food companies try to hide the trans fat contents of their products by reducing the serving sizes so that each serving has less than a half gram of trans fats. If a food falls within this parameter, the U.S. Food & Drug Administration (FDA) allows the company to describe the food as being free from trans fat. The resulting serving sizes are generally so unrealistically small that you could end up consuming multiple servings, putting more of these trans fats into your body than you thought because you assumed the product was devoid of trans fats. Disgusting! Yet companies get away with these marketing manipulations every single day, and your health suffers the consequences.

CHOLESTEROL'S BAD RAP

Although it has been demonized over the past fifty years, cholesterol is not the enemy in our health. In fact, just the opposite is true. Cholesterol is an extremely important nutrient in our bodies. Although many people believe that having high cholesterol puts them at a greater risk of heart disease, in truth the problem is elevated levels of blood sugar and insulin that raise inflammation in the body and can lead to heart attack, stroke, and cardiovascular disease. High insulin levels act like steel wool on your arteries and veins, which leads to irritation and damage that raises inflammation. Consequently, the liver squirts out more cholesterol to help heal the arteries and veins from the damage. That's right; cholesterol serves as a healing agent in the body, which should make you want to have more of it, not less.

For a much more comprehensive look at cholesterol, read Jimmy's book written with Dr. Eric C. Westman, *Cholesterol Clarity*.[15]

Over time, repeating this process of damage and healing over and over again creates a scab that begins to restrict the pathway through which blood needs to flow. If nothing changes, then eventually the artery will become either partially or completely blocked, and this is what leads to a heart attack. The cholesterol or saturated fat didn't lead to the heart attack. It was high insulin that resulted from consuming a diet high in carbohydrates. We have vilified the wrong thing while the real bad guy that leads to heart-health issues, namely refined sugar and carbohydrates, has gotten a free pass. It's time to reverse this wrongful conviction of saturated fat and arrest the true culprit in cardiovascular disease—carbage!

HOW TO AVOID THE BAD FATS AND GET THE GOOD FATS

Now that you understand a little more about the various kinds of fats and the clear quality differences between them, it's time to get practical about how to purchase the fats you'll be including in your low-carb, high-fat, ketogenic diet. Avoiding heavy chemical processing is the key to skirting the bad stuff, and it's pretty easy to do. If you see the words *refined, hydrogenated, partially hydrogenated,* or *cold-processed* (not to be confused with *cold-pressed*) in the ingredients list of a food product, then run for the hills. These are the worst of the bad fats, and you never want to eat them. On the flip side, if you see the terms *organic, cold-pressed, expeller-pressed, unrefined,* and *extra-virgin,* then you have found the perfect fats for your *Real Food Keto* diet. This minimal processing that keeps the fat on low heat and allows for very little light exposure maintains all the amazing health benefits of the real food fats we've discussed in this chapter. This naturally creates antioxidants that prevent the fats from going rancid.

THE TRUTH ABOUT CANOLA OIL

You may have heard that canola oil is a healthy fat to include in your diet. It's low in saturated fat and high in polyunsaturated fat, especially omega-3 fatty acids. Some dietitians and nutritionists have deemed it the world's healthiest fat. We hate to burst their bubble, but it's not even close to being a healthy fat. It comes from rapeseed oil (it already sounds dastardly, right?), which is inedible because of the bitter compounds in it. Canadian scientists worked out a way to remove the bitterness by genetically modifying it. The heavy processing includes deodorizers to remove the pungent smell; it also involves the use of solvent cleaners with a toxic chemical called hexane. If you're still on the fence about canola oil, look on YouTube for a video entitled "How Canola Oil Is Made"—you'll thank us later.

So what are the best fats for cooking? Saturated fats like grass-fed butter, lard, organic and virgin coconut oil, and ghee (clarified butter) work best for frying and sautéing foods. But you also can use healthy omega-6 polyunsaturated-rich chicken fat, half monounsaturated/half saturated tallow (beef or lamb) or organic and virgin red palm oil, and the mostly monounsaturated duck fat and goose fat. So, when you're cooking, and you want to add flavor and healthy nutrition to your dish, consider using these fats. They're the best of the best. Other fats that are appropriate for use in low- to medium-heat cooking or for drizzling on top of foods include mostly monounsaturated expeller-pressed sources such as unfiltered olive oil (if it's high quality, it should be yellow to green in color and cloudy), avocado oil, macadamia nut oil, and sesame oil.

Finally, there are some truly horrible oils that you should avoid if you're following the principles of *Real Food Keto*. Many people are unaware that not all fats are appropriate for use in cooking. You can damage the following fats if you heat them: vegetable (seed) oils, corn oil, flax oil, hemp oil, pine nut oil, pumpkin oil, safflower oil, sunflower oil, and grapeseed oil.

PRACTICAL TIPS FOR ADDING MORE FAT TO YOUR DIET

We've given you a lot of great information about fat in this chapter, and some of it may seem a bit overwhelming. Go back and reread this chapter several times to truly absorb everything we communicated here. *Real Food Keto* is all about getting you to eat more whole-food fats in a much more deliberate way than you probably ever have before. To that end, we want to give you some practical tips for adding more fat to your low-carb, moderate-protein, high-fat lifestyle that incorporates lots of fresh, real foods to nourish your body. That includes plenty of F-A-T!

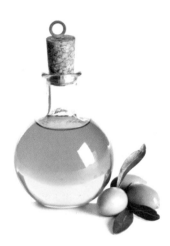

Remember, you want to get a good mix of saturated fat (30 percent), monounsaturated fat (60 percent), and the right kinds of polyunsaturated fats (10 percent), including omega-3, omega-6, and omega-9 fats, into your daily meals. If you don't get the proper mix of these fats or use the wrong types of fats (you know what they are by now!), then you'll experience higher levels of inflammation and a disturbance in your immune response. That ain't good! Remember: Be sure to look for keywords such as *virgin, cold-pressed, organic,* and *grass-fed* on your fat sources to ensure that you're getting the best fats.

FAT AND YOUR DIGESTIVE SYSTEM

You might not relish the idea of ramping up your fat intake because you've had issues in the past (and maybe even right now) with digesting dietary fat. You can find more information in Chapter 10, which is entirely about digestion. For now, you need to know that it's imperative to get your digestion working well, or you won't be able to absorb any of the healthy fats in your diet. A properly functioning liver and gallbladder are necessary to digest the fats you eat. After Christine had her gallbladder removed in 2006, she found it challenging to handle any fats other than butter and coconut oil (these fats work well because they don't require bile to break them down) for about a year. Using digestive enzymes will help you break down the foods you eat so you can eventually reintroduce other fat sources. Be patient with yourself and give it some time.

Another practical tip for adding more fat to your diet seems obvious: choose fattier cuts of meat. It's so incredibly delicious to eat something like bacon or pork belly (yes, these foods are considered healthy when you're eating keto), and you feel satiated for hours after eating it. For less-fatty meats, such as chicken breast, turkey breast, lamb, lean ground beef, kangaroo, goat, veal, and shrimp, add fat to them. We love topping our steak with grass-fed butter instead of steak sauce; it's *divine*. While you're looking for ways to add more fat, don't forget that the primary purpose of eating vegetables is to be a conduit for fat. Cheese on your broccoli, butter on your cauliflower, or avocado oil drizzled on top of a bed of spinach—nothing beats adding fat to these healthy carbohydrates to make you feel satisfied. Is this truly a diet? Nope, it's a way you can eat for the rest of your life to be healthier than you ever could have imagined.

Finally, a fantastic healthy fat that you should be supplementing with is good-quality fish oil. For those of you who don't necessarily like eating fish or have a difficult time getting enough of it into your diet, there are liquid fish oils that don't taste fishy at all. We use a brand called Carlson's, which is available from Amazon.com and from most vitamin shops; it has a nice lemon flavor. If liquid fish oil still makes you squeamish, then there are pharmaceutical-grade fish oil gel caps that you can take. We use the ones from Keto Living (KetoLiving.com), but beware of the kinds you find in vitamin stores, drugstores, and discount stores. If you take them and start to experience fishy burps shortly thereafter, then that fish oil is likely rancid and no longer health promoting. Quality always matters.

In Chapter 5, we move away from the importance of fat and shift to another essential macronutrient: protein. However, the *Real Food Keto* approach is not a high-protein one, and you'll quickly learn why we advocate for moderating protein intake for optimal health. We have a few fancy-schmancy words to share with you about this (with plenty of translation to help you understand them).

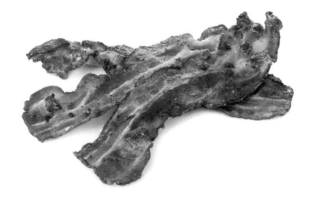

REAL FOOD KETO TAKEAWAYS FROM CHAPTER 4

- The fear of fat was set in motion by the flawed Seven Countries Study conducted by Ancel Keys.

- The sugar industry paid Harvard researchers to hype negative health implications of fat.

- The Dietary Guidelines for Americans codified fat-phobia and ushered in the low-fat-diet era.

- The benefits of consuming dietary fat are endless, including increased energy, better satiety, optimized brain health, improved cardiovascular health, and lower inflammation, to name just a few.

- The negative implications of fat deficiency far outweigh any supposed risks of consuming too much fat.

- The three types of prostaglandins are interconnected by the kinds of fat you're eating.

- The three major kinds of fat are saturated, monounsaturated, and polyunsaturated.

- The essential polyunsaturated fats—linoleic acid and alpha-linolenic acid—are critical in your diet.

- Properly balancing the omega-6 to omega-3 ratio to get it as close to 1:1 as possible is the goal.

- Hydrogenated oils and trans fats are truly the worst of the worst fats you could consume.

- The demonization of cholesterol rising as a result of eating fat is completely unnecessary.

- Avoid fats that use the terms *refined, hydrogenated, partially hydrogenated,* or *cold-processed.*

- Embrace fats that use the terms *organic, cold-pressed, expeller-pressed, unrefined,* and *extra-virgin.*

- The best fats for cooking tend to be saturated fats like grass-fed butter, lard, coconut oil, and ghee.

- Never cook your food in vegetable (seed) oils, corn oil, flax oil, hemp oil, pine nut oil, pumpkin oil, safflower oil, sunflower oil, or grapeseed oil.

- Adding more fat to your diet is as simple as eating fattier cuts of meat, putting fat on your meat and vegetables, and regularly taking fish oil supplements.

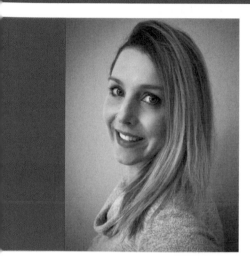

KATIE NEWMAN, NTP AND FITNESS TRAINER

www.katienewman.com

I don't veer too far from the foundational approach we learned in the NTA because it works! The results I get with my clients by implementing a high-fat, low-carb diet are astounding! I have transformed more lives in the past two and a half years by emphasizing nutrition than I did in eighteen years of personal training. I take a bioindividual approach to tailoring my clients' nutrition, fitness, and lifestyle recommendations to fit their mind and body. Utilizing the nutritional assessment questionnaire and the functional evaluation have been valuable assessment tools in optimizing my clients' success. Here's a testimonial from one of my clients:

"Katie has been instrumental to me on my keto journey. After months of trying the keto way of eating on my own, with minimal success, Katie helped me fine-tune my diet while adding certain supplements tailored to help with issues specific to me. Katie's knowledge, thorough instruction, and follow-up have given me the confidence to push through my plateau. Now I am truly enjoying the benefits of a high-fat, low-carb lifestyle. I feel great, and my weight is on the downswing again. Thank you, Katie!"

CHAPTER 5

Protein
(But Not Too Much)

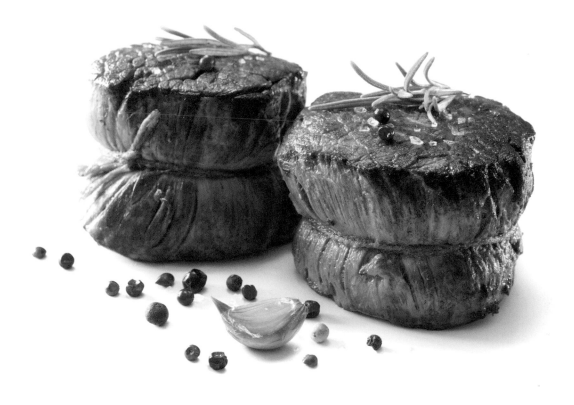

Protein has become something of a media darling within nutritional health circles (except among vegans) as food manufacturers push lean protein for muscle growth and vitality. But is a high-protein diet a good idea? After reading about the importance of fat in Chapter 4, you realize why you need copious amounts of that essential macronutrient. Although protein also is essential (meaning the body can't make protein on its own), it's important to make sure you're not eating too much of it on your *Real Food Keto* plan. What "too much" means varies from person to person because of bioindividuality. You need to test your blood sugar to find out how varying levels of protein affect you and determine what works best for you.

Things can get a little confusing when you hear one person talking about boosting protein intake on Instagram, and then you hop over to Facebook and see someone else telling you to limit it. Who do you believe? The ketogenic diet we outline in this book is a *low-carb, moderate-protein, high-fat diet.* It's not a high-protein diet and never has been. You should dismiss anything you see from someone claiming to be ketogenic but promoting a high protein intake. You'll find out why excessive protein in the diet is the antithesis of being in a state of nutritional ketosis later in this chapter.

Lest you misunderstand us, we want to be very clear about something—consuming some protein is extremely important because your body's makeup comprises about 18 percent protein. Proteins are the basic building blocks of your body, and the human body has about 50,000 different proteins that form four specific things for the body to operate well: nerves, muscles, organs, and flesh. There even are proteins that have specialized functions like enzyme production and the creation of antibodies. The key point we want to underscore is that consuming too much protein can cause blood sugar problems (among other things) because the body can't store protein and has to convert any excess to glucose (sugar). When you're trying to become a fat burner, creating sugar is your kryptonite!

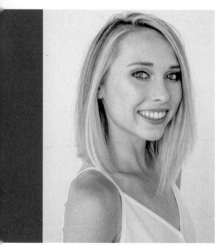

CHRISTINA RICE, NTP, PRIMAL HEALTH COACH
www.christinaricewellness.com

I once had a client who spent seven years visiting a number of doctors and trying every supplement under the sun after being diagnosed with a rare autoimmune condition that left her with chronic joint pain and frustrating brain fog while she also dealt with extreme bloating, minimal bowel movements, and intense sugar cravings. She had gotten to the point of barely being able to walk around outside because she was in so much pain, and she couldn't sleep through the night. She had given up hope, but once we shifted her to a high-fat, low-carb, ketogenic approach, her joint pain and bloating slowly went away, her brain fog lifted, her bowels regulated, her sugar cravings vanished, and she was able to sleep through the night for the first time in years. Watching this change in diet give my client her life back is a true testimony to how therapeutic proper nutrition can be, and that story will stick with me forever.

AMINO ACIDS
AND THEIR ROLES IN THE BODY

We just shared with you that the body has about 50,000 different proteins that make up every part of what makes you human. These proteins combine to make twenty different amino acids that are building blocks for humans and animals, and two that aren't in the human body, which are called nonstandard amino acids. (One of these, pyrrolysine, has been found in a gutless marine worm. Try sharing that fun fact at the water cooler at work!) The seven other amino acids serve a variety of purposes in the body. A total of ten of the twenty-two amino acids are considered essential, and the key roles they play in the body include helping with neurotransmitter production, muscle production, hormone production, and RNA and DNA regulation. The following table is a complete list of the twenty-two essential and nonessential amino acids. In addition, we've listed seven compounds that the body can make that are classified as amino acids, plus two nonstandard amino acids that aren't present in the human body.

AMINO ACIDS[1]

Essential Amino Acids	Nonessential Amino Acids	Other Amino Acids	Nonstandard Amino Acids (Not Found in the Human Body)
Isoleucine	Alanine	Carnitine	Selenocysteine (discovered in 1986)
Leucine	Asparagine	Citrulline	Pyrrolysine (discovered in 2002)
Lysine	Aspartic acid	Gamma-aminobutyric acid	
Methionine	Cysteine	Glutathione	
Phenylalanine	Glutamine	Ornithine	
Threonine	Glutamic acid	Taurine	
Tryptophan	Glycine	Cystine	
Valine	Proline		
Histidine	Serine		
Arginine	Tyrosine		

One thing to remember when you're trying to focus on your protein intake is you need to get *complete proteins*. Complete proteins contain adequate proportions of all the essential amino acids. Despite what you may have heard from people in the plant-based eating world, eating a vegan diet will not give you an adequate amount of complete proteins because plants are composed of incomplete proteins. The two best sources of protein from plants are legumes and cereal grains, but neither of these foods is on the menu when you eat keto.

Besides getting complete proteins and natural fats, animal-based products also give you the best source of zinc and vitamin B12 (cobalamin).

Animal-based foods are the *only* source of complete proteins because they have a mix of all the essential amino acids and many of the nonessential ones, too. The body can't properly use these proteins unless you combine them with dietary fat. Foods like eggs, full-fat dairy, fish, and fatty meats are perfect for people on a ketogenic lifestyle. Don't forget, our hunter-gatherer ancestors consumed mostly meat (eating nose to tail) and then supplemented their diets with vegetables, fruits, nuts, and seeds.

THE BENEFITS OF EATING THE RIGHT AMOUNT OF PROTEIN

Now that you understand the roles of amino acids, it's time to look at what happens in your body when you eat the right amount of protein. Enzymes are proteins that have very specific functions in every single biochemical process. One of these specialized functions of proteins (called *immunoglobulins*) is that they serve an antibody purpose as a means of fighting infection and destroying foreign invaders. The hemoglobin protein also plays a key role in blood health, specifically through the red blood cells that deliver oxygen throughout the body.

Proteins compose some key hormones in the body—including the master hormone insulin as well as human growth hormone (HGH)—which help maintain a healthy metabolism and virtually every other important function in the body. Growing kids need protein, and even adults need proper amounts for tissue growth. When you cut your arm, protein acts as the super glue to clot the blood, so you don't bleed out.

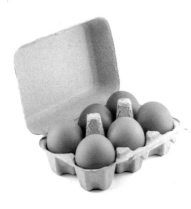

One of the cool benefits of proteins is their ability to control the pH balance of the tissues and blood, which prevents the blood from becoming too acidic or alkaline. Proteins have the Goldilocks effect on the pH balance— they keep things just right. The specific protein called adenylyl cyclase can sense changing bicarbonate levels in the blood and adjust the pH back to normal levels on the fly. The amino acid cysteine, which is in red meat, is essential for a healthy immune system. The sulfur-rich cysteine is needed to make glutathione, a powerful antioxidant that prevents cells from becoming damaged by free radicals and oxidative stress.[2]

THE PROBLEM WITH EATING TOO MUCH OR TOO LITTLE PROTEIN

With all these benefits, you might think consuming protein in your diet is a virtual free-for-all. But remember, a ketogenic diet is low in carbohydrates, high in fat, and *moderate* in protein. Why moderate? Because a high-protein diet can be counterproductive to your goal of becoming a lean, mean, fat-burning machine. Excess protein cannot be stored by the body, so it gets sent to the liver where it's converted to glucose. That's the opposite of what you want to happen when you're pursuing nutritional ketosis. This process of gluconeogenesis (we explain that long G word in greater detail in Chapter 11) is something you need to avoid when you eat keto. It's not enough just to cut carbs. You must, must, must moderate your protein to avoid having these negative effects kick in.

Testing your blood sugar is the perfect way to see how your body reacts to the amount of protein you're eating. Excessive protein consumption can raise blood sugar levels in some people because of gluconeogenesis (the mechanism that the body uses to convert excess dietary protein to glucose through the liver).

Also, a high-protein, low-fat diet is known to activate the IGF-1 hormone that speeds the growth of cells. When cells are pushed to divide rapidly, disease-causing DNA damage is likely to occur, and the cells age at a rapid pace. That ain't good! High protein intake also depletes the body of two key fat-soluble vitamins—A and D—as well as some minerals, such as calcium. The biggest danger of eating too much protein is that it can lead to a condition known as *hypercalciuria,* which involves the inability to absorb calcium. Your body gets rid of it all through your urine, which leads to osteoporosis and other bone-related diseases of old age. Makes you think twice about that 20-ounce porterhouse steak now, doesn't it?

What about the flip side of this—are there problems that can happen if you don't eat *enough* protein? Absolutely. You don't want to impact your metabolism negatively, but that's exactly what you do when you don't get enough protein. The result is that you have trouble losing weight, building muscle, maintaining energy, and more. Your immunity will become compromised, your brain won't function properly, you'll likely have fits of anger, blood sugar dysregulation will occur—we don't need to go on. You get the idea. Eat enough protein to take care of your body's needs. Remember, even though you're moderating protein as part of your *Real Food Keto* approach, you still need this essential macronutrient in the right amount.

SOURCES OF PROTEIN

We've learned that proteins make up the amino acids that play so many roles in how the body functions. And we've also learned about the many benefits that protein conveys and why you want to avoid eating too much protein. Now let's take a look at the best sources of protein to make sure you're getting the highest quality to benefit your health.

- Choose wild-caught fish and seafood whenever possible. Keep in mind that the smaller the fish (think sardines), the less exposure they have had to heavy metal toxins.
- Organic and 100 percent grass-fed and grass-finished beef, lamb, buffalo, elk, and goat.
- Organic and 100 percent pasture-raised poultry, such as chicken, turkey, and duck, as well as their eggs.
- Organic and 100 percent pasture-raised dairy products like full-fat cheeses, full-fat raw milk and cream, full-fat yogurt, and (our favorite!) full-fat grass-fed butter.
- Soaked and sprouted nuts and seeds, including almonds, pecans, macadamia nuts, pili nuts, pistachios, pumpkin seeds, and sunflower seeds.

WHAT IF I CAN'T AFFORD THOSE HIGHER-PRICED PROTEINS?

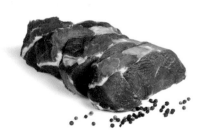

You might be highly skeptical of those hifalutin, fancy-schmancy protein sources we suggested and wonder why you can't just go to your local grocery store and get the meat sold there. We understand; we've been in that situation where all we could afford were whatever grain-fed meats were available at our local supermarket. We're not expecting you to be absolutely 100 percent perfect in your food choices for every meal, but we want you to know the goal is to get the best possible foods to nourish your body. As we stated at the beginning of the book, this journey is about progress—not perfection.

When you first begin eating keto and incorporating real food proteins into your diet, it might be difficult to shell out two or three dollars more per pound for these higher-quality foods without justifying it in your budget. We get it. However, when you start adding them into your regular rotation, you'll find that you'll end up spending less money on food overall because you'll be properly nourished, and you won't want to eat out as often. There's nothing more satisfying to your body than feeding it real food, and we only wish we had learned this a whole lot sooner in life. You'll see once you embrace it fully.

Now that you've learned all about the role of healthy fats and moderate amounts of protein in your diet, it's time to take a look at the macronutrient that you'll be eating the least of on your ketogenic diet. In the next chapter, we explain how to make the most of the few carbohydrates that you eat.

REAL FOOD KETO TAKEAWAYS FROM CHAPTER 5

- Protein is an essential macronutrient, but that doesn't make it a free-for-all.

- Protein makes up 18 percent of your body.

- There are 50,000 different proteins used to create nerves, muscles, organs, and flesh.

- Twenty amino acids keep the body running efficiently when consumed in adequate amounts.

- Only animal-based food products contain complete proteins. Plants contain incomplete proteins.

- Many biochemical pathways run on proteins that help make the body run efficiently.

- Protein intake that is too high or too low can cause serious health problems.

- Choose organic, grass-fed/grass-finished, pasture-raised foods as your protein sources.

- Do the best you can in choosing the proteins that are right for you and purchase the best quality possible.

CHAPTER 6

Carbohydrates Customized to You

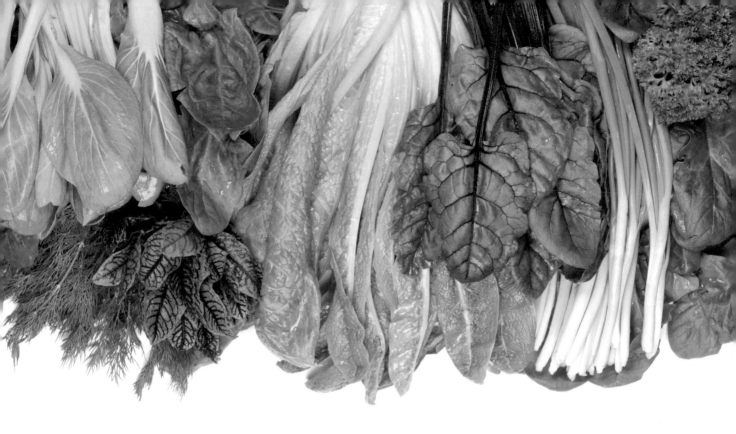

Now that you've learned all about the importance of getting a high amount of healthy fats and a moderate amount of protein into your ketogenic lifestyle, it's time to turn to the macronutrient that many people think you avoid entirely when you go keto—carbohydrates! In a book called *Real Food Keto,* it might seem strange that we would dedicate an entire chapter to this subject given that carbs are reduced so significantly when you're pursuing a state of nutritional ketosis. However, it's a *low*-carb way of eating, not a *no*-carb way of eating. Although there's no such thing as an essential carbohydrate in your diet (unlike essential fatty acids and essential amino acids), there's still value in consuming certain carbs from whole food sources.

The goal of being ketogenic is to minimize the negative effects that come from eating more glucose than your body can handle. Some very healthy people can consume large amounts of real food–based carbohydrates—100 to 150 grams per day—while perfectly maintaining their health and weight. Unfortunately, these people are a great minority of the population. In the real world, most of us—estimated to be as much as 85 percent of the population—fall on the spectrum of insulin resistance, which you learn more about in Chapter 11. Let's look a little closer at insulin resistance and why proper carbohydrate intake for people with this condition is so important.

INSULIN RESISTANCE

Your body has a perfectly natural way to handle the real food carbohydrates that you eat when you're metabolically healthy. The way it's supposed to work is that when you consume these kinds of carbs, your blood sugar rises, which provokes the pancreas to squirt out just enough of the hormone insulin to push the glucose into the cells to be stored for energy and to keep your blood sugar level within a tight range. It's an elegant system that's like a well-oiled machine when it works properly.

But most people are not consuming real food carbohydrates—they're eating crappy carbage like cookies, biscuits, snack cakes, fast food, and other less-than-ideal carbohydrates. When these kinds of carbs make up the preponderance of what you're eating, the natural ability of the pancreas to produce insulin to push glucose into the cells becomes impaired over time. Specifically, the beta cell function is overworked as it tries to keep up with all the extra glucose (sugar) floating around in your bloodstream from the excessive carbohydrates you've consumed. After a while, the insulin can't keep up with the overload of glucose, and your body converts the glucose that isn't used into stored body fat. Elevated glucose leads to hyperglycemia and the beginning stages of insulin resistance. If left unchecked, this situation can turn into type 2 diabetes down the road.

A person who consumes a diet rich in carbohydrates, especially refined ones, over a period of years and decades will start to damage their beta cell function in the pancreas more and more until the cumulative effects won't heal quickly. The insulin production has to go higher and higher to try to keep up with the demand you're putting on your body with all that excessive glucose. Like anything you stress beyond its original purpose, this process totally unravels as insulin continues to rise. Type 2 diabetes is the manifestation of many years of allowing this process to replicate on a daily basis through a junk food carb diet (also known as the standard American diet).

The damage of consuming these non-nourishing carbohydrates doesn't stop there. Massive increases in sugar consumption, as well as non-sugary foods that turn into sugar in the body (such as refined grains and starches), can lead to *glycation,* a process in which glucose reacts with proteins and causes them to become sticky. *Advanced glycation end products (AGEs)* form, and they are a surefire way of aging your body rapidly and hardening your cells so that they lose their ability to function properly. Not good.

It's through this prism of understanding of the difference between a healthy response to carbohydrates and an unhealthy one that we want you to look at this macronutrient for yourself and others in your life. We're not all just a bunch of lemmings. Each of us is uniquely bioindividual in the way we respond to food and lifestyle, as we've discussed throughout this book, and that bioindividuality applies abundantly in this discussion. Realizing that there are people all along the spectrum—from insulin sensitive (able to handle more carbohydrates) to full-blown type 2 and type 1 diabetics (not able to handle very many carbohydrates)—will help you understand why we can't all consume the same amount of carbohydrates and achieve similar weight and health goals.

Knowing about insulin resistance should give many of you a sense of relief because you've wondered why your health and weight haven't been as optimal as you would like despite your doing what you believed was a pretty good job with your diet. You're not alone, and in these pages we hope to offer you lots of clues to unlock the barriers to attaining your health goals. Keep reading, because we have so much more to share with you.

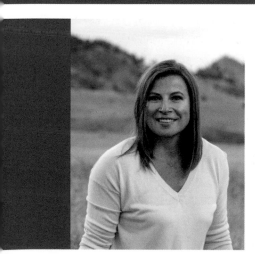

SHAWN MYNAR, NTP, RWP

www.shawnmynar.com

I teach women how to implement a low-carb, high-fat, ketogenic diet to gain control of their health and happiness. I empower them to learn about their individual bodies and take the necessary actions to reach their health goals. One of the most important steps in this process is to make the dietary changes necessary to produce ketones and get maximum healing potential for their bodies.

A TUTORIAL ON CARBOHYDRATES

What is a carbohydrate? Carbohydrates are pretty much composed of carbon, oxygen, and hydrogen. And even though some nutritional health experts recommend that our diets consist of upward of 60 percent carbohydrates, the fact is we don't need that many because our bodies are a mere 2 percent carbohydrate. It will likely come as a shock to learn that inside the human body there is only *one teaspoon* worth of glucose. ONE TEASPOON! That's not a lot, and it underscores the insanity of overloading the body with unnecessary carbohydrates.

Again, this is not to say we should avoid carbohydrates altogether. Instead, the key is to budget carbs to just the amount you can tolerate without negatively affecting your blood sugar while still reaching your health goals. The kind of carbohydrates you consume also is significant because not all carbs are created equal. Keto-friendly complex carbohydrates—such as leafy green vegetables, squash, broccoli, and tomatoes—contain longer chains of sugar molecules called *polysaccharides.* These complex carbs generally have things in them like fiber that can slow their impact on your blood sugar as compared with simple carbohydrates. Simple carbs, such as fruits, fruit juice, table sugar, and corn syrup, contain shorter chains of sugar molecules called *monosaccharides* and *disaccharides.* The body easily and rapidly digests and absorbs simple carbs to use as energy. Unfortunately, there usually is little fiber or anything else to slow the blood sugar impact, and the negative results are profound, especially in people with insulin resistance.

Sugar (carbohydrates that have names that usually end in *-ose*) has been getting a lot of attention in recent years as being a culprit in the demise of our health. As we shared earlier in the book, sugar was pretty much given a free pass by mainstream health experts for a long time while they focused almost all their attention on vilifying fat. We now realize just how incredibly wrong that was, and people are becoming wise to reducing sugar. It's this carbohydrate that's wreaking the most havoc on people's weight and health. Especially when sugar goes through the refining process, it's stripped of any nutrients that it might have had. This is why those who consume excess sugar develop various nutrient deficiencies; their bodies have to pull nutrients from their bones and other parts to get what they need. Yikes!

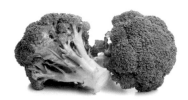

Jimmy was a major sugar addict before he shifted to a ketogenic diet, drinking sixteen cans of soda and eating whole boxes of snack cakes at a time. I also dealt with sugar addiction, which I fed with M&Ms, Skittles, and Dr. Pepper. This explains why both of us became so deficient in various nutrients and why we're now so passionate about warning others not to fall down the same trap. Trying to overcome sugar addiction is a bear, and we know the challenge you face if you're in the same situation. That's why we're writing this book: to show you that there's hope for you to overcome it once and for all.

FORMS OF CARBOHYDRATES

Now that you have an idea about what a carbohydrate is and the positive and negative effects carbs can have on your body, let's take a look at the various kinds and forms of carbohydrates:

THE KINDS AND FORMS OF CARBOHYDRATES[1]

SUGARS		LARGER CARBOHYDRATES	
Monosaccharides	**Disaccharides**	**Oligosaccharides***	**Polysaccharides**
Fructose (fruit sugar)	Sucrose	Inulin	Starch
Glucose	Lactose		Dextrin
Galactose	Maltose		Cellulose
			Pectin
			Glycogen

*These are made up of 2 to 10 monosaccharides.

Okay, maybe that table made your head spin, so we'd like to elaborate on each of these carbohydrates to better explain them to you.

- *Monosaccharides* are the most basic form of sugar, and they're water-soluble. They taste sweet and form crystals.

- *Disaccharides* are two monosaccharide residues (sometimes referred to as double sugars) and are also water-soluble.

- *Oligosaccharides* contain two to six (and sometimes as many as ten) monosaccharides. These play some positive roles in the body, most notably in aiding the immune response. Oligosaccharides also are water-soluble and sweet to the taste.

- *Polysaccharides* are complex carbohydrates that are long chains of monosaccharides bound together, and they are not water-soluble. These get broken down in the mouth and small intestine as simple sugars. (If you want to test this for fun, place a small piece of whole-grain bread on your tongue and firmly press it against the roof of your mouth for about a minute. Despite there not being any sugar in the bread, it will begin to taste sweet on your tongue. It's a telling example of how all carbohydrates are broken down into sugar, beginning in the mouth.)

Because this book is about eating a ketogenic diet, we don't recommend consuming sugar and sugary foods (duh) that are simple carbohydrates. We also don't recommend consuming bread, potatoes, pasta, rice, yams, corn, and all the other grain-based and starch-based foods that make up even the supposedly "better" complex carbohydrates. Leafy green and nonstarchy vegetables are your go-to sources for complex carbs. You should avoid most sugar-based carbohydrate foods altogether.

Some experts often make the argument that consuming complex carbs is healthy for you because of the nutrients you get from them, but there's not one single nutrient in a complex carbohydrate that you can't get from other food sources that only minimally impact your glucose. Defenders of complex carbs also say that the body handles them better than it handles simple carbs because complex carbs don't raise blood sugar levels as quickly. People with insulin resistance can attest that even these "healthy" carbs will likely continue the damage that's been done. The bottom line is that complex carbs can still negatively impact you—only at a much slower rate. It's like saying filtered cigarettes are good for you because you absorb the toxins more slowly than from cigarettes without filters. Does that make filtered cigarettes healthy? Not even close.

Here's a fun fact: If you don't eat carbohydrates, your body can make sugar on its own. The concept of gluconeogenesis (GNG) is that your body converts

When you eat fruit, add a source of fat to the fruit to help get more fat into your diet. We like double cream with our berries. The added fat slows the impact of the carbohydrates you do eat.

the protein and some fats you consume to glucose to create sugar. (This process takes place in the liver. We go into great detail about gluconeogenesis in Chapter 11.) Because of GNG, there is no such thing as an essential dietary carbohydrate. Your body can very efficiently make the glucose it needs for the few glucose-dependent functions it has.

Properly balancing the right kinds of carbohydrates, like leafy green vegetables, nonstarchy veggies, and the occasional berries, can provide your body great benefit when you're consuming a ketogenic diet. If you're more insulin sensitive and occasionally want to have a starchy vegetable like sweet potatoes, then that's fine. We're not about making *all* carbohydrates the bad guy. Getting the appropriate amounts in your body where you are today sets you up to attain the health you've always wanted. In fact, we want to point out some of the positive roles healthy carbohydrates, namely leafy green and nonstarchy vegetables, play in the body:

- Healthy carbohydrates can provide a quick fuel source for the brain and muscles.
- Healthy carbohydrates, especially fiber, can help you feel fuller to regulate your fat and protein intake.
- Healthy carbohydrates are an excellent source of fiber, which helps keep bowels regular.
- Healthy carbohydrates help lubricate joints.
- Healthy carbohydrates feed your good gut bacteria to optimize and grow your microbiome.

THE CARBOHYDRATES YOU WANT TO AVOID

Maybe you're starting to get a handle on your carbohydrate intake. To help you get a firmer grasp on it, we want to emphasize the kinds of carbohydrates you want to avoid at all costs if attaining optimal health is your goal. These are the types of carbs you need to keep out of your diet altogether. Unfortunately, they're the very ones that far too many people in Western cultures still gravitate to day after day after day because they're oblivious to the serious negative consequences of their dietary choices. We refer to them as crappy carbage throughout the book: the refined carbohydrates (cue the Darth Vader theme music).

When you walk into any grocery store, convenience store, drugstore, or big-box store, this stuff is impossible to miss. At our local Sam's Club, the first eight aisles of shelves are loaded with candy, cakes, cookies, gummies, crackers, and more. We think our blood sugar rises at least 20 points as we walk past all those sugary and grainy foodlike disease agents. Can you imagine how devoid food stores would be if they had to eliminate the junk carbs they currently sell? The middle aisles of the grocery store would be completely barren because all the good food is arranged around the perimeter of the store. It's saying something about how far from real food we've strayed when the products that we consume the most (and that have the most prominent placement) are those that our ancestors would not have recognized as food. Scary thought, huh?

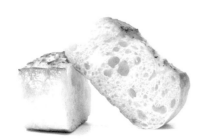

These highly refined and processed carbohydrates are devoid of the natural nutrients that you can easily get from whole foods because manufacturers have stripped out the nutrients. In fact, the manufacturers reintroduce synthetic forms of various vitamins and minerals to fortify the products with a little something your body can use. Otherwise, the foods would be the epitome of empty calories that offer no nourishment to your body. Despite this fortification, the refined carbohydrates turn right around and strip your body of the vital nutrients—which is something that most people don't realize. It's sobering to think back to all those years we mindlessly ate our fair share of these kinds of foods before our eyes were opened to the harmful effects they were having. It's much worse than anyone wants to admit. That's why we're sounding the alarm in *Real Food Keto* so you know and can make informed decisions moving forward.

It should almost go without saying that the carbohydrates you want to avoid as much as humanly possible are refined sugars like white sugar and high-fructose corn syrup (sometimes referred to as corn sugar). However, you also should avoid sugary foods that are promoted as "healthy," like fruit juice, agave, maple syrup (sorry to all our Canadian friends), and even honey. Yes, these sugars tend to come from natural sources, but they also very naturally raise your blood sugar and insulin levels the same way as any other sugar. Sugar is sugar is sugar, and your body can't tell the difference. This is especially important for the insulin-resistant population that tends to need a ketogenic diet to be healthy. Sugar simply cannot be a part of your healthy lifestyle.

Other carbohydrates to completely avoid include refined grains like bread and pasta. Don't fall for the slick marketing gimmicks that attempt to glorify the whole-grain content of a loaf of whole wheat bread, a seven-grain bagel, or anything labeled whole-grain (which runs the gamut from pancake mix to

We're not saying that there are *no* good, real foods that come in a package. We've found quite a few packaged foods that do things the right way. We've included a list of the *Real Food Keto*–approved food companies in the Resources section at the end of the book.

Hamburger Helper). The truth about most of these whole-grain foods is they have been highly refined; what's left are just a few bits of whole grains so that the manufacturer can market the product as "whole-grain." These products aren't foods that are health-promoting. Remember that many people eating keto can't tolerate eating grains at all. If you can tolerate grains, then make sure you consume them in their true whole form and prepare them properly by soaking and sprouting them. It's the way traditional cultures used to do it before Big Food took over and people stopped investing time in preparing the food they eat.

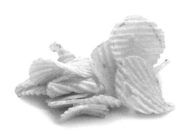

As a general rule, if a refined carbohydrate comes in a package, then it's not going to be one you should eat. Most of these foods have an ingredient list that's a mile long, and they're full of things that you can't even pronounce. (Usually many of the ingredients are a result of the fortification the manufacturer has to do to reintroduce vitamins and minerals that processing has stripped out.) The products include man-made chemicals, additives, and preservatives that our bodies were never meant to consume; think about just how toxic those things are to your body. Furthermore, most of these very bad carbohydrates are combined with the worst of the worst fat we discussed earlier—vegetable oils. (It's like a double whammy!) So you have refined grains, refined sugar, and refined fat in virtually every single packaged food—chips, cookies, crackers, and even frozen meals, just to name a few.

THE CARBOHYDRATES YOU WANT TO EAT

Throughout this chapter, we've shared information about the various kinds of carbohydrates and the concerns of consuming the truly unhealthy kind. Because we advocate for carbohydrate *reduction* rather than carbohydrate *elimination* in *Real Food Keto,* you might be wondering which carbs should be part of your diet to help you get all the micronutrients you need while also helping you achieve a healthy state of nutritional ketosis. Never fear, friends. We've created a list to guide you. You'll probably find yourself referring to the next page often if you get confused by the advertising and marketing that accompanies most carbohydrate-based foods.

CHOOSING KETO-FRIENDLY CARBOHYDRATES

1. STICK WITH LEAFY GREEN AND NONSTARCHY VEGETABLES.

Try to eat as many colors of vegetables as possible when they're in season and incorporate raw veggies now and then. Don't get lured in by the beautiful display of vegetables at your grocery store in January when many vegetables are out of season. Our bodies were designed to consume only foods that grow in the current season. Shop farmers markets and even grow your own vegetables in a greenhouse (like we do) for access to these healthy carbs. Check out the "How We Eat Carbohydrates" section on the next page for some of our favorite leafy green and nonstarchy vegetables.

2. EAT WHOLE FRUITS IF YOU CAN TOLERATE THE CARBOHYDRATES.

As we previously mentioned, some people with insulin resistance can't eat fruit and should treat it as nature's candy; in other words, those people need to avoid it. But for those of you who tolerate more carbohydrates (sugar) in your diet, try to stick with the fruits that are lowest in sugar, like berries. You should consume only the fruits that are in season (just like we recommend with vegetables). Also, never, ever drink fruit juice. Although the juice might provide a few of the nutrients of the fruit it contains, the concentrated sugar content is generally just as bad as drinking a sugary soda!

3. MAKE SURE YOU CHOOSE THE VEGETABLES THAT ARE THE LOWEST IN STARCH, LIKE ZUCCHINI AND YELLOW SQUASH.

Spaghetti squash is one of our favorites, but we consume it less often than other vegetables because of its higher carbohydrate content. Try to avoid butternut squash and acorn squash; their carbohydrate counts are considerably higher than zucchini or yellow squash, which makes them a poor choice for your ketogenic approach.

4. INCORPORATE FERMENTED FOODS INTO YOUR MEALS.

Many people who eat keto neglect the critical role fermented foods play in replenishing your intestines with good healthy bacteria for creating all sorts of health-boosting vitamins like thiamine (B1), riboflavin (B2), cobalamin (B12), and the ever-important fat-soluble vitamin K. (Find out more about the wonderful benefits of these and other vitamins in Chapter 9.) Fermented foods help your body absorb minerals properly as well.

The very best sources of fermented carbohydrates that should *always* be refrigerated include kombucha (fermented tea), kefir (fermented milk), sauerkraut (fermented cabbage), pickles (fermented cucumbers), and kimchi (a Korean dish using fermented vegetables, spices, and seasonings). Never buy any of the foods in the preceding list if they're in the center aisle. They need to be refrigerated to preserve the healthy bacteria.

If you prefer to eat a more plant-based ketogenic diet, try tempeh (fermented soybeans), miso (fermented soybean, barley, or brown rice with koji, which is a fungus), and natto (Japanese dish with fermented soybeans). Some people avoid some fermented foods because of the higher carbohydrate content in these foods. Remember, however, that the buggers in your gut feed on the sugar that's in fermented foods. Ideally, you don't want the fermented carbohydrate to taste overly sweet and so fermenting them longer reduces the carb content even more.

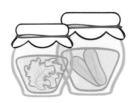

HOW WE EAT CARBOHYDRATES

Because Jimmy has been so well known as a low-carb advocate for many years, people often think we sit around every day gnawing on meat and butter and doing shots of raw eggs from our backyard chickens. The reality is that we consume the kind and amount of carbohydrates that is right for our unique bodies. We know our carbohydrate tolerance level is very low because we've tested our blood sugar response after we've eaten carbs; that biomarker and others show that we need to restrict carbs. Jimmy can have about 30 grams of total carbohydrates daily. Christine can have a bit more, but if she has much more than 40 grams, issues creep up in her weight and health. Carb tolerance is highly individualized, and you're going to have to figure out how much is the right amount for you through trial and error and testing with a glucometer. We wish we could issue a grand carbohydrate edict and state that everyone who wants to be ketogenic should consume 50 grams of carbohydrates a day! Sadly, it doesn't work that way. Fret not, though; you'll find your groove.

So what limited carbohydrates do we eat? Jimmy's favorite leafy green vegetable is baby spinach; Christine's choice is mixed greens. We also like keto-friendly nonstarchy veggies like squash, zucchini, bell peppers, cauliflower, green beans, and broccoli. Cook these in a bit of grass-fed butter and bone broth, and you've got an amazing side dish to go with your meals. Christine also likes munching on raw veggies, such as celery, cauliflower, and broccoli, that she dips in some homemade Ranch Dressing (page 347). Yummers!

You might be wondering about fruit. For the most part, we don't eat fruit. The only exceptions are our favorites: Christine's is strawberries, and Jimmy's is blueberries. To blunt the sugar impact of the berries on our blood glucose, we tend to eat small quantities of these fruits and add a healthy fat, such as heavy whipping cream, to them. (Check out the Strawberries and Cream Smoothie recipe on page 276 for an example.) When we travel outside the United States to places like Australia, New Zealand, and Europe, we enjoy this glorious high-fat real food called double cream, which makes an excellent complement to the berries with just a hint of 87 percent dark chocolate. Oooooh, it's so good!

Honestly, Christine still loves having an occasional sweet potato in her diet. Even though she rarely treats herself to one, she almost always pays the consequences for the indulgence in her blood sugar. Christine also has tried some of the so-called "resistant starches" that are promoted as healthy for

If you have gut-health issues, start slowly incorporating fermented carbohydrates and other fermented foods into your meals. Adding too many at once can cause gas and bloating.

your gut bacteria, but after trying them and testing her blood sugar, she found they weren't something she could tolerate. For example, at various times she's tested her blood sugar after consuming sweet potatoes or a resistant starch, and she experienced high blood sugar readings of almost 200 mg/dL, she felt jittery and shaky, and her heart started to race. The rise in heart rate indicates that the body has problems with the particular food consumed and could indicate a food sensitivity.

NOTE FROM CHRISTINE

Cassava flour is one of the popular resistant starches that is not supposed to affect blood sugar, and I tried it a few years back to see how my body would react. When I tested after eating it, I found my blood sugar had shot up to nearly 200 mg/dL within a half hour, and it remained significantly elevated for the next six hours. Holy crap! These results indicated to me that, resistant or not, this carbohydrate most definitely could not be a part of my diet. If I hadn't tested my blood sugar response, I wouldn't have known this starch wasn't good for me. So, if you're not already testing, get a blood glucose meter (BestKetoneTest.com is one place to find them) and start testing right away as you begin applying the principles of *Real Food Keto* to your life.

Last but not least, we love having fermented carbohydrates in our diet, but we don't have them with every single meal. However, to optimize your gut health, you should strive to have fermented carbohydrates at every meal. The good news is that it takes only about a tablespoon of sauerkraut, pickles, kimchi, and more to benefit your diet. Even better, try making fermented foods at home so that you can control what ingredients are in the food and the quality of those ingredients. It can be a fun project to do with your children, who might be curious about what you're doing with cabbage and cucumbers. Getting your kids to embrace real food before they become adults could be a real game-changer in their health and longevity down the road.

So that's what you need to know about carbohydrates. Yes, we keep them minimized with a purpose in mind when we eat ketogenic, but we hope this chapter helped you understand that carbohydrates serve a purpose in a healthy diet. You don't need to eliminate them completely. You just need to be selective about which carbohydrates you include.

Now that we've discussed the three primary macronutrients—fats, proteins, and carbohydrates—it's time to talk about what many people consider the fourth macronutrient: water. In the next chapter, we get into all the ins and outs of why proper water consumption and hydration is as important, if not more important, than the food you eat.

REAL FOOD KETO TAKEAWAYS FROM CHAPTER 6

- If you have a healthy metabolism, you should be able to handle the glucose effects of real food.

- People with insulin resistance can no longer tolerate even real food sources of carbohydrates.

- Carbohydrates make up just 2 percent of the body.

- There is no such thing as an essential carbohydrate, but you still want to consume some for the benefits they provide.

- Refined sugars and grains are wreaking havoc on health because they strip your body of key nutrients.

- The four major carbohydrates are monosaccharides, disaccharides, oligosaccharides, and polysaccharides.

- Your body can very efficiently make carbohydrates through a process called gluconeogenesis.

- Benefits of carbs include energy, fiber, healthy bowel function, lubricating joints, and gut health.

- Avoid refined, processed, and packaged carbohydrates at all costs.

- Choose low-starch veggies, low-sugar fruits, and fermented sources of carbohydrates. Leafy green and nonstarchy vegetables are your go-to sources for complex carbohydrates.

- Test your blood sugar often with a glucometer to see what effect carbohydrates have on you.

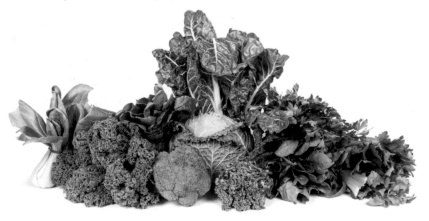

CHAPTER 7

Water: The Fourth Macronutrient

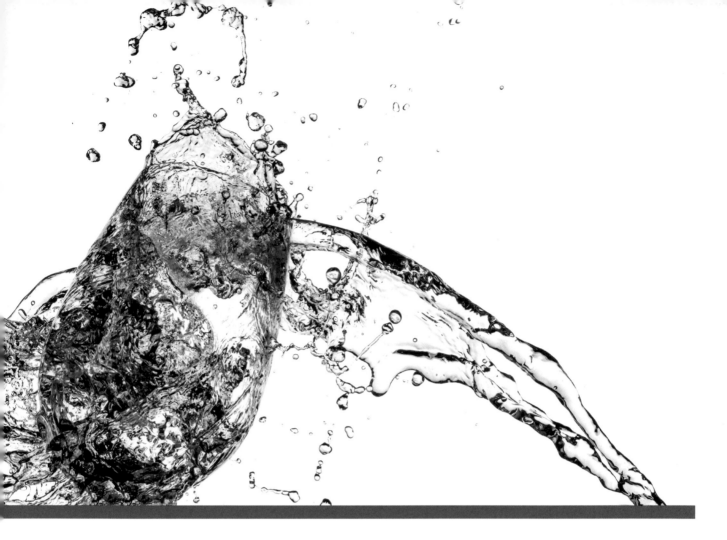

Everybody knows you have to drink water every day, and you probably grew up hearing that you need to be consuming eight 8-ounce glasses of water daily. We uncover the whole truth about this old wives' tale in this chapter. We also discuss what happens when you don't drink enough water. Most people don't realize that dehydration can happen very quickly and can manifest in a string of symptoms that impact you physically and mentally.

The body is 55 to 60 percent water! It's literally found in every single tissue. Although it's not necessarily a macronutrient in the way that fat, protein, and carbohydrates are, the critical role of water in keeping the body functioning optimally qualifies it as the honorary fourth macronutrient.

We've already discussed quite a few nutrient deficiencies in this book, but by far, the most common deficiency in the United States is good old H_2O. By the time you feel the first tinge of thirst, the process of dehydration has already begun. When the amount of water in your body is off by even a little, the minerals and electrolytes that keep your body in tiptop shape are directly affected. Your body can make water from metabolic processes like cellular respiration, but the amount produced is a mere 8 percent of your daily water need; the rest must come from the foods and beverages you consume.

A forty-seven-year-old British woman who was hiking through the Grand Canyon in October 2015 was found dead after she had consumed so much water that it depleted her body of sodium and caused her brain to swell.[1] Getting too much water can lead to *hyponatremia,* which is a condition where sodium in the blood becomes too diluted. Of course, this kind of "water intoxication" is very rare, and it's certainly the exception rather than the rule. So how much water is enough without being too much? How do you calculate when enough is enough? Let's explore that question further.

HOW TO CALCULATE YOUR DAILY WATER NEED

There's a perfect formula for determining how much water you should be drinking on a daily basis: simply take your current body weight and cut that number in half. The result is the number of ounces of water you should be consuming. For example, a 240-pound man needs 120 ounces of water a day. The maximum water intake for everyone is 128 ounces (1 gallon). Here's what that equation looks like:

$$\frac{\text{YOUR BODY WEIGHT}}{2} = \text{DAILY WATER INTAKE IN OUNCES}$$

However, there's a little glitch in this calculation that you need to be aware of because it requires you to drink even more water to offset it. (You knew it couldn't be *quite* that easy, right?) The monkey wrench in the works is this thing called a *diuretic*. Common beverages like coffee, caffeinated and herbal teas, alcohol, soft drinks (even diet ones), and boxed fruit juices can suck water out of your body, which means you need to replenish that water in addition to consuming the recommended amount of water from the formula. To account for the negative impact that diuretics have on your water intake, multiply the number of ounces of diuretics that you drink by one and a half; the result is the number of additional ounces of water you need to consume that day. For example, if you drink an 8-ounce cup of coffee, then you need to offset the water that diuretic pulled out of you by consuming an extra 12 ounces of water. However, you still don't want to exceed 128 ounces of water in a day. Here's what that equation looks like:

$$\text{OUNCES OF DIURETIC X 1.5} + \frac{\text{YOUR BODY WEIGHT}}{2} = \text{DAILY WATER INTAKE IN OUNCES}$$

As you can see, finding the amount of water that isn't too much or too little is a bit tricky, but being purposeful in getting what you need is vital. If you drink more water than your body needs, you'll experience unpleasant symptoms, including confusion, nausea, bloating, and headaches. These come on because the kidneys are unable to properly deal with the excess liquid, which leads to water buildup in the body.

Too much water intake causes the cells in your body to swell, which directly impacts your brain, which can start swelling as well. Tamara Hew-Butler, DPM, PhD, an associate professor at Oakland University, says that the brain has to swell only 8 to 10 percent before it reaches the skull and begins pushing out the brain stem.[2] Brain swelling can lead to significant neurodegenerative damage and very possibly death. The biggest concern with overconsumption of water is the loss of electrolytes, which leads to muscle spasms and cramping. If you find that this is happening to you, grab some pink Himalayan salt or an electrolyte supplement like Keto Vitals (www.ketovitals.com) to replenish your supply of magnesium, sodium, potassium, and calcium.

Even though we know all about the importance of consuming enough water, we still struggle to drink enough of it because we get busy and forget. It's almost like you need to set the alarm on your phone to go off every fifteen or twenty minutes to remind you to stop and drink water. One helpful tip is to not drink all your water at once. Have a big cup that you can carry around with you and sip from throughout the day. We have Yeti brand cups that keep our water cold all day long.

When Christine becomes dehydrated, she really notices because her blood pressure drops sharply. She even keeps a bottle of water in bed with her at night, like a teddy bear that's ready to quench her thirst when she needs it most. The heavy respirations that occur while you're sleeping cause you to lose a lot of water at night. That's why it's recommended that you drink a tall glass of water shortly after you wake.

We enjoy using a countertop water dispenser, especially in the heat of the summer. We add slices of fresh fruit like lemons, limes, blueberries, and strawberries—as well as the occasional cucumber—to infuse a hint of flavor to encourage more drinking. The extra flavor makes drinking water more interesting, and you might find that it increases your water intake. We also like flavored sparkling waters, such as LaCroix, in place of diuretic soda pop.

It's okay to drink sparkling water on occasion, but don't make a habit of it. Carbonated water contains phosphoric acid, which can inhibit stomach acid production as well as interfere with your body's ability to use calcium. The more plain water you drink, the better.

IS DISTILLED WATER GOOD TO DRINK?

Drinking distilled water may not be good for some people, specifically those who are already mineral deficient. It can pull trace minerals like magnesium from the body, so people who are already deficient in these minerals will become even more deficient. Consuming distilled water also can deplete your electrolytes, including sodium, potassium, and chloride, which can lead to irregular heartbeat, high blood pressure, muscle cramps, weakness, confusion, and seizures, depending on which trace minerals and electrolytes are lacking. Distilled water can lower the pH in your body, making it more acidic. When pH goes down, the parathyroid produces parathyroid hormone (PTH), which stimulates osteoclast activity (the breakdown of bone) to release calcium from the bones into the blood in an attempt to normalize pH levels. If this happens too often, the result is osteoporosis.

THE BENEFITS OF APPROPRIATE WATER INTAKE

Water is and always will be the most important nutrient you can get. Eat all the high-fat, moderate-protein, low-carb food you want, but if your water intake is off by even a little, it can lead to some serious health issues. Our bodies were made to be nourished by water, and the reasons for and benefits of getting just the right amount of water are plentiful. Let's take a look at some of them:

- Every single tissue in the body needs water.
- Water helps improve the delivery of oxygen to your cells.
- Water aids digestion by removing waste through regular bowel movements.
- Water dumps toxins out of the body through perspiration and urination.
- Water absorbs shocks to the organs and joints.
- Water is crucial in helping regulate body temperature.
- Water transports nutrients to where they're needed all across the body.
- Water appropriately thins bodily fluids to prevent them from becoming too viscous or thick.
- Water moistens oxygen and is required for proper breathing.
- Water plays an important role in helping the body heal from injury.
- Water assists cells in communicating effectively.
- Water balances the electrical properties of cells (electrolytes).
- Water boosts energy and prevents fatigue.
- Water promotes feelings of fullness, reduces hunger, and raises metabolism.
- Water moisturizes the skin and smooths wrinkles.
- Water boosts the immune system to fight disease.
- Water helps relieve and prevent headaches.
- Water lubricates the joints and maintains the elasticity of muscles.
- Water boosts mental health and makes you feel happy.
- Water is the least expensive nutrient you can get.

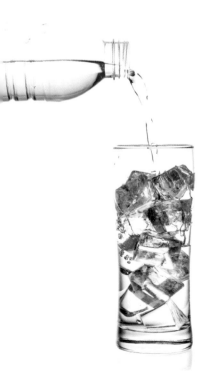

THE EFFECTS OF THE RIGHT WATER INTAKE ON SPECIFIC SYSTEMS IN THE BODY

Now that's an impressive list of benefits of drinking adequate amounts of water! We hope that it motivates you to dial in this aspect of your health so you can unlock all these remarkable improvements. Now that you have the big picture of the fourth macronutrient and know why you want to pay as much attention to it as you do fat, protein, and carbs, let's take an in-depth look at the effects of proper water intake on specific functions of the systems in the body.

ENDOCRINE FUNCTION

The endocrine system (a hormonal messenger system that we cover in great detail in Chapter 12) needs enough water to help hormones move efficiently around the body. If there's a lack of hydration, then the blood and bodily fluids become too thick, and this transportation system of the hormones becomes like a river made of molasses. Not good. So drink up to prevent this from happening.

IMMUNE FUNCTION

Because the immune system is active every time we breathe, the lungs need water to keep the air passages moist from the nose all the way to the lining of the lungs and even into the mucosal lining from the stomach to the digestive tract. Consequently, proper hydration, digestion, and immune function are interrelated. Because mucus consists of 98 percent water and just 2 percent inorganic salts, antiseptic enzymes, immunoglobulins, and glycoproteins (which are all designed to trap foreign invaders), water intake is crucial to your immune system working as intended. Additionally, when you're drinking enough water, the lymphocytes (white blood cells that are part of the immune system) are allowed to free-flow because you have proper blood and lymph viscosity (which helps fight infections). Finally, proper hydration can help prevent asthma attacks and allergy symptoms because it acts as a potential antihistamine. Buh-bye, Benadryl!

VASCULAR FUNCTION (HEART HEALTH)

You probably didn't realize that your water intake could affect your heart health, but it can have a profound influence on various precursors to heart attack, stroke, and cardiovascular disease. If the body becomes dehydrated, the vascular system selectively closes some of the vessels, which in turn raises blood pressure to the point of hypertension. Getting the right amount of water also plays a role in how efficiently proteins and enzymes (specifically taurine, L-carnitine, creatine, troponin, and others) function in your overall heart health.

DETOXIFICATION

Water plays an especially vital role in flushing toxins out of the body on a daily basis through sweat, urine, feces, and breath. Water keeps the bodily fluids from retaining toxins, which helps the lymph shuttle them to the liver for excretion out of the body.

We highly recommend that you read the book *Your Body's Many Cries for Water* by Fereydoon Batmanghelidj, MD, if you want to learn more about the positive role water plays in making your body work well. Batmanghelidj notes that many of today's most common diseases are nothing more than dehydration and that doctors are treating patients' symptoms with needless prescription medications when they should be recommending that they drink more water.[3] The list of diseases for which people take drugs when they could possibly solve the problem by drinking more water include dyspeptic pain (indigestion or irritability), rheumatoid arthritis, headaches, depression, high blood pressure, high cholesterol, asthma, and allergies. If a problem arises with any of these, then it's likely a result of dehydration.

TIPS FOR RELIEVING CONSTIPATION

Constipation is a condition in which it is difficult to empty the bowels, and it can result from dehydration. A person who has less than one bowel movement a day is probably suffering from constipation. When a person is constipated, stools (feces) are usually hard and broken up. Other symptoms include gas, abdominal pain, stomach bloating, and loss of appetite. The Bristol Stool Chart (which you can easily find through a search on the Internet) shows you the different types of stools and what they mean. Following are some suggestions for preventing and relieving constipation.

TAKE SUPPLEMENTS

- Vitamin C, if taken in excess, can cause diarrhea. But taking a little extra vitamin C can help relieve constipation.

- Vitamin B1 (thiamine) aids digestion.

- A derivative of vitamin B5 (pantothenic acid) known as dexpanthenol stimulates muscle contractions in the digestive system, which helps move stools along.

- Vitamin B9 (folate/folic acid) helps stimulate digestive acids. If you have trouble metabolizing folic acid due to an MTHFR gene mutation, try methylated folate instead.

- Vitamin B12 (cobalamin) deficiency can lead to constipation.

- You can simplify things by taking a B complex rather than taking the individual B vitamins.

- Magnesium citrate can help relieve constipation.

INCREASE WATER INTAKE

Make sure to drink plenty of water during the day. If you consume beverages that have a diuretic effect (see page 121), you need to drink extra water to counteract the effects of the diuretics. You should not drink more than 128 ounces (1 gallon) of water daily.

LOOK AT MEDICATIONS

Certain medications, like opioids, can cause constipation. Make sure to drink plenty of water when taking these meds.

LOOK AT YOUR DIGESTION

Usually, something going on further down in the digestive tract is a result of something going on higher up in the digestive tract. If you're not producing enough stomach acid to digest the foods you eat, undigested food can clog the ileocecal valve, which can cause stools to back up.

Proper hydrochloric acid production in the stomach stimulates the secretion of pepsin, which we need to digest proteins.

If you're in a sympathetic or stressed state, you won't be able to digest foods correctly, which can lead to constipation.

SIGNS OF DEHYDRATION

How do you know if you've become dehydrated? What are the early signs, and which ones come along later if you keep ignoring the signals your body is giving you to drink more water? Most people have no idea that if the body's water content falls by as little as 2 percent, many early signs manifest themselves. If you ignore those signals and dehydration progresses a little further (to about a 10 percent water loss), then you suffer more significant symptoms. And if you continue to ignore those more advanced symptoms and dehydration is pushed to more than a 10 percent loss of water, then death is the only other sign you'll get. The following list is a result of inadequate water intake. Do you suffer from any of these symptoms?

SIGNS OF DEHYDRATION

EARLY SIGNS	LATER SIGNS
Fatigue	Heartburn
Anxiety	Joint pain
Irritability	Back pain
Depression	Migraines
Cravings	Fibromyalgia
Cramps	Constipation
Headaches	Colitis (inflammation of the colon)
	Heart palpitations
	Asthma/allergies

KETOACIDOSIS VERSUS NUTRITIONAL KETOSIS

People tend to fear getting ketoacidosis when they go on a low-carb, high-fat diet because this type of diet produces ketones in the body. However, as long as your pancreas can still make even a little insulin, developing ketoacidosis is nearly impossible. The primary concern with ketoacidosis is for someone with type 1 diabetes who eats a high-carbohydrate meal and then doesn't take insulin afterward. The result is that blood glucose levels rise higher than 240 mg/dL, which makes the body think it's starving, which then causes a simultaneous rise in blood ketone levels to more than 20.0 mmol/L. This puts a type 1 diabetic into a highly acidic state, and they drop into a coma and could die without insulin and electrolytes. Someone eating keto who is not a type 1 diabetic can develop ketoacidosis if they get severely dehydrated or work the body beyond exhaustion and overheat, but these cases are very rare. In these extraordinary instances, dehydration can impact the pancreas negatively and cause muscle to be broken down, leading to acidity in the blood. Now you have another reason to drink up when you're eating a ketogenic diet.

Remember: Nutritional ketosis is safe for the body. The range for blood ketones when a person is in nutritional ketosis is 0.5 mmol/L to 3.0 mmol/L.

We're sure you've experienced a few of these symptoms at some point in your life. Even we experience these issues when we get out in the garden in the middle of the day in summer and forget to drink enough water. The primary symptoms we've experienced are later signs of heartburn and back pain, which means we blew right by cravings, headaches, and fatigue without giving them a second thought. The body is a very intelligent system and tells us what it needs; we just have to pay attention to the signs it gives us.

HOW TO STAY PROPERLY HYDRATED

Because dehydration is a much bigger problem than water overload, we want to provide some helpful tips for staying hydrated as you begin your *Real Food Keto* journey. The best thing you can do right away is to limit the number of diuretic drinks you consume in a day, including coffee, black and green tea, diet soda, fruit juice (which is not recommended on keto anyway), and alcohol. Every single one of these beverages pulls more water from your body than it provides. Thus, you need to use the equation we shared on page 121 to make sure you're replenishing what you need. Better yet, limit or eliminate these diuretics.

We carry water bottles or insulated cups with us everywhere, and we still struggle to drink enough plain water because we get bored with it. A big reason why many people get dehydrated is that they simply can't stomach drinking the recommended daily amount. One trick we've come up with is adding fresh fruit to a large water dispenser so that we can drink from it throughout the day. We add sliced strawberries and blueberries for a refreshing cold drink of homemade flavored water. If you haven't tried cucumber water yet, you need to try it; you'll thank us later.

Another tip for drinking enough water is to sip a little bit throughout the day. A lot of people like to chug-a-lug their water, and that's not a good strategy. We suggest the Quarter Hour Solution (QHS): Whenever the clock hits 15, 30, 45, or 60 minutes (the turn of a new hour), it's time to take a sip. Of course, if you feel thirsty, you can take a sip at any time, but our proven QHS strategy will give you approximately 8 ounces of water an hour plus whatever you drink when you feel thirsty. This method allows your body to be properly hydrated without becoming overly hydrated to the point that it starts dumping electrolytes and suffering the fate of that British woman at the Grand Canyon (see page 120).

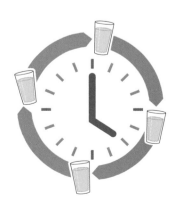

Another tip for getting more water into your body is to sleep with a water bottle. As we mentioned earlier, Christine does this, and it drives Jimmy nuts, but it helps her get that extra little bit of water to reach her hydration goal. Whenever she wakes up in the middle of the night to go to the bathroom, she grabs that bottle of water and takes a sip. Okay, honestly sometimes she chugs because she's really thirsty. In this case, chugging is okay because her body is sending her signals to drink more, and so she does. Plus, don't forget that you lose water throughout the night when you breathe more heavily. Because you can't stop breathing (unless you're a zombie), replenishing the water you lose from respiration during sleep is crucial.

Finally, if you know you're going to be working in the garden, mowing the grass, or in direct sunlight for some time (especially during the heat of summer), make sure you have plenty of water with you. It will quench your thirst and help you maintain the proper body temperature so you don't become overheated and possibly get heatstroke. Don't play the hero if you don't feel well when you get hot. Drink, drink, drink . . . water, that is.

We should all drink a toast to water right about now, but it's time to shift gears and move into what's perhaps the most exciting part of this book. Before Christine studied to become a Nutritional Therapy Practitioner, she had no idea about many of the concepts you'll be reading about in Part 3. The first thing we share with you is the role of minerals in your diet, which many people have no clue about. We make it all understandable for you, so put your thinking cap on and get ready to have your mind blown.

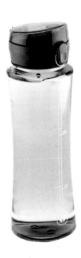

REAL FOOD KETO TAKEAWAYS FROM CHAPTER 7

- Water makes up 55 to 60 percent of your body.

- Dehydration is the most common nutritional deficiency in the United States.

- The maximum daily water intake for everyone is 128 ounces (1 gallon).

- Drinking too much water can be just as harmful as being dehydrated.

- Minimize your intake of diuretic beverages like coffee, tea, soda, fruit juice, and alcohol.

- There are myriad benefits that come from appropriate water intake.

- The endocrine, immune, vascular, and detoxification systems in the body all rely on water.

- The early signs of dehydration start at as little as a 2 percent loss of water.

- The later signs of dehydration kick in at up to a 10 percent loss of water.

- Losing more than 10 percent of your body's water can result in death.

- Sip water throughout the day using our Quarter Hour Solution (QHS) method.

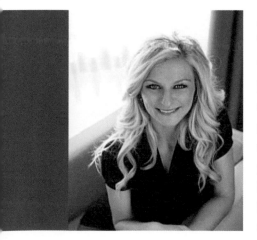

JESSICA TYE, NTP

www.jessicatye.com

Through my knowledge of nutritional therapy, I have been able to go from just having faith that my keto lifestyle is what is responsible for how amazing I feel to truly understanding the mechanisms and physiology behind it. I am able to go from mere correlation to actual causation! With that professional understanding and knowledge, I am able to serve my clients better and continue to educate the public so that they too can see and feel these amazing health benefits in their lives and the lives of their family and friends. I am blessed to be living what I believe I was called to do and serving others—nutritional therapy has made that a reality for me.

part 3
APPLYING NUTRITIONAL THERAPY

So far in this book, you've learned about why we advocate for a real, whole foods–based diet combined with the therapeutic effects that come from consuming a low-carb, moderate-protein, high-fat diet. Whereas much of that information probably wasn't brand-new to you (unless you're new to keto), Part 3 dives deeply into areas of nutritional health that are rarely talked about as part of the health discussion. However, the chapters in this part cover the things that we believe are the foundation for truly healing your body so that the *Real Food Keto* concepts you learned in Parts 1 and 2 can make a lasting impact.

To that end, we're going to start applying the principles of nutritional therapy to what you've already learned. What's *nutritional therapy*? It's using food and lifestyle changes to bring about optimal health. It's really no more complicated than that.

Christine began studying nutritional therapy through the Nutritional Therapy Association (www.nutritionaltherapy.com) so that she could learn about the role the food we eat plays in balancing hormones, improving digestion, and regulating blood sugar. She ended up learning so much more, and that's what we share with you in this part. If you are inspired to learn even more about these incredible concepts or are interested in becoming a Nutritional Therapy Practitioner (NTP), we share some helpful information in the Call to Action at the end of this part.

Now let's start applying nutritional therapy to a low-carb, high-fat, ketogenic diet.

CHAPTER 8

Minerals and How to Get Them

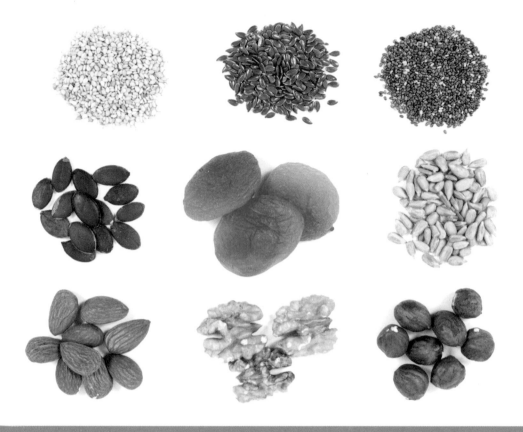

We're starting this section about the application of nutritional therapy with a topic that's extremely important in your health, even though hardly anyone ever talks about it—minerals! Minerals are especially relevant for people who eat keto because of some common issues that can crop up as you begin to switch from being a sugar burner to a fat burner. You might feel fatigued, get leg cramps, have headaches, and experience other symptoms of what people in the keto community affectionately refer to as the "keto flu." It's not actually the flu; it just feels like the flu. The symptoms are a result of an electrolyte imbalance that occurs when specific minerals—like magnesium, potassium, sodium, and calcium—get dumped from the body when the glycogen stores are released. Consequently, replenishing minerals when you're eating keto is a vital part of being successful.

We know about mineral deficiencies all too well. When Jimmy first started a low-carb lifestyle as he followed the Atkins diet in 2004, he dealt with some of the most excruciating nighttime leg cramps that he'd ever experienced. He'd wake up screaming and writhing in pain in the middle of the night, and we had no idea the reason was that the salt and other minerals in his body needed to be replenished to normalize his electrolytes. Now we try to warn others as they start keto so that they can prevent these symptoms from developing by consuming 3 to 5 grams of sodium from pink Himalayan salt or some other quality salt that includes lots of minerals. You also could try a supplement. Keto Vitals (www.ketovitals.com) is one that includes a variety of electrolytes to help keep your minerals properly balanced.

When we talk about consuming more salt, we're not referring to commercial table salt (like Morton Salt). Those products aren't real salt, and you should avoid them because they're produced with chemicals in factories. We're talking about sodium from natural sources of salt, such as sea salt.

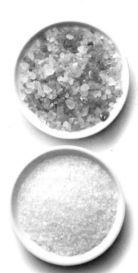

Of course, part of the challenge with getting enough salt when you're following a well-formulated ketogenic diet and eating whole foods is that those foods lack large amounts of sodium. Most processed foods contain very high levels of sodium to make them more palatable and to cover up the junk ingredients in them, so when you eat a diet that includes a lot of processed foods, you get plenty of sodium. When you switch to real food, you're eating minimally processed foods that don't contain the same levels of sodium. As a result, you need to pay more attention to your salt intake.

But sodium is only one of the many minerals the body needs to run well. The 103 known minerals make up about 4 percent of the body. Because the body can't make these minerals and you have to obtain them through food and supplementation, they're considered essential. At least eighteen minerals must come from your diet for you to maintain proper health.

The body is extremely resourceful in maintaining the proper levels of minerals. If you get an overabundance of minerals, your body stores them in places where it can use them and then excretes the extra. When you're getting insufficient amounts of minerals, your body seeks them out to keep this balance. However, if you experience a complete deficiency in any one particular mineral, your entire mineral balance is thrown off kilter, which can lead to a whole host of health issues that we'll cover in just a moment.

THE BENEFITS OF MINERALS

Ask most people about the benefits of having minerals in the body, and you'll likely get blank stares in return. This topic is completely off the radar of most people, including Christine until she studied to become an NTP. We want to bring this topic to light so you can understand why minerals play such an integral role in a healthy lifestyle. What you're going to learn is that each mineral needs to be at the proper level to assist your body in performing its various functions. Let's take a look at some of the general benefits that come from minerals.

- **Minerals assist in making enzyme reactions possible.** You might think to yourself, "So what? Why should I care about this?" Well, you should care because, without these enzymatic reactions in the digestive system, you can't properly break down food and absorb the nutrients into your body, and it's a pretty big problem if you can't absorb nutrients from your food.

- **Minerals help maintain proper pH balance.** Blood pH needs to stay within a small range of between 7.35 and 7.45, and stomach pH should fall between 1.5 and 3.0 on a scale of 0 (pure acidity) to 14 (pure alkalinity).[1] Here's a diagram to help you visualize this better:

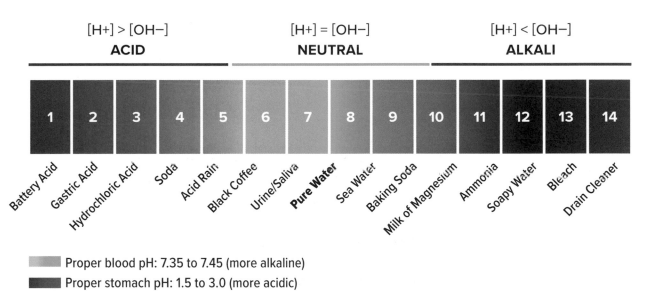

$[H+] > [OH-]$					$[H+] = [OH-]$				$[H+] < [OH-]$				
ACID					**NEUTRAL**				**ALKALI**				
1	2	3	4	5	6	7	8	9	10	11	12	13	14
Battery Acid	Gastric Acid	Hydrochloric Acid	Soda	Acid Rain	Black Coffee	Urine/Saliva	**Pure Water**	Sea Water	Baking Soda	Milk of Magnesium	Ammonia	Soapy Water	Bleach	Drain Cleaner

Proper blood pH: 7.35 to 7.45 (more alkaline)
Proper stomach pH: 1.5 to 3.0 (more acidic)

How do minerals help maintain this proper pH balance in the blood and stomach? The parathyroid hormone called calcitonin helps regulate blood pH by taking calcium out of the bones and depositing it into the blood, which normalizes the blood pH when it's too acidic. On the flip side, if the blood pH is too alkaline, then the exact opposite takes place—the body uses calcitonin to take calcium out of the blood and deposit it back into the bones. (It's like transferring money between two bank accounts that you own.) Likewise, adequate levels of zinc help with the production of hydrochloric acid (HCl), which results in proper stomach pH for good digestion.

- **Minerals help transport nutrients across cell membranes.** Sodium, potassium, calcium, and chloride (which you might recognize as the electrolytes we've discussed a few times throughout the book) help maintain the proper fluidity of cells, which is what enables minerals to cross cell membranes. Getting the nutrients exactly where they need to go helps prevent nutritional deficiencies that manifest as chronic disease.

- **Minerals aid in proper nerve conduction.** Nerve cells transmit and receive signals to and from the other neurons in the body that transmit electrical impulses to control movement and other basic functions. The nerves function correctly when electrolytes are balanced. Hydration plays a key role in this process because the electrolytes need adequate water to do their jobs. (Read more about this in Chapter 7. Also, this would be a good time to take a sip of water.)

- **Minerals help the endocrine system function well.** Chapter 12 is all about the endocrine system; for now, suffice it to say that it is the chemical messenging system of the body. Each hormone and endocrine organ and gland has a mineral that it relies on for functioning. The graphic on the next page shows each organ of the endocrine system and the corresponding mineral that it needs to work properly. (A more comprehensive list appears in Chapter 12.)

- **Minerals are necessary for proper immune health.** Minerals play a key role in shoring up your immunity. You need ionized calcium, for example, to support white blood cell activity. Zinc aids in wound healing; a telltale sign that you're deficient in zinc is an inability to heal quickly. For a immune system boost, taking a zinc supplement does the trick because the zinc serves as an antioxidant and protects against free radicals. Iodine is an excellent antibacterial and antiviral agent that helps protect the body from foreign invaders.

A. The thyroid depends on iodine.

B. The prostate depends on zinc.

C. The pituitary depends on manganese.

D. The pancreas depends on chromium.

E. The gonads depend on selenium.

F. The adrenals depend on copper.

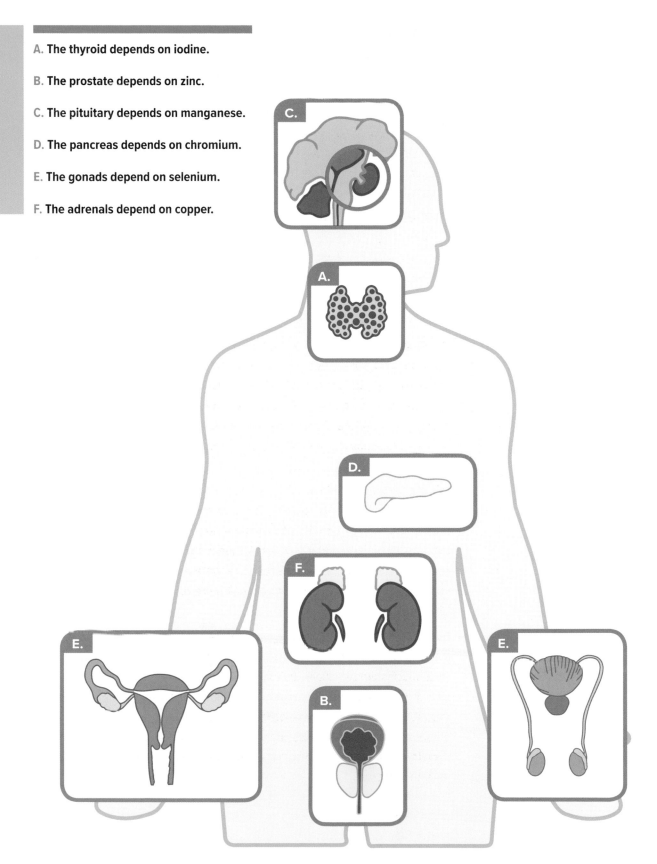

- **Minerals help maintain heart health.** The cardiovascular system requires two important minerals to function well: magnesium and calcium. Calcium triggers the contraction and relaxation of the heart and all the other muscles in the body, but without magnesium, the calcium wouldn't work as intended. Getting the appropriate calcium-to-magnesium ratio is critical for preventing conditions such as an irregular heartbeat (a sign of magnesium deficiency).

We'd be remiss if we didn't mention the key role of one particular vitamin and its connection to calcium—vitamin K2, which is also known as Activator X. Vitamin K2 tells calcium where it needs to go in the body so that calcium isn't deposited in places where it's not needed, such as the coronary arteries. Vitamin K2 deficiency can lead to osteoporosis and bone spurs because calcium doesn't know where to go.

The cardiovascular system also requires appropriate amounts of sodium to function well. Yep, you read that right: If you want a healthy heart, you'd better get salt *into* your diet. Many people fear salt because of what they've heard about sodium raising blood pressure levels. However, the truth is that only about 5 percent of the population has a sensitivity to salt. Someone with a healthy blood pressure level would have to consume a disgusting amount of salt—close to 7.5 grams, which is about one and a half teaspoons—to get anywhere close to making salt intake an issue. Boy, just thinking about it is making us thirsty! If you're eating a real food–based, ketogenic diet, then it would be extremely difficult to consume too much salt. Balancing your sodium intake with proper levels of potassium will flavor your foods well and keep your heart functioning optimally.

- **Minerals help lower the acidity of the blood from the detoxification process.** Calcium helps directly buffer the acidity that develops in the blood during detoxification. Toxins deplete several important minerals, such as magnesium, which can lead to a lack of the enzymes required for healthy Phase 1 liver detoxification. Additionally, certain minerals keep heavy metals from piling up in the tissue. Technically, heavy metals like lead, mercury, cadmium, and aluminum are considered minerals, but they're the toxic kind. The proper balance of healthy minerals in your body is necessary to keep these bad boys from harming you. (Christine has had heavy metal toxicity, and she underwent intravenous chelation therapy to remove those minerals and to replenish other minerals that had been depleted.) Finally, the minerals molybdenum and manganese help activate enzymes that aid in detoxifying the metabolism.

As you can see, minerals play an integral role in your health, and you should not ignore them. The problem is that too many people don't know what minerals are or their two major classifications. We're going to educate you on that now.

TWO MAJOR CLASSIFICATIONS OF MINERALS

Just as nutrients come in two primary classifications—macronutrients and micronutrients—minerals are divided into two groups. There are macrominerals, which are found in the body in greater amounts because the body needs more of them to function well, and microminerals (also known as trace minerals), which are present in much lower quantities in the body because they're needed in smaller amounts. We've created a list of macro- and microminerals that the body requires for optimal health.

MACROMINERALS	MICROMINERALS	
Calcium	Boron	Manganese
Chloride	Chromium	Molybdenum
Magnesium	Cobalt	Rubidium
Phosphorus	Copper	Selenium
Potassium	Germanium	Silicon
Sodium	Iodine	Vanadium
Sulfur	Iron	Zinc
	Lithium	

Perhaps you recognize a few of these terms. Some other terms on this list might sound like they came from the planet Krypton. (Molybdenum, anyone?) Don't worry; we are going to explain all the critical information to help you understand why these minerals are so incredibly important in your pursuit of health. Let's take a closer look at each of these macro- and microminerals and the roles they play. This is eye-opening stuff that will make you a lot more conscious of ensuring that you are getting minerals into your diet.

Adequate stomach acid (hydrochloric acid) is required to absorb calcium in the body. If you don't have enough stomach acid, then you can develop osteopenia and even osteoporosis. (Read more about the underproduction of stomach acid in Chapter 10.)

HEALTH BENEFITS OF MACROMINERALS

Calcium is the most prominent mineral in the body. Upward of 93 percent of the calcium in our bodies is in our bones. Calcium helps give bones their inflexibility.

Calcium also helps with transmitting nerve impulses, contracting and relaxing the muscles, regulating the pH balance in the blood, assisting with blood clotting, aiding in insulin production, facilitating enzyme reactions, and providing strength to the entire skeletal system.

CALCIUM COFACTORS

Calcium has several cofactors (meaning dependence on something else) for it to work properly, including the following things:

- Blood pH levels in the 7.35 to 7.45 (normal) range
- Proper hydration and electrolytes like sodium and potassium
- Well-functioning parathyroid hormone
- Other minerals such as chloride, magnesium, and phosphorus
- The fat-soluble vitamins (A, D, E, and K)
- Essential fatty acids
- Good digestion (see Chapter 10 for information about digestion)

Chloride balances the quantity of fluid both inside and outside the cells, maintains proper blood volume and blood pressure, stabilizes body pH, enables the electrical impulses in the nervous system, and aids in the digestion of food (because it's in the gastric juices).

Magnesium plays a key component in the transmission of nerve impulses, regulates body temperature, boosts energy production, assists the body in detoxification, builds strong bones and teeth (because it helps make calcium work correctly), prevents the blood from becoming too thick, and is used in the metabolism of fats and in synthesizing protein.

Phosphorus is the second most abundant mineral in the body. It's good for bone health, helps nerve function, makes muscles contract, and is an essential part of the structure of the DNA and cell membranes.

When you combine foods with plenty of magnesium (like avocado and spinach) with foods that contain vitamin B6 (eggs and pork, for example), you have the perfect recipe for preventing kidney stones from developing. Spinach, bacon, and avocado omelet, anyone?

Phospholipids are fats that contain phosphorus and help with certain cellular functions. They form the membrane that makes up the outer level of the cell wall, and they also control what goes in and out of the cell by maintaining the fluidity of the cell membrane. What does this mean? Your body can get the nutrients it needs in the places that they're needed.

Potassium is a key electrolyte that conducts electricity in the body, which controls nerve impulses and other bodily functions. Potassium is essential for heart function, plays a role in skeletal and smooth muscle contraction for normal digestion and muscular function, converts blood glucose (sugar in the blood) into glycogen stores (stored glucose in the muscles), and maintains proper cellular fluid levels (like radiator fluid for the body).

Be careful with supplementing with potassium because taking too much can be very harmful to your body—or even fatal. Talk to your healthcare provider about checking your potassium levels before you start taking supplements of this mineral.

Sodium maintains healthy blood pressure, keeps normal fluid balance in the body, and transmits nerve impulses.

Sulfur is the third most abundant mineral in the body. It's in vital amino acids used to create protein for cells, tissues, hormones, enzymes, and antibodies.

MICROMINERALS

Boron is critical to building strong bones; enhances the metabolism of steroid hormones like testosterone, estrogen, and DHEA; and is essential for the conversion of vitamin D into its active form of 1.25 dihydroxycholecalciferol. Studies indicate boron could be useful in cell membrane function.

Chromium improves insulin sensitivity and blood sugar management by enhancing the function of hormones that improve carbohydrate, protein, and fat metabolism.

Cobalt is necessary for vitamin B12 absorption, which helps in the digestion of iron. However, too much cobalt increases T4 (thyroxine) production, which is detrimental to thyroid health and the metabolism.

Copper is necessary for your adrenals to work. It's involved in the conversion of dopamine in the brain into the neurotransmitter norepinephrine (which is what happens when you're in fight-or-flight mode). It's also essential for the repair and synthesis of connective tissue, is used for the breakdown of estrogen in the liver, has anti-inflammatory properties, and is needed to metabolize iron from the liver.

BALANCING COPPER AND ZINC

Copper and zinc have an inverse relationship like two sides of a scale. If the body becomes deficient in zinc, copper tries to compensate by increasing and tilting the scale heavily on the side of copper. Conversely, if the body becomes deficient in copper, zinc rises correspondingly. Both these microminerals compete for the same metabolic pathway, which is the reason there's an antagonistic relationship between the two. Keeping the proper balance between copper and zinc prevents ramifications that you'll read about later in this chapter.

Germanium supports the immune system.

Iodine is a major micromineral because it exists in every cell of the body, is the primary mineral component of the thyroid, and is important for estrogen metabolism in breast tissue.

Iron builds red blood cells.

Lithium stabilizes mood and improves brain health.

Manganese helps repair bone, connective tissue, and joints. It aids in the conversion of blood glucose to glycogen (stored glucose); is necessary for a healthy pancreatic function; and is used in the synthesis of cholesterol and fatty acids.

Molybdenum helps rid the body of toxins by removing the chemical compounds that are found in petroleum products. It also acts as a catalyst for enzymes to help break down sulfur-containing amino acids that we need for optimal health.

Rubidium provides no known essential functions in the body, but some studies have shown that it helps reduce tumor growth in animals and has a tranquilizing effect.

Selenium is a mineral antioxidant that protects against oxidative stress and is key in healthy thyroid function because it converts thyroxine (T4) into the active form triiodothyronine (T3). Selenium is important for adrenal function, it supports immune function, and it's necessary for sexual function (hey, Baby, pass the Brazil nuts!).

Silicon strengthens bone and connective tissues such as joints and cartilage.

Vanadium regulates blood sugar because it contains an insulin-like property to help address prediabetes, diabetes, low blood glucose, elevated cholesterol, heart disease, and water retention.

Zinc is another important micromineral because of all the things it does. It improves mental function, immune function, and sexual function. It's also essential for stomach acid production, and it regulates the release of the fat-soluble vitamin A from the liver. Furthermore, zinc helps synthesize cholesterol, fats, and proteins; is good for prostate health; and is needed for appropriate taste perception.

THE IMPORTANCE OF PROPER MINERAL BALANCE

You might never have thought about minerals before reading this book, but we hope the list of the various benefits of having the appropriate amounts of minerals in the body wakes you up to how critical these are to your overall health. Remember, it's the balance of the minerals that matters most—like the balance between sodium and potassium or calcium and magnesium. Too much of any one mineral in the body can cause a chain reaction that causes another mineral to become deficient and various consequences to occur. A perfect example of this is when excessive iron and copper levels in the body can prevent the body from absorbing zinc (and you'll recall that excessive levels of zinc can lead to a copper deficiency).

Wondering where you're going to get your minerals isn't something to get overly worked up about. Most people simply want to eat food without obsessing over every little mineral that's in their diet, and that approach usually works out okay. If you're concerned about whether your minerals are properly balanced, ask your doctor to run a vitamin and mineral status test to see where you stand. However, be aware that a deficiency can negatively affect your health. Most doctors prescribe medication for the symptoms of the mineral deficiency rather than helping you obtain mineral balance, but an NTP can help you work through deficiencies to make your health as robust as it can possibly be. Read the information at the back of the book to learn more about real food sources you can include in your diet to get the minerals you need to keep your system in balance.

For information about finding an NTP to consult with you about your nutrition, see the list of NTPs in the Resources section or visit the Nutritional Therapy Association website at www.nutritionaltherapy.com.

HORMONE REPLACEMENT THERAPY AND MINERALS

We have a word of warning for women of childbearing age who take birth control pills or women who are on hormone replacement therapy (HRT). Both birth control and HRT have been shown in research to increase the risk of vitamin and mineral deficiencies. Taking birth control pills or HRT for long periods of time can deplete critical nutrients from the body and/or cause a major imbalance in the minerals.[2] If you fall into one of these groups, you need to be aware of the potential for issues so you can take the appropriate steps in preventing these deficiencies from becoming a problem. Taking a good iron-free multivitamin (unless you've been diagnosed with low iron or you don't consume enough red meat) and fixing your digestion can play a big role in avoiding problems. You also can try adding some healthy, keto-friendly real foods, such as eggs, spinach, seafood, cashews, tomatoes, and dairy, to replenish the deficiencies. Since she had a hysterectomy in 2016, Christine uses an estrogen patch for HRT. Needless to say, she keeps a very close check on her vitamin and mineral status.

We're not suggesting you stay away from hormone replacement therapy altogether. HRT does have benefits, such as easing perimenopausal and menopausal symptoms like hot flashes, night sweats, mood changes, weight gain, and metabolism issues. There is something called *bioidentical hormones* that are a good option if you need HRT. These bioidentical hormones are manmade from plant estrogens that are identical to what the body produces, which means the body can easily use them. Bioidentical hormones have other benefits, as well, such as improving gut health, helping with mineral absorption, and improving metabolism. It can be tricky to find a practitioner who knows a lot about using bioidentical hormones and is comfortable doing so, but if you can find someone who does use these hormones in their practice, they could have great benefits for you.

For further information on this subject, you can read the PubMed article, "Oral Contraceptives and Changes in Nutritional Requirements."[3]

SIGNS OF MINERAL DEFICIENCIES

When you read through the following information about minerals and signs of their deficiencies, you might notice some symptoms that you might be experiencing and that your general practitioner may have diagnosed as some disease that requires you to take a medication. If so, perhaps it's time to have the discussion with your doctor about determining whether you have any of these specific mineral deficiencies. If you do, you want to address them rather than letting them fester any longer.

You also might ask the obvious question—what can I do to prevent a mineral deficiency? We're so glad you asked! Take a look at the list of mineral-rich foods that we've provided at the end of the book. Consuming a wide variety of those on a consistent basis should do the trick, but the next section gives a few tips for preventing mineral deficiencies.

BORON
Certain types of arthritis may be associated with a deficiency in boron.

One Moore Thing: Very little toxicity is associated with boron.

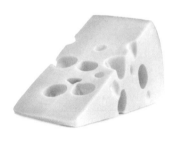

CALCIUM
- A huge sign of calcium deficiency is osteoporosis, which is a loss of bone mass. Drinking soft drinks can increase the risk of osteoporosis because they contain phosphoric acid. Phosphoric acid interferes with our body's ability to absorb and use calcium.

- Muscle cramps and muscle spasms can occur.

- A person might experience insomnia or hyperactivity if they're deficient in calcium.

- Periodontal disease is associated with calcium deficiency.

- Anxiety might result from a calcium deficiency.

One Moore Thing: Excess calcium levels can cause imbalances with other minerals.

CHLORIDE
- A chloride deficiency can lead to excessive fatigue.

- Muscle weakness can occur.

- Breathing problems might arise.

- Frequent vomiting might occur.

- A person can experience prolonged diarrhea.

- Excessive thirst can be a sign of chloride deficiency.

- If you have high blood pressure, it might be due to chloride deficiency.

- High levels of sodium in the blood are associated with a chloride deficiency.

One Moore Thing: Hyperchloremia is an electrolyte imbalance that occurs when there's too much chloride in the blood. Signs of hyperchloremia include fatigue, muscle weakness, excessive thirst, dry mucous membranes, and high blood pressure. Some people may not experience any symptoms at all and don't know they have hyperchloremia until a blood test reveals it. Be aware that hypochloremia (low levels of chloride in the body) and hyperchloremia (too much chloride in the body) have some of the same symptoms listed, so talk with your healthcare provider to determine which you might have.

CHROMIUM

Deficiencies of chromium can lead to blood sugar dysregulation.

One Moore Thing: Chromium deficiency is common in America due to poor availability of chromium and difficulty in absorbing it. A large intake of sugar and refined carbohydrates can increase chromium needs.

COPPER

- Blood cells can break down (hemolytic anemia), which includes symptoms of dark urine, yellowing of the skin and whites of the eyes (jaundice), heart murmur, increased heart rate, an enlarged spleen, and an enlarged liver.

- A person with copper deficiency can experience symptoms of anemia, including fatigue, headache, shortness of breath (especially when exercising), dizziness, pale skin, leg cramps, insomnia, and difficulty concentrating.

- A person can have a lowered number of white blood cells, which could lead to an increased propensity for infection.

- Depigmentation of skin can occur.

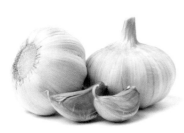

One Moore Thing: Things that can cause a copper deficiency include a genetic inability to absorb copper in the intestines and low-functioning adrenal glands. Signs of copper toxicity are nausea and vomiting, and long-term supplementation of copper can cause liver cirrhosis. If you cook with copper cookware or if you have old plumbing, you might be at increased risk of copper toxicity.

IODINE

- Iodine deficiency can lead to delayed development in children.

- Hypothyroidism is related to iodine deficiency. Symptoms include weight gain, sensitivity to cold, hair loss, fatigue, chronic indigestion, irritability, depression, constipation, muscle weakness, dry and itchy skin, infertility, heavy or irregular periods, and high cholesterol.

One Moore Thing: Iodine deficiency usually takes the form of a swollen thyroid gland, called goiter, which is more common in women. A deficiency in iodine is a worldwide problem. Despite the prevalence of iodized salt, deficiencies of iodine remain a problem in the United States. Certain foods block iodine from being absorbed and used. These foods are known as goitrogens, *and they include broccoli, cabbage, peanuts, and turnips. You also can get too much iodine, which results in iodine toxicity. Symptoms include increased heart rate, skin irritation, diarrhea, nervousness, and headaches. Iodine has a generally wide range of safety, but consuming high doses (20 to 30 mg/day) for a long time may suppress thyroid function.*

IRON

A person deficient in iron can become anemic. Signs of iron-deficiency anemia include a sense of fatigue and being overly tired or drowsy, weakness, breathlessness, coldness in extremities, pallor (an unhealthy pale appearance), swollen tongue, and spooning of the nails.

Things that can cause iron-deficiency anemia are a decreased intake of iron, insufficient levels of stomach acid, and blood loss (either externally or internally). Excess menstrual bleeding is a common cause of iron-deficiency anemia in women.

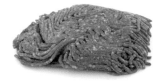

One Moore Thing: Excess amounts of iron in the body can cause tissue damage. Ten percent of the population has a genetic problem in which iron deposits form in the tissues, especially the liver. Iron toxicity is more common in men than in women because men don't have a menstrual cycle. Vitamin C in excess amounts can lead to iron toxicity because it enhances iron absorption.

LITHIUM

Influence of lithium deficiency is not known or proven.

One Moore Thing: Too much lithium can interfere with iodine uptake by the thyroid gland and may block thyroxin release or thyroid-stimulating hormone (TSH). Anyone with kidney disease must take lithium with caution. Therapeutic doses of 500 to 1,500 mg/day are prescribed only by doctors, who also must closely monitor blood lithium levels. Symptoms of lithium toxicity include nausea, vomiting, diarrhea, thirst, increased urination, tremors, drowsiness, confusion, delirium, skin eruptions, and hair loss. With further toxicity, staggering, seizures, kidney damage, coma, and even death may occur.

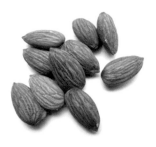

MAGNESIUM

- People who are deficient in magnesium can experience heart palpations.
- Magnesium deficiency can cause a person to have stinky feet.
- A deficiency in magnesium can cause muscle spasms and painful menstrual cramps.
- A person can have high blood pressure if they're deficient in magnesium.
- An increase in blood triglycerides and cholesterol can result from a magnesium deficiency.

One Moore Thing: If you take too much magnesium, you can experience diarrhea.

MANGANESE

- Someone can experience fat and carbohydrate synthesis problems with a deficiency in manganese.
- People can experience glucose intolerances because of a manganese deficiency.
- Impaired growth can result from manganese deficiency.
- Reproductive difficulties can happen with a deficiency in manganese.
- A person can have skeletal abnormalities with a deficiency in manganese.
- Weak ligaments can be a result of manganese deficiency.

One Moore Thing: If you get too much manganese (more than 100 mg/day), you might experience nausea or gastric upset.

MOLYBDENUM

Molybdenum deficiency is uncommon.

One Moore Thing: Molybdenum increases the excretion of copper. Doses of greater than 500 mcg/day may lead to lower copper levels in the body.

PHOSPHOROUS

- A person can experience a loss of appetite with a phosphorous deficiency.
- Bone pain and stiff joints can happen with this deficiency.
- People can experience fatigue and weakness if they're deficient in phosphorous.
- Irregular breathing and numbness can occur.
- A person can experience irritability if they are deficient in phosphorous.
- Weight changes can be a sign of a phosphorous deficiency.

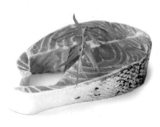

One Moore Thing: Phosphorus is so abundant in the Western diet that deficiency in this mineral isn't common. Things that can cause a deficiency in phosphorous are the use of antacids, alcoholism, and certain vegetarian diets. Phosphorous deficiency also can happen during the treatment of diabetic acidosis.

POTASSIUM

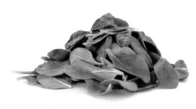

- A person can experience fatigue if they're deficient in potassium.

- Mental confusion can happen as a result of a deficiency in potassium.

- Muscle cramps and weakness can occur with a deficiency in potassium.

- A person might experience cardiovascular problems with a potassium deficiency.

One Moore Thing: Many people are deficient in potassium. Potassium is often leached out of cooked food because potassium is water-soluble. On the flip side, taking too much potassium can be very harmful to your health—possibly even fatal. We recommend that you talk to your healthcare provider about determining your potassium status before you start any potassium supplementation.

RUBIDIUM

There is no known deficiency or toxicity for rubidium.

One Moore Thing: Given that there are no known issues with rubidium deficiency, all we have to say is this: Don't worry; be happy!

SELENIUM

- Arthritis can be a sign of selenium deficiency.

- A person might experience painful muscles with selenium deficiency.

- Anemia might result from a deficiency in selenium.

- Growth retardation in children might occur with a selenium deficiency.

- Cardiovascular disease might be a result of selenium deficiency.

One Moore Thing: Selenium deficiency is becoming more widespread due to the depletion of selenium in soil, which also means it's depleted from our food supply. Selenium has a narrow therapeutic dosage range and margin of safety. Selenium toxicity may happen at doses greater than 800 mcg/ day. Symptoms of toxicity include a metallic taste in the mouth, damage to fingernails, depression, nervousness, mental instability, a garlic smell to sweat and breath, gastrointestinal irritation, and hair loss.

SODIUM

If a person is deficient in sodium, it's likely that the addictive pathways will be turned on, causing a person to crave other things, such as carbohydrates like sugar or alcohol. Read *The Salt Fix* by James DiNicolantonio for outstanding science-based information on the importance of salt.[4]

One Moore Thing: The adrenal glands produce a hormone called aldosterone, which helps the body retain valuable sodium. Someone with adrenal dysfunction doesn't produce enough aldosterone and therefore dumps sodium out of the body through urination.

SULFUR

- A deficiency in sulfur may cause a reduced ability to synthesize protein.

- The sulfur-containing amino acid cysteine is necessary for making glutathione, which is a powerful antioxidant that helps prevent cell damage.

- When deficient in sulfur, a person might experience fatigue, depression, and an increased sensitivity to physical and psychological stress.

One Moore Thing: Methylsulfonylmethane (MSM) is the only bioavailable form of sulfur that's a macromineral. It's found in good amounts in cultured or raw foods. It can be destroyed easily when you cook and process foods. It's good for the formation of collagen and in helping reduce the visibility of wrinkles. It's anti-inflammatory in nature, so it helps with arthritis and can also help athletes with post-workout soreness. MSM can help flush toxins from the muscles and can help with food allergies. In people with multiple sclerosis (MS), it helps heal the myelin sheath around nerves.

VANADIUM

Because vanadium aids in blood sugar metabolism, a deficiency might lead to hypoglycemia or diabetes.

One Moore Thing: Too much vanadium can cause conjunctivitis, pneumonia, anemia, and irritation of the respiratory tract. It may also cause dizziness, lethargy, vertigo, anxiety and sadness, or melancholy feelings.

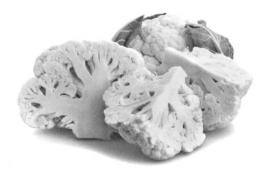

ZINC

- People with a zinc deficiency don't taste or smell as well as a person who has enough zinc in their body. As a result, people with a zinc deficiency often don't have much of an appetite.

- Zinc deficiency leads to hypochlorhydria (a deficiency in stomach HCl).

- Someone with a zinc deficiency can have an aversion to meat.

- A zinc deficiency can cause a depressed immune system, so a person deficient in zinc might get sick often or their wounds might not heal promptly.

- Zinc deficiency can lead to skin disorders and white spots on the fingernails.

- Children can experience growth retardation if they're zinc deficient.

One Moore Thing: Doses of zinc greater than 20 mg on an empty stomach can lead to nausea and stomach upset. This is more common in people who have low stomach acid. Long-term zinc supplementation in doses greater than 50 mg/day can lead to copper deficiency. Zinc is depleted by stress, refined carbohydrates, caffeine, alcohol, and sexual activity (in men).

TIPS FOR PREVENTING MINERAL DEFICIENCIES

There's been a recurring theme for most of the book: Make sure your digestion is working right. Having a well-functioning digestive system is so important that Chapter 10 focuses on digestion. For now, know that getting the proper amount of stomach acid (enough to maintain a stomach pH between 1.5 and 3.0) prevents these mineral deficiencies from happening. However, if you produce too little stomach acid, which is the case in a startling nine out of ten people right now, then the foods you eat can't be digested properly, and your body can't absorb the nutrients from even the best foods. Ask your doctor to run what is called the Heidelberg Gastrotelemetry test to determine your level of stomach pH. Read more about issues with insufficient stomach acid in Chapter 10.

BEWARE OF FOOD SENSITIVITIES

One of the goals of *Real Food Keto* is to encourage you to consume a variety of foods so you don't run the risk of developing food sensitivities. Jimmy experienced this in 2017 when he discovered through a food sensitivity panel that his sensitivity to egg yolks and egg whites was five times higher than the norm. With a ton of backyard chickens giving us fresh free-range organic eggs on a daily basis, this was a tough sensitivity to deal with. Although eggs are incredibly healthy for someone eating a ketogenic diet, because of the sensitivity Jimmy developed, he had to give up eggs for a while. After abstaining for about five months, he slowly started working them back into his diet; he just doesn't eat them every day anymore! Now he can eat eggs every few days with little to no trouble. See, there *can* be too much of a good thing!

A person with a normal blood pressure of 120/80 mmHg would have to consume 7.5 grams of salt to raise the blood pressure five or six points in the systolic (top number) reading, which would still be considered normal blood pressure. As we mentioned earlier, 7.5 grams is *a lot* of salt! It's equivalent to 1.32 teaspoons. We love salt, but that much sounds gross.

Another great tip for preventing mineral deficiencies is to consume a wide range of real foods that contain lots of different vibrant colors. When you purchase food directly from a local farmer or farmers market, you know where it comes from, and it generally tastes better than anything you could get from those fluorescent-lighted, temperature-controlled, fake-food-selling places most people call grocery stores. Don't forget to buy foods when they're in season. (In North America, strawberries aren't available in January, ya know?!)

One mineral deficiency that far too many people still deal with is sodium because they skimp on their salt intake. Remember, salt is an incredibly healthy part of your diet, just as saturated fat is. Despite salt being vilified as harmful to your cardiovascular health, the truth is that it's an essential aspect of making sure your body functions well. The only exception to this is for those very few people who are salt sensitive (and most of you already know who you are). For the rest of us, make sure you're getting a good-quality pink Himalayan salt or another mineral-rich natural salt. (Remember, avoid the blue-and-white container with the girl holding an umbrella—that ain't salt!)

Finally, especially for people who are on a ketogenic diet like we advocate for in this book, electrolyte balance is crucial to preventing some pretty painful side effects that come from mineral deficiency—specifically sodium, potassium, magnesium, chloride, and calcium. If you reduce your carbohydrate intake, moderate your protein consumption, and eat more healthy fats, then you shift your body from being primarily a sugar burner to mostly being a fat and ketone burner. When you do this, the glycogen stores—including all the electrolyte minerals—are dumped. So replenishing them prevents you from experiencing the typical leg cramps that come from adapting to nutritional ketosis. See the Resources section for information on some brands of electrolytes that we recommend.

In Chapter 9, we turn to the cousins of the minerals—the vitamins. Most people think vitamins come in a supplement bottle, but we have an entirely different take on what your primary source of vitamins should be. Gee, we wonder what that could be in a book called *Real Food Keto*?

REAL FOOD KETO TAKEAWAYS FROM CHAPTER 8

- The symptoms of the so-called "keto flu" are actually signs of electrolyte deficiency.
- Minerals provide many benefits to the body when they're in the proper balance.
- Macrominerals and microminerals are the two primary classifications of minerals.
- The specific health effects of the individual macro- and microminerals is significant.
- Ask your doctor to run a vitamin and mineral status test to know where you stand.
- Real, whole foods are chock-full of a variety of minerals for the body.
- Many doctors mistake physiological signs of mineral deficiency as other diseases.
- Be sure to eat a wide variety of foods to get a full range of the minerals your body needs.

CHAPTER 9

Vitamins and How to Balance Them

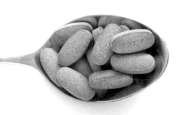

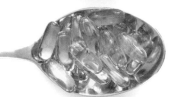

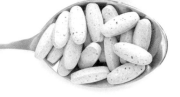

In Chapter 8, we told you about the various minerals that the body needs to function well. We now shift our attention to a subject many people are aware of without having a full understanding of—vitamins. For most people, vitamins are a pill they take in the morning with water because they know it's "healthy" for them to do. But have you ever thought about *why* vitamins are good for you? Surely there's a reason beyond because-that's-what-I've-always-done, right? Keep reading this chapter to learn about compelling reasons to not only prioritize your vitamin intake but to seek out real food sources of these vitamins.

Vitamins make up approximately 1 percent of the entire body. Each of the various vitamins play an important and specific role inside the body to work in perfect harmony with one another to adapt to shortfalls. The goal of this chapter is to help keep you properly balanced in the various vitamins so that you don't become deficient in any one area; when you become deficient, health problems can start to rear their ugly heads. You see, vitamins don't exist as single compounds. Instead, they're in groups that work as teams in perfect symbiotic harmony to improve your body. Ahhhhhhh.

For example, did you know that seventeen separate B vitamins have been identified, but all of them function together to work in you? With vitamin D, there are as many as twelve different components at work, and several of them are considered active. The lesser-known, but still important, vitamin P (which is also known as a bioflavonoid) contains at least five compounds. This indicates that our bodies are extremely complex with mechanisms in place to glean the nutrients from the food we eat and supplements we take to impact how we function day to day.

Not surprisingly, most of the vitamins function best when they're paired with trace minerals (as discussed in Chapter 8), enzymes, coenzymes, and, of course, other vitamins. These are *cofactors*, and they require proper digestion and hydration (remember the fourth macronutrient—water?) to absorb and transport the vitamins where they need to go. It's like the whole system was created by some sort of intelligent design or something.

Like minerals, there are two major classifications of vitamins: the fat-soluble vitamins and the water-soluble vitamins. The fat-soluble vitamins require that you consume fat with them so they can be absorbed and used by the body. Examples include vitamin A, vitamin D, vitamin E, and vitamin K. The water-soluble vitamins have to be taken with some water and include all the B vitamins, vitamin C, inositol (which is often referred to as vitamin B8 but is a pseudovitamin), and choline (which is considered to be part of the B-vitamin complex but is an organic compound).

There are five vitamins the body can make endogenously (inside the body): the fat-soluble vitamins D and K and the water-soluble vitamins B1 (thiamine), B2 (riboflavin), and B12 (cobalamin). (Other vitamins must be taken exogenously.) Many people know vitamin D is the "sun vitamin" because our bodies can create it when we expose our skin to bright sunlight. The gut microbiome produces Vitamin K. Cool! And the three B vitamins that are made by the body are also the result of healthy bacteria in the intestines. See, feeding those little buggers the right way is critically important to your health—more than you even knew!

GUT HEALTH

Minding your gut health is something we hope this book inspires you to do for perhaps the first time in your life. Gut health is important to discuss in this chapter on vitamins because the good bacteria located in our intestines are what produce the ever-important and critical vitamin K2 as well as the B vitamins biotin, cobalamin, and folate. The body can store most fat-soluble vitamins, but it can't store vitamin K, which is why it's important that you keep your vitamin K2 at appropriate levels for your overall bone health. A healthy liver and gallbladder assist the body in properly absorbing vitamin K. Even still, most of the vitamin K2 needed by the body needs to be added either through supplementation or by consuming foods rich in it. If you still fear the effects of consuming real food fats (despite all we've said), here's one more pitch: Without the fat, your body can't absorb or use vitamin K or any of the other fat-soluble vitamins (A, D, and E).[1] Eat some butter already!

You might be interested in knowing that the way food is grown and farmed can affect the vitamin content in the foods that end up on your dinner table. Nitrogen-based fertilizers can strip the minerals out of the soil, which affects the mineral content of the foods grown in that soil—even to the point of being entirely depleted of minerals. How do we know? Buy a commercially raised orange in your local supermarket and have it tested for its vitamin content. It will come back devoid of any vitamin C! An orange is generally synonymous with vitamin C, but the composition of the fruit is changing because the farming methods used (especially by big, commercial factory farms) are ruining the vitamin content in the soil. So sad. It's why we love taking care of our soil in our front yard garden and our backyard greenhouse; we want to be able to reap the nutrient density that comes from getting quality vitamins in the foods we grow and consume.

At this point in *Real Food Keto,* you already know we aren't fans of consuming sugar, refined carbohydrates like flour, pasta, and bread, and inflammatory vegetable oils and hydrogenated fats if your goal is to consume whole foods through the template of a low-carb, moderate protein, high-fat diet. But there's a vitamin connection to why you want to avoid these foods, too. These foods are well-known to deplete your body of various vitamins and minerals, leaving you deficient and causing all sorts of trouble in your health. When you add lifestyle choices of using and abusing alcohol, tobacco, and many drugs—which also deplete the body of vitamins and minerals—you have a recipe for undermining your goal of being healthy.[2]

If you'd like to learn more about when the various vitamins were discovered and other vitamin facts, we recommend you visit www.thoughtco.com/history-of-the-vitamins-4072556 to read "The History of the Vitamins."

Vitamins are a critical part of your health journey. We encourage you to get them as much as possible from whole food sources. But when that's not enough, it can give you peace of mind to know that you can supplement to get what you need.

Let's get our hands dirty now and take an in-depth look at all the vitamins and the benefits they play in the body. This is good stuff, so soak it all in and come back and read this section often as you continue learning!

VITAMINS AND THEIR BENEFITS

In this section, we go over the different vitamins and the benefits each vitamin has for the body. Vitamins, just like minerals, play a vital role in how well our bodies function. If you are deficient in one or more of these vitamins, you could experience some health problems, which we cover later in this chapter. For a great list of real food sources of the vitamins covered in this chapter, see the list that starts on page 355.

WATER-SOLUBLE VITAMINS	FAT-SOLUBLE VITAMINS
Vitamin B1 (thiamine)	Vitamin A
Vitamin B2 (riboflavin)	Vitamin D
Vitamin B3 (niacin)	Vitamin E
Vitamin B5 (pantothenic acid)	Vitamin K
Vitamin B6 (pyridoxine)	
Vitamin B7 (biotin)	
Vitamin B8 (inositol)	
Vitamin B9 (folate/folic acid)	
Vitamin B12 (cobalamin)	
Vitamin C	
Vitamin U	

Vegetables and fruits provide this thing called *carotene,* which is the vitamin A precursor. Animal-based foods are a great source of vitamin A, especially when you consume the organ meats.

INULIN (POLYSACCHARIDE BASED ON FRUCTOSE)

We previously discussed this polysaccharide, which is based on fructose, when we discussed carbohydrates in Chapter 6. It plays a big role in feeding your gut flora (which in turn increases the absorption of calcium and magnesium), relieving constipation, and curbing appetite by making you feel more satiated (full). Inulin is often used as an alternative to sugar in ketogenic foods because it has a sweet flavor.

VITAMIN A

This vitamin combined with other nutrients from real food sources is perfect for maintaining healthy immunity, promoting cardiovascular health, developing adrenal hormone and activity, helping grow strong bones, boosting fertility, and improving eczema and acne (by helping the skin repel bacteria and viruses). Vitamin A also possibly slows retinal decline, aids in wound healing, and promotes night vision. The cones of the eyes (which help you see color) rely on this vitamin for proper function, and getting an adequate amount prevents color blindness. (Jimmy likely has a vitamin A deficiency because he can't distinguish blue from purple.)

VITAMIN B1 (THIAMINE)

Thiamine pyrophosphate requires magnesium to turn it into a biologically active form of the vitamin that the body can use. Vitamin B1 is excellent for carbohydrate metabolism and protein breakdown (which are good things when you eat keto), energy production (especially in the brain), nerve cell function and conductivity, mucous membrane health, mental function, anemia prevention, and blood sugar regulation.

VITAMIN B2 (RIBOFLAVIN)

Vitamin B2 helps with breaking down carbohydrate, protein, and fat so the body can use the nutrients as energy. It allows the oxygen you breathe in to be used well by the body, boosts eyesight, is necessary for converting vitamin B6 (pyridoxine) into its active form, helps convert niacin into tryptophan, minimizes migraine headaches, reduces cataracts, lowers high blood pressure, and is necessary for phase 1 detoxification. (Read Chapter 13 for information about detoxification.)

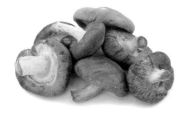

VITAMIN B3 (NIACIN)

This vitamin helps with carbohydrate metabolism, helps produce adrenal steroid hormones, reduces the risk of developing heart disease, lowers LDL and raises HDL cholesterol, helps create essential fatty acids, alleviates coldness and numbness in the extremities (known as Raynaud's syndrome), lowers blood sugar levels, and improves arthritis, acne, muscle weakness, indigestion, diarrhea, and vomiting.

VITAMIN B4

Vitamin B4 used to refer to the substance adenine, which was named in 1885 by German biochemist and genetic pioneer Albrecht Kossel. The root is the Greek word *aden*, which refers to the pancreas. However, it has since been discovered that the body can make adenine endogenously, which means you don't have to obtain it from food sources, so it's no longer considered a part of the B vitamins. That said, it plays a huge role in the development of human DNA and RNA. It also acts as a cofactor with other vitamins to produce adenosine triphosphate (ATP, which is the usable energy for the cells). Adenine, which is water-soluble, has been shown to be beneficial in reducing insomnia, anemia, headaches, high cholesterol, indigestion, gallstones, and wrinkles; stabilizing blood sugar levels; and controlling acne.

VITAMIN B5 (PANTOTHENIC ACID)

This vitamin helps produce adrenal hormones, assists the body in using fats and carbohydrates, improves asthma and allergies, and reduces hair loss. It also lowers stress and anxiety, contributes to improving breathing and cardiovascular conditions, and aids in hemoglobin synthesis for healthy blood. In addition, vitamin B5 boosts healthy cholesterol production in the body (a very good thing!), contributes to developing steroid hormones and fatty acids, and lowers triglyceride levels (another fantastic thing, because triglycerides are the truly "bad fat" in the blood).

VITAMIN B6 (PYRIDOXINE)

Vitamin B6 helps create body proteins, balance hormones, create chemical transmitters, stimulates coenzyme activities in the body, boosts immunity, alleviates premenstrual syndrome (PMS), prevents kidney disorders, treats anemia, increases stomach acid production (since most people are dealing with insufficient stomach acid levels), helps with depression, decreases nausea and vomiting in pregnant women, and enables vitamin B12 to be absorbed.

VITAMIN B7 (BIOTIN)

This vitamin improves nerve, digestive, and cardiovascular function; aids in fatty acid, amino acid, and glucose metabolism; plays a key role in the synthesis of insulin; and can help naturally lower cholesterol levels.

VITAMIN B8 (INOSITOL)

Inositol is often referred to as a vitamin, but it's a simple carbohydrate that occurs naturally in animal and plant tissue to promote the export of fat from the liver; thin the bile; promote cell growth and survival; help brain neurotransmitters, serotonin, and acetylcholine to work properly; and help control liver disorders, depression, diabetes, and panic attacks.

NOTE FROM CHRISTINE

I think back on that decade I took prescription medication for regular panic attacks when I simply could have boosted my inositol vitamin levels. I wish I had known then what I know now.

VITAMIN B9 (FOLATE/FOLIC ACID)

Folic acid helps with cell division, DNA and other genetic material creation, and red and white blood cell production; converts homocysteine into methionine; improves restless leg syndrome and depression; and reduces gastrointestinal inflammation.

METHYLATED FOLATE

In the Introduction, Christine talked about the methylenetetrahydrofolate reductase (MTHFR) gene mutation (and we discuss it in more detail in the "MTHFR? What did you call me?!" sidebar later in this chapter), which has a connection to vitamin B9 (folate/folic acid). If you run the genetic test for MTHFR and you have the mutation from one or both of your parents (which means you're missing this enzyme in your body), then you need to be taking methylated folate, which is the active, natural form. The folate found in food is not considered biologically active, so you must supplement with methylated folate if you have MTHFR. The KetoEssentials Multivitamin available from www.ketoliving.com contains 5,000 mcg of methylated folate.

VITAMIN B12 (COBALAMIN)

The final B vitamin we have to share with you keeps nerves healthy; improves the health of red blood cells and prevents megaloblastic anemia; aids in carbohydrate metabolism; is used in the creation of DNA; is required for the conversion of homocysteine into methionine; and improves acne, allergies, and depression.

BUGS BE GONE!

One of the unheralded benefits of eating a whole foods–based ketogenic diet is it acts as a natural insect repellent. People spray toxic chemicals on their skin to keep biting insects at bay, but wouldn't it be better to do it in a non-toxic way by eating keto-friendly foods such as fish, beef liver, chicken, eggs, and dairy? What do these foods have in them that help repel insects naturally? The exact cause isn't known, but it's thought that the B complex that includes vitamins B1, B2, B3, B5, B6, B7, B9, and B12 does the trick because they, especially B1, are eliminated through the skin and produce an odor that's unpleasant to bugs but undetectable to humans. While everybody else is swatting at the family picnic, you'll be smiling and enjoying yourself bug-bite free.

One of the best and cheapest sources for getting more vitamin D into your body is from standing in the sun with as much of your skin exposed as possible. You don't have to be outside a long time to develop thousands of international units' worth of vitamin D. Just spend ten to fifteen minutes in the sun without sunscreen. (Sunscreen inhibits your body's ability to create the vitamin D.)

VITAMIN C

This vitamin improves digestion, can act as a laxative, improves mineral absorption, fights free radical damage (it's a natural antioxidant), boosts immunity, and promotes healthy teeth and gums. Vitamin C also is vital for proper blood circulation and heart health, is necessary for converting tyrosine into the neurotransmitters norepinephrine and epinephrine, and helps absorb dietary iron. But that's not all! It's required for steroid hormone synthesis, helps detox from drug addiction, lowers triglycerides, promotes wound healing, and removes heavy metals during the detoxification process.

VITAMIN D

This key vitamin helps regulate calcium and phosphorus absorption; maintains strong bones and teeth; protects against developing cancer, multiple sclerosis (MS), and type 1 diabetes; prevents osteoporosis; normalizes immune function; is the gold standard treatment for the skeletal disorder known as rickets; contributes to healing broken bones; and mobilizes excess calcium out of the body.

VITAMIN E

This vitamin serves as a powerful antioxidant to protect against nerve and muscle cell damage, shields the liver from oxidative damage, protects nerve and muscle cell function, and prevents the peroxidation of cholesterol and other blood fats (which damages the cells). It also keeps blood platelets from clumping together, improves the symptoms of restless leg syndrome, decreases the muscle cramps induced by exercise, alleviates painful menstrual cramps, helps with menopausal symptoms, and clears chronic acne. You can use Vitamin E in a topical application to heal burns and remove scar tissue.

VITAMIN K

We shared a lot about this fat-soluble vitamin earlier. You might remember that it's outstanding for improving heart health, shuttling calcium where it needs to go (including to the bones to help prevent osteoporosis), protecting the kidneys from forming calcium stones, promoting healthy blood clotting, relieving pregnancy-induced nausea and vomiting, reducing annoying floaters in the eyes, and helping heal fractures and bruises.

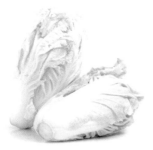

If you improve your gut health, then the good bacteria in your intestines can produce solid amounts of vitamin K2, which you need because the body doesn't store K2. If you have compromised gut health, perhaps you should consider supplementing with K2 as a means for boosting the benefits to your health as you heal.

VITAMIN U (METHYLMETHIONINE)

You probably haven't heard of this vitamin, and technically it's the enzyme methylmethionine, which isn't a vitamin per se. However, methylmethionine acts in the same way as a vitamin, which is why we've listed it here. It helps heal ulcers in the stomach and duodenum, kills viruses, helps with the symptoms of acid reflux, and improves sensitivity in those who are sensitive to cigarette smoke and strong smells like perfume and bleach. (Jimmy suffers from these sensitivities.)

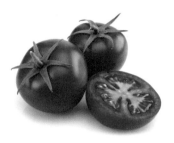

Now that you know about all the vitamins and why they're crucial to maintaining optimal health, let's examine the accessory nutrients that help make those vitamins work the way they're supposed to.

NOTE FROM CHRISTINE

A FEW VITAMINS, SO MANY BENEFITS

I can tell you from personal experience that extra vitamin and mineral supplementation has helped improve several numbers of my bloodwork and made me healthier. Despite getting serious about eating a ketogenic diet in 2011, some of my lab work remained less than optimal. Since becoming a Nutritional Therapy Practitioner, I've applied what I learned to take various vitamins, digestive enzymes, supplements for healing my stomach and providing adrenal support, zinc, and phosphatidylcholine for fatty acids, and I'm already reaping the benefits of these changes.

My fasting insulin dropped from 16.4 in August 2017 to 11.7 in March 2018, and the only change I had made was adding vitamins to my routine. My fasting blood glucose went from slightly above normal (at 104 mg/dL) in January 2017 to within normal range at 85 mg/dL in March 2018. My GGT (gamma-glutamyl transpeptidase), which is a test to check liver function, was 189 U/L in August 2017. By March 2018, it had gone down to 116 U/L. My hemoglobin A1c, which is a blood test that gives the average blood glucose over the previous three months, fell from 5.7 in February 2017 to 5.1 in March 2018. Controlling blood sugar levels is a key aspect of the *Real Food Keto* approach, and the fact that I can see how vitamins are working in conjunction with my ketogenic diet to make me healthier is a real confidence booster that I'm doing the right thing for my health.

My NTP colleagues and I can help you identify what kind of supplementation you need. For your convenience, we've included a list of some NTPs who support a ketogenic diet in the Resources section.

ACCESSORY NUTRIENTS AND THEIR BENEFITS

The nutrients in this section aren't vitamins, but without them the vitamins couldn't do what they're designed to do in the body. We've listed the accessory nutrients and the benefits they play in the body. (The real food sources for these accessory nutrients are included in the list at the end of the book that starts on page 355.) Sometimes these are viewed as the unwanted stepchildren of nutrients because they get so little attention compared to vitamins and minerals, but these oft-overlooked nutrients are some of the most important that you could possibly have in your body.

CHOLINE

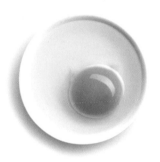

This water-soluble, vitamin-like essential nutrient plays an important role in the manufacturing of the neurotransmitter acetylcholine. It also comprises the primary components of the specific cell membranes phosphatidylcholine (lecithin) and sphingomyelin, is required for proper fat metabolism, increases production of acetylcholine in the brain, supports brain-related processes such as memory (don't forget this one), and supports proper detoxification.

BETAINE

Choline oxidizes into betaine, and betaine helps with detoxification, healthy blood, optimal intestinal and liver health, and fat metabolism. It also thins out thickened bile, eases constipation, lowers the inflammation marker homocysteine by converting it to methionine, and improves cellular health. This one is a biggie you don't want to neglect!

CHOLINE AND NAFLD PREVENTION

Although the body can make choline from the amino acids methionine and serine, it was recognized in 1998 as an essential nutrient by The Institute of Medicine. If the body has a choline deficiency, fats can become trapped in the liver, which leads to a condition known as nonalcoholic fatty liver disease (NAFLD). A ketogenic diet helps alleviate this disease, but choline plays a big role in preventing NAFLD.

COENZYME Q10 (UBIQUINONE)

Commonly referred to as CoQ10, Coenzyme Q10 is an essential component of the mitochondria and is involved in the manufacture of adenosine triphosphate (ATP, which is the energy currency of every single process in the body). CoQ10 is like the spark plug for your car because it makes everything in the body work, acts as an antioxidant to protect against lipid peroxidation (where free radicals steal electrons in the cell membranes of cholesterol that damage the cells), and works with vitamin E to prevent damage to the fat and cholesterol in the blood.

STATIN MEDICATIONS AND COQ10

As Jimmy wrote in his book *Cholesterol Clarity,* CoQ10 is one of the substances in the body that becomes a victim when you take a cholesterol-lowering statin medication like Lipitor or Crestor. Statin drugs have become so notorious for depleting the body of CoQ10—a key heart-health nutrient—that many doctors now recommend that patients who take statin medications supplement with extra CoQ10. Some pharmaceutical formulations of statin medications even include CoQ10. Jimmy had to take 400 mcg CoQ10 supplementation daily for many years after coming off his cholesterol medications to help restore healthy levels of CoQ10 in his body.

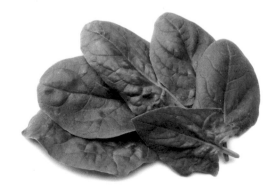

FIBER SUPPLEMENTS

Plant compounds and residues that are indigestible by the human digestive system serve some incredible purposes, including bulking and shuttling fecal waste out of the body, acting as a natural laxative to promote regularity, protecting against degenerative diseases, protecting against certain kinds of cancer-causing agents in the intestines, lowering total cholesterol in the blood, slowing digestion for the body to properly absorb the nutrients, and increasing pancreatic enzyme secretion to help control the rise in blood sugar levels as you consume food.

The composition of plant cell walls varies according to the plant species; consequently, the type of dietary fiber in each plant varies. Most of the commercially available dietary fiber supplements are single components or combinations of insoluble fibers and soluble fibers, which include mucilage, gums, and pectin substances. The water-soluble fiber (meaning you need to take it with water before meals) forms a gelatinous mass that increases satiety (a feeling of being full), which can be beneficial for people who want to lose weight. Fiber supplements are well-known to have anticancer, antibacterial, antifungal, and antiviral properties.

FLAVONOIDS

This group of plant pigments is the reason there are colors in fruits and flowers. Flavonoids are known to help with the treatment of venous and capillary disorders, such as varicose veins and capillary fragility; disorders of the retina, including diabetic retinopathy and macular degeneration; and inflammatory and allergic conditions like asthma, rheumatoid arthritis, and lupus. They also reduce bruising, swelling, and nosebleeds, and they're used in the long-term care of people with type 2 diabetes because of their ability to properly manage blood sugar levels.

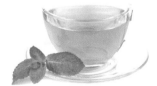

It's the flavonoid content of food, certain juices, herbs, and bee pollen (which isn't recommended if you're on keto, but it is rich in flavonoids) that provide the many medicinal actions that naturopaths, functional medicine practitioners, and other natural healthcare providers seek for their patients. The specific flavonoids include PCO (proanthocyanidins or procyanidins), quercetin, green tea polyphenol, and citrus bioflavonoids (including rutin).

GLUCOSAMINE

Glucosamine, which is manufactured by the body, is a molecule composed of glucose and an amine (nitrogen and two molecules of hydrogen) that stimulates the production of glycosaminoglycan—the key structural components of cartilage—and promotes the incorporation of sulfur into cartilage (which is why using glucosamine sulfate is known as the best source for supplementation).

LIPOIC ACID (THIOCTIC ACID)

This sulfur-containing, vitaminlike substance is involved in the conversion of carbohydrates into energy, is an effective antioxidant against both water- and fat-soluble free radicals, and may help improve energy metabolism (especially for those who have a compromised immune function).

MELATONIN

The pineal gland secretes this hormone. Production of melatonin is stimulated by darkness and suppressed by light. This hormone plays a key role in regulating circadian rhythms and may have antioxidant and anticancer effects.

CAVEAT ABOUT MELATONIN SUPPLEMENTATION

Liquid melatonin supplements are the fastest acting, best-absorbed form of melatonin. However, we have a word of caution about using these supplements too often or in doses that are too high: Your body will shut down production of melatonin as a result of frequent and higher-dosage use of a melatonin supplement. Jimmy ran into this issue when he was trying to normalize his sleep a few years ago, and after he stopped taking melatonin supplements, his body needed many months to begin making melatonin naturally again.

One of the best ways to boost your melatonin is to consume foods that contain the precursor to its production. Try consuming foods with the amino acid tryptophan In your last meal of the day because they induce the production of serotonin, which leads to the production of melatonin that will help you get into the four stages of sleep required for optimal health. (We share more on this in Chapter 11.) These *Real Food Keto* foods include full-fat dairy products (avoid fake cheese products like American cheese—they're not cheese), nuts, seafood, turkey (think Thanksgiving coma), chicken, eggs, sesame seeds, pumpkin seeds, and sunflower seeds.

When the body is deficient in what is called *methyl donors,* including folic acid, vitamin B12, SAMe (described later in this section), and/or essential fatty acids, the brain simply cannot produce enough phosphatidylserine. Getting enough of these methyl donors in the form of minerals, vitamins, and accessory nutrients is critical to optimizing your health.

PHOSPHATIDYLSERINE

This major phospholipid is a fat-containing phosphorus component of the cell membrane whose role is to play the traffic cop for allowing the nutrients to go in and out of the cell. It covers and protects the cells in the brain and easily crosses the blood-brain barrier to play a key role in determining the integrity and fluidity of cell membranes, and that contributes to keeping your brain health as sharp as a tack. We met a woman in Indiana a few years back who gave her husband phosphatidylserine as a supplement, and it helped improve signs of his Alzheimer's disease.

PROBIOTICS

Probiotics are considered the good bacteria in a healthy gut. The gastrointestinal tract comprises at least 400 different species, including *Lactobacillus acidophilus* (you're not born with this one; colonization begins once you are born) and *Bifidobacterium bifidum* (which is first introduced to the body naturally during breastfeeding). Most of the good bacteria in the body is in the gut, so increasing the quantity of good bacteria by consuming probiotic foods and supplements inhibits the growth of detrimental organisms, helps produce those vitamins (K2, B1, B2, and B12) that are key for optimal nutritional health in the gut, and directly affects the function of the immune system.

ANTIBIOTICS AND GOOD BACTERIA

If you've taken antibiotics during your lifetime (and most of us have), then you need to know that the way they work to help you when you get sick is by destroying the bad bacteria that caused the sickness to begin with. The problem is that they also attack and eliminate much of your healthy bacteria, which is why probiotic foods and supplementation is so critical. If, like us, you've been on many rounds of antibiotics in your lifetime (for example, more than thirty rounds for Christine and more than twenty-five rounds for Jimmy), your overall gut health is likely compromised.

Although there are foods that contain high doses of methionine in them that are friendly to the ketogenic diet, that does not necessarily mean they will automatically increase the levels of SAMe. The body must have proper amounts of folate, vitamin B12, vitamin B2, zinc, choline, and magnesium for it to convert homocysteine to a usable form of SAMe and glutathione. If you're deficient in any of these vitamins and minerals, then your body cannot convert homocysteine into mood-stabilizing SAMe.[3]

S-ADENOSYL METHIONINE (SAME)

This compound, which is found naturally in the body, is formed by combining methionine (an essential amino acid) and ATP and is required in the manufacturing of all sulfur-containing compounds in the human body. It helps support proper detoxification and aids the body in dealing with depression, osteoarthritis, fibromyalgia, liver disorders (like cirrhosis), and migraine headaches.

GLANDULAR PRODUCTS

The use of glandular therapy is the oldest known form of medicine and is necessary when a regular function of the human body is no longer producing the required hormones for optimal health. Most glandular products come from either a cow or a pig because those animals' organ anatomy is most similar to human anatomy. Glandular products help with adrenal disorders, liver disorders, atherosclerosis, arterial and venous disorders, thyroid disorders (like Christine's Hashimoto's disease, for which she takes a desiccated pig thyroid medication called Armour), endocrine and exocrine pancreatic dysfunction, immune complex diseases, viral infections, and other autoimmune disorders.

CAUTION: Toxins build up in the organs of animals. Make sure your organ meats are from quality grass-fed, organic animals that are free from hormones and antibiotics and that aren't subjected to inferior feeding methods.

SYMPTOMS OF VITAMIN DEFICIENCY

We just shared in great detail all the vitamins and accessory nutrients required for optimal health. At this point, you might be wondering what happens if you fall short of getting adequate levels of these vitamins and what signs and symptoms might show that you're dealing with a vitamin deficiency. These are the perfect questions for us to address next. In this section, we list the vitamins and accessory nutrients and the most common signs that indicate a deficiency. Some symptoms show up for several different vitamin deficiencies, so you need to confirm in which areas you are deficient by running the vitamin and mineral status test with your doctor.

BETAINE

- Bloating, belching, and flatulence immediately after meals
- Heartburn
- Indigestion
- Undigested foods in stools
- Acne
- Rectal itching
- Chronic candida

INULIN (POLYSACCHARIDE BASED ON FRUCTOSE)

No known signs of deficiency, but an excess can lead to gas and bloating

VITAMIN A

- Trouble distinguishing between blues and purples
- Sensitivity to bright lights at night
- Dry eyes
- Dry skin
- Frequent infections due to decreased immune function
- Night blindness

VITAMIN B1 (THIAMINE)

- Loss of appetite
- Weakness
- Pain in the limbs
- Shortness of breath
- Swollen feet or legs
- Enlarged heart or fast heart rate

VITAMIN B2 (RIBOFLAVIN)

- Anemia
- Nerve damage
- Sluggish metabolism
- Mouth or lip sores
- Skin disorders
- Sore throat

VITAMIN B3 (NIACIN)

- Skin disorders
- Apathy
- Swollen mouth and bright red tongue
- Headache
- Fatigue
- Depression
- Disorientation

ADENINE DEFICIENCY

Although there isn't any such thing as vitamin B4 (read more about this in the "Vitamin B4" sidebar earlier in this chapter), there are still serious consequences to your health if you're deficient in adenine. Here are the signs that your body isn't producing enough of this:

1. Nausea
2. Gastrointestinal problems
3. Depression
4. Poor immune function
5. Muscle weakness
6. Slow physical growth
7. Anemia

VITAMIN B5 (PANTOTHENIC ACID)

- Fatigue
- Depression
- Irritability
- Insomnia
- Stomach pains
- Vomiting
- Burning feet
- Upper respiratory infections

VITAMIN B6 (PYRIDOXINE)

- Irritability
- Anxiety
- Depression
- Confusion
- Muscle cramps
- Fatigue
- Worsening PMS symptoms
- Worsening anemia symptoms

VITAMIN B7 (BIOTIN)

- Hair loss
- Skin rashes
- Depression
- Lethargy
- Hallucination
- Numbness and tingling of the extremities
- Ataxia (loss of full control of bodily movements)

VITAMIN B8 (INOSITOL)

- Poor brain function
- Vision problems
- Hair loss
- Fatty liver
- Constipation
- High LDL
- Eczema
- Atherosclerosis

VITAMIN B9 (FOLATE/ FOLIC ACID)

- Anemia
- Poor growth
- Inflammation of the tongue
- Loss of appetite
- Shortness of breath
- Diarrhea
- Irritability
- Forgetfulness
- Fatigue
- Mouth sores
- Pale skin

Deficiency in inositol is rare, but there are a couple of things that can deplete the body of it. The first is long-term use of antibiotics, and the second is long-term use of lithium.

MTHFR? WHAT DID YOU CALL ME?!

There are a lot of acronyms in the nutritional health world that you have seen us use quite often throughout this book, but there's only one that looks like a dirty word. The technical term is Methylenetetrahydrofolate Reductase—but we'll never spell that out again; you just need to know it as the MTHFR gene mutation. When you have this gene mutation, your body simply cannot turn folic acid into folate, which means you must consume a methylated form of folate. You have to take a one-time genetic test (which is expensive if your insurance doesn't cover it) to see if you inherited the gene mutation from one or both parents.

The two different gene mutations are C677T and A1298C. No, these aren't *Star Wars* characters; they refer to specific genetic issues passed on by either one parent (homozygous) or both parents (heterozygous). People with the C677T mutation can have increased inflammation levels as measured by their homocysteine, which leads to an increased risk for heart disease, but the A1298C mutation does not. However, the A1298C mutation increases ammonia and decreases neurotransmitters, but the C677T mutation does not. Christine has the C677T mutation, and Jimmy has the A1298C mutation.

We were fortunate enough to have this genetic test done and covered by insurance because it was a part of the labs our primary care physician ran. Knowing that we have these gene mutations leads us to believe this is part of the reason we were never able to have children of our own, and we think it's a contributing factor to why Christine struggled with depression at one point.

It's possible that you can have both the C677T and A1298C gene mutations. In these cases, your chances are greater for having high homocysteine levels, thrombosis (local clotting of the blood in part of the circulatory system), cardiovascular disease, migraines, depression, chronic fatigue syndrome, Raynaud's syndrome, schizophrenia, bipolar disorder, dementia, Alzheimer's disease, defects developing during pregnancy, and recurrent miscarriages. If you're not able to convert folic acid into folate, the folic acid can build up in your system, and it could lead to the development of cancer. Consuming dairy can worsen the problem when you have these gene mutations because dairy can block the folate receptors, especially in the brain.[4] Ask your doctor about running the MTHFR gene mutation test to find out where you stand.

VITAMIN B12 (COBALAMIN)

- Fatigue
- Anemia
- Breathlessness
- Poor balance
- Memory issues
- Tingling feet

VITAMIN C (ASCORBIC ACID)

- Bruising
- Bleeding gums
- Weakness
- Fatigue
- Rash
- Fever
- Loss of appetite

VITAMIN D

- Thin, brittle, or misshapen bones
- Joint pain
- Fatigue
- Muscle weakness
- Getting sick often
- Depression
- Impaired wound healing

VITAMIN E

- Muscle weakness
- Loss of muscle mass
- Abnormal eye movements
- Vision problems
- Having trouble walking

VITAMIN K (K2)

- Easy bruising
- Excessive bleeding from wounds
- Heavy menstrual periods
- Blood in the urine or stool

VITAMIN U (ENZYME METHYLMETHIONINE)

Possible signs of deficiency can be sensitivity to tobacco smoke or pollution in the air.

As we mentioned before, vitamin K2 is necessary to help other vitamins and minerals get where they need to go. If someone is K2 deficient, they could have a deficiency of calcium in the bones (osteoporosis) while also having too much calcium in the arteries. The result is a hardening of the arteries known as *arteriosclerosis*.

People with high homocysteine levels are often deficient in vitamins B2, folate, and betaine. These vitamins are needed to process homocysteine.

SYMPTOMS OF ACCESSORY NUTRIENT DEFICIENCY

Accessory nutrients are substances that aren't essential to human life like vitamins and minerals are, but they do play important roles in many biochemical reactions by working with vitamins and minerals. Although accessory nutrients aren't classified as vitamins or minerals, they do promote optimal health.

CHOLINE

A choline-deficient diet can lead to liver and kidney disorders.

One Moore Thing: A high dose might lead to gastrointestinal upset, but it's generally well tolerated. High-dose phosphatidylcholine supplementation can worsen depression in some cases.

COENZYME Q10

A deficiency may be a result of impaired CoQ10 synthesis due to nutritional deficiencies, a genetic or acquired defect of CoQ10 synthesis, or increased tissue needs for CoQ10. A deficiency mostly affects the heart and leads to heart failure.

One Moore Thing: No serious adverse effects have been reported related to CoQ10 toxicity; supplementation with CoQ10 is generally well tolerated. Please note that some medications, such as cholesterol-lowering statin drugs like Lipitor and Crestor, deplete the body of CoQ10, requiring supplementation of this accessory nutrient to prevent deficiency.

FIBER SUPPLEMENTS

A lack of dietary fiber contributes to intestinal exposure to cancer-causing agents. A low-fiber diet increases the risk of diverticula, hemorrhoids, and varicose veins by creating stress, strain, and pressure during defecation.

One Moore Thing: Individuals with esophageal disorders should avoid fiber supplementation in pill form because they can be hard to swallow and can further irritate the esophagus. Adequate amounts of water are important when taking any fiber supplement.

FLAVONOIDS

A deficiency in flavonoids can lead to susceptibility to bruising, nose bleeds, hemorrhoids, and frequent colds or infections.

One Moore Thing: Most flavonoids are extremely safe and well-tolerated. Green tea, a source of flavonoids, contains caffeine, and overconsumption may cause a stimulant reaction. Most individuals, however, don't experience these reactions.

GLUCOSAMINE

The inability to produce sufficient glucosamine results in loss of shock-absorbing cartilage. In affected weight-bearing joints, cartilage destruction is followed by hardening and formation of bone spurs in the joint margins. Pain, deformity, and limitation of motion in the joints results.

One Moore Thing: Side effects of taking glucosamine supplements are rare, but you might experience light to moderate gastrointestinal symptoms. If these symptoms occur, try taking glucosamine sulfate during a meal.

LIPOIC ACID

Experimental studies show low levels of lipoic acid results in reduced muscle mass, failure to thrive, brain atrophy, and increased lactic acid accumulation. In some conditions, like diabetes, cirrhosis, and heart disease, individual lipoic levels are lower than normal.

One Moore Thing: There are no reported side effects or toxicity associated with supplementing with lipoic acid.

MELATONIN

Disruption of pineal function, and consequently melatonin production, may be a major reason for seasonal affective disorder and jet lag.

One Moore Thing: There appear to be no serious side effects at recommended dosages of supplemental melatonin, but taking a high dosage or using it for a prolonged period may disrupt normal circadian rhythms. Some cases of depression get much worse when a person is given melatonin during the day.

PHOSPHATIDYLSERINE

Low levels of phosphatidylserine are associated with depression and poor mental function in the elderly.

One Moore Thing: There are no reported side effects or toxicity associated with supplementing with phosphatidylserine.

PROBIOTICS

A deficiency of friendly bacteria eventually leads to a potentially toxic bacteria overgrowth and compromised immune function.

One Moore Thing: Probiotics are extremely safe and not associated with any side effects.

S-ADENOSYL METHIONINE (SAME)

The body manufactures all the SAMe it requires from methionine. When there's a deficiency of methionine, vitamin B12, or folic acid, a decrease in SAMe might result.

One Moore Thing: No significant side effects have been reported with oral use of SAMe, other than occasional gastrointestinal upset. Individuals with bipolar depression should not take SAMe unless under strict medical supervision.

GLANDULAR PRODUCTS

Source, quality, dosage, and type of glandular product affect the level of safety when using glandular therapy, and you should talk with a healthcare practitioner to determine what's right for you.

THE IMPORTANCE OF VITAMINS D AND B

Getting out in the sun every day helps regulate your circadian rhythm (the natural biological process that regulates the wake and sleep cycles). Christine's circadian rhythms are way off, but Jimmy tends to go to bed and wake up at the same times every single day.

In this chapter, we've given you an overview of the major vitamins and accessory nutrients that you need for optimal health. However, there are two extremely important vitamins that we'll refer to as DAB (vitamin D and vitamin B). You should be especially mindful of these as you pursue shoring up your vitamin levels because they play such vital roles in the body. You'll be doing the dab dance if you nail these two crucial vitamins.

VITAMIN D

Interestingly, vitamin D is not a vitamin at all. It's a steroid hormone whose role is to maintain and repair various functions in the body. As we've previously stated, vitamin D is one of the few vitamins you can get exogenously by exposing your skin to the sun. It has been estimated that 85 percent of Americans are deficient in vitamin D, even in geographical areas where there's adequate sunlight. Photon rays from the sun, especially in the middle of the

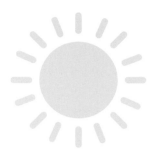

day, work with cholesterol to create vitamin D. Part of the issue is that many people lack the levels of cholesterol required to convert the sun that hits the skin into vitamin D. If you can't get adequate sun exposure, you might need to supplement with a vitamin D3 gel cap to keep your body at healthy levels.

BENEFITS OF VITAMIN D

- Helps us remain disease free
- Helps with weight control
- Aids in counteracting hypertension
- Aids in optimal absorption of calcium
- Helps prevent autism
- Aids in dealing with autoimmune issues
- Acts as a potent antibiotic
- Helps keep us safe from heart disease

- Aids during flu season
- Slows down the aging process
- Reduces inflammation
- Aids in fertility
- Helps prevent macular degeneration
- Helps with athletic performance
- Helps with mental disorders

WAYS TO TEST VITAMIN D

There are two ways to test for vitamin D:

- Mass Spectrometry Analysis or Mass Spec Test: Mass spectrometry is a very sensitive test that uses a specific analytical technique to measure the quantities of substances in the body, even very small amounts.

- Radioimmunoassay (RIA) Test: A Radioimmunoassay test is a very sensitive method for measuring very small amounts of a substance (for example, hormone levels) in the blood. LabCorp (www.labcorp.com) offers this test.

If you have one of the tests run, use the following guidelines for interpreting the results:

1. A result of less than 50 ng/ml indicates a deficiency.
2. A result between 50 and 65 ng/ml is optimal.

Too much vitamin D in the body raises the calcium score in the body. Always test vitamin D before taking a vitamin D supplement, and test again four to six weeks after you start supplementing.

LIPOTROPIC FACTORS AND BETAINE

Lipotropic factors describe the action of choline in the prevention and treatment of fatty livers. Lipotropic factors are produced naturally in the body. They are substances that remove and prevent fatty deposits, such as homocysteine, in the body. They promote the flow of fat and bile through the liver to help keep it from getting congested with fat. Lipotropic factors *and* B vitamins are necessary for estrogen conjugation.

Betaine is created by choline in combination with the amino acid glycine. Just like some B vitamins, including B9 (folate/folic acid) and vitamin B12 (cobalamin), betaine is considered to be a "methyl donor." This means it aids in liver function, detoxification, and cellular functioning within the body.

VITAMIN B: IT'S REALLY TWO DIFFERENT COMPLEXES

There are two different types of vitamin B complexes. The first, known as the "B" complex, is based on vitamin B1 (thiamine) and contains other B vitamins that are soluble in alcohol, including adenine, B6 (pyridoxine), and B12 (cobalamin). The second, referred to as the "G" complex, is based on vitamin B2 (riboflavin) and contains other B vitamins that aren't soluble in alcohol, such as B3 (niacin), B8 (inositol), B9 (folate/folic acid), para-aminobenzoic acid or PABA (found in folic acid), the lipotropic factors, choline (similar to the B vitamins), and betaine (methyl donor). Here are a few of the primary differences between the B and G complexes:

B COMPLEXES	G COMPLEXES
Alcohol-soluble	Alcohol-insoluble
Heat stable	Unstable with heat
Stimulating	Relaxing
Helps carbohydrate metabolism	Helps metabolize fats

Here are the symptoms a person can experience with B- and G-type deficiencies:

SYMPTOMS OF DEFICIENCIES

B-TYPE DEFICIENCY: PERSON NEEDS B1, ADENINE, B6, AND B12	G-TYPE DEFICIENCY: PERSON NEEDS B2 AND ASSOCIATED B VITAMINS
Is hypotensive (has low blood pressure)	Is hypertensive (has high blood pressure)
Craves sugar	Craves alcohol
Feels bad or run-down a lot	Feels good or pumped up most of the time
Gets sick often	Does not get sick often
Tends toward congestive heart failure (CHF)	Tends toward myocardial infarction (MI)

TIPS FOR PREVENTING VITAMIN DEFICIENCIES

Vitamin deficiencies can be serious business, so addressing any shortfalls is critical to maintaining your health. How do you make sure you're getting enough of all the vitamins? We have some tips to share with you as we close out this chapter.

First, make sure you have adequate stomach acid. We've mentioned this before in this book, but it bears repeating because it's so fundamental to ensuring all the other things in your body work properly. Having the right amount of stomach acid makes it possible for you to digest, break down, and absorb the nutrients you eat. If you have a stomach acid deficiency, then you can take HCl supplementation or digestive enzymes to aid in digestion. Make sure to consult with an NTP or another healthcare provider to see if you might need to supplement to bring your stomach acid level up. (Read more about testing for stomach acid production in Chapter 10.)

Second, eat a wide variety of foods. The more colors you eat, the better. Try to get your foods from the local farmers market or directly from farms; even better, grow some of your food. Knowing where your food came from and how it was grown boosts your confidence that you're getting good vitamin intake. We love our garden, greenhouse, and backyard chickens that give us real, whole foods that nourish our bodies.

Finally, consider taking a good multivitamin to help with any deficiencies you have. KetoLiving.com has a great multivitamin that even has the methylated folate to address the MTHFR gene mutation we discussed earlier. In Christine's case, she needs to take B vitamins in addition to a multivitamin because it's easier for her to become deficient because both her mom and dad passed along the MTHFR gene mutation.

Now that you're all geeked out about vitamins, Chapter 10 shifts the attention to an area that we've touched on quite a bit throughout the book—digestion. Many people think when they eat food, digestion starts in the stomach and then continues in the intestines. However, did you know that digestion actually starts in the brain? Oh, yeah, get ready to have your mind blown with the next chapter. We have plenty for you to digest.

REAL FOOD KETO TAKEAWAYS FROM CHAPTER 9

- Vitamins make up about 1 percent of the entire body.

- There are two major classifications of vitamins: fat-soluble and water-soluble.

- Real, whole foods can be the primary source of nearly every vitamin the body needs.

- Certain accessory nutrients can be combined with vitamins to make the vitamins work better.

- Signs of vitamin deficiency are easy to spot and correct with proper food and supplementation.

- It's important to ask your doctor about running the MTHFR gene mutation test to see how your body handles folate.

- Don't neglect the DAB (vitamin D and vitamin B), which are the two major vitamins to zero in on.

- It's not difficult to follow a few quick and easy tips for preventing vitamin deficiencies.

CHAPTER 10

Digestion Starts in the Brain

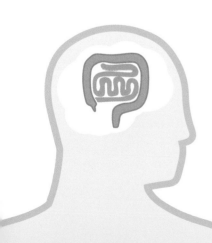

One of the biggest themes we have harped on again and again in this book is the importance of digestion in literally every aspect of health. If that part of your body isn't working well, then nothing will function as intended. Most people are oblivious to just how important this process is. Digestion happens 24 hours a day, 7 days a week, 365 days a year for a lifetime. We never even think about it because it's a part of the autonomic response of the body. That is, we don't think about it until things start to go haywire, such as when you have too much *Helicobacter pylori (H. pylori),* which leads to the development of stomach ulcers, gastroesophageal reflux disease (GERD), bloating, constipation, diarrhea, and many more gastrointestinal problems. By the time you finish reading this chapter, you'll be armed with so much knowledge about digestion that you won't be able to stop talking about it.

When I first started learning about digestion in my training as a Nutritional Therapy Practitioner (NTP), I would mention some of the terms I had been taught (and that we share with you in this chapter), such as *cholecystokinin, secretin,* and *duodenum.* Jimmy would give me a funny look and joke with me for using $10,000 words that he didn't know. After years of listening to him blabber on about keto this and beta-hydroxybutyrate that, it was neat to finally expose him to concepts about health that are complex but important.

One of the hallmarks of being in a healthy state of nutritional ketosis is that the foods you consume are incredibly satisfying for your hunger. Most people discover this benefit almost immediately once their body begins to stabilize blood sugar and insulin levels and is nourished by all the real, whole foods that we've talked about throughout this book. There may be a certain segment of the population that doesn't have an appetite; however, the lack of appetite doesn't have anything to do with the satiating properties of the fats they're consuming.

Satiation is a major clue in determining whether you're well nourished, but it doesn't give you the whole picture, as you will soon find out. One of the first indicators that you lack an appetite because of something other than being well keto-adapted is that you feel bloated after a meal or have no desire to eat at all. This could be a result of low stomach acid (another common theme we've shared throughout *Real Food Keto*), which means food sits in the stomach for long periods. Excessive gas usually accompanies this issue. Not fun. Additionally, having vitamin and mineral deficiencies might reduce your appetite, but not in a good way. This is why listening to what your body is telling you is critically important, and we hope we've hammered on this enough through these pages so you're becoming more aware of how your health is going.

Let's start by discussing how digestion is supposed to work and function well.

PROPER DIGESTIVE FUNCTION

So many people deal with digestive disorders nowadays that it may be difficult to comprehend what normal digestion is supposed to look like in a healthy person. Every cell depends on your digestion working well so you can absorb all the nutrients that help your body function optimally. This can happen only when

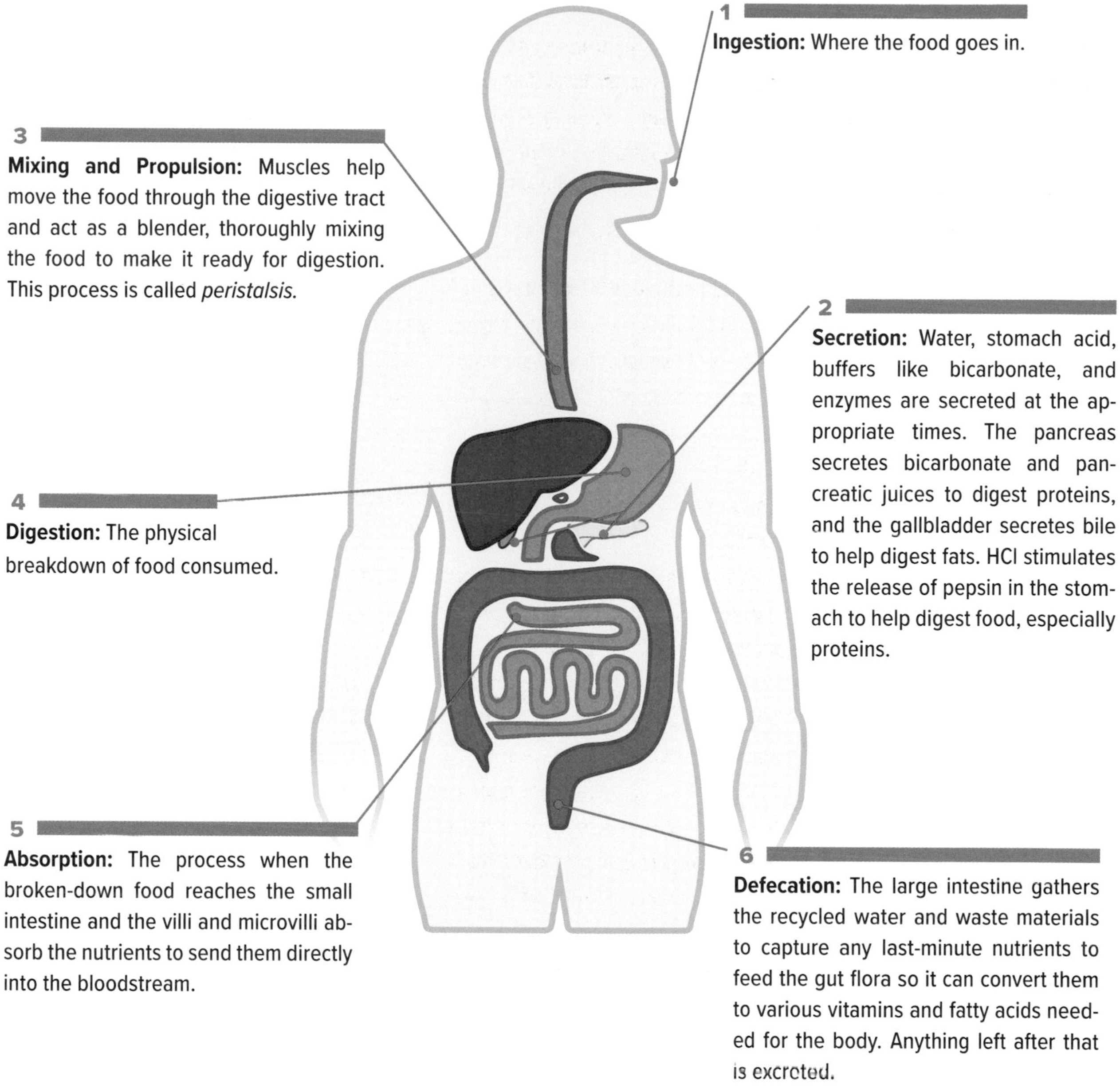

1

Ingestion: Where the food goes in.

3

Mixing and Propulsion: Muscles help move the food through the digestive tract and act as a blender, thoroughly mixing the food to make it ready for digestion. This process is called *peristalsis.*

2

Secretion: Water, stomach acid, buffers like bicarbonate, and enzymes are secreted at the appropriate times. The pancreas secretes bicarbonate and pancreatic juices to digest proteins, and the gallbladder secretes bile to help digest fats. HCl stimulates the release of pepsin in the stomach to help digest food, especially proteins.

4

Digestion: The physical breakdown of food consumed.

5

Absorption: The process when the broken-down food reaches the small intestine and the villi and microvilli absorb the nutrients to send them directly into the bloodstream.

6

Defecation: The large intestine gathers the recycled water and waste materials to capture any last-minute nutrients to feed the gut flora so it can convert them to various vitamins and fatty acids needed for the body. Anything left after that is excreted.

you're in a parasympathetic state, which means you're relaxed, stress-free, and focused on the dining process. The lost art of eating together at a dining table sorely needs to be rediscovered in the twenty-first century.

The digestive system is required to break down the foods we consume into small enough molecules that the nutrients can be gleaned, absorbed, and then used by the cells for the areas of the body where they're needed. Understanding the six digestive functions shown in the illustration can help you know why you might run into problems down the road.

Most people assume that digestion starts the moment we put food in our mouths, but it actually begins much sooner than that. Think about a food you love that reminds you of your childhood, like cotton candy at the state fair. Did you notice your mouth suddenly getting flooded with saliva? This is the brain signaling the salivary glands to produce saliva with the anticipation that it will be needed to break down the carbohydrates that you would ostensibly be consuming if you ate the cotton candy. Just the thought of food or the smell of food can trigger the salivary glands to start producing saliva. Nobody ever thinks about this, but this is a part of why we say that digestion starts in the brain. You don't have to have food sitting in front of you for that natural process to kick in automatically.

Each macronutrient has a primary area where digestion takes place:

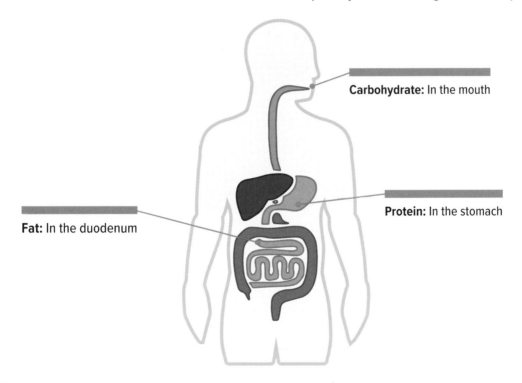

Carbohydrate: In the mouth

Protein: In the stomach

Fat: In the duodenum

Once the brain signals the salivary glands to start producing saliva, the mouth is ready for the food to begin being digested. The mouth is the physical starting point for our entire digestive tract. In the mouth, we physically break down food by chewing, and the saliva moistens the food so it's easier to swallow. Saliva is 99.5 percent water and 0.5 percent solutes, including the enzyme salivary amylase, which aids in the digestion of carbohydrates, and the simple act of chewing begins the process of digesting all three macronutrients—carbohydrates, proteins, and fats. This is why we encourage you to chew your food for at least thirty seconds to ensure that it's properly broken down as it works its way into your stomach and through your digestive tract.

pH stands for the Power of Hydrogen. The scale runs from 0 to 14, with 0 being pure acidity and 14 being pure alkalinity. The lower the number on the pH scale, the more acidic the fluid. That's why your stomach pH needs to be between 1.5 and 3.0 to have enough acidity to break down the food you consume.

Okay, it's time to get a little nerdy and tell you the fancy word for food once it's swallowed. That term is *bolus.* The bolus travels through the esophagus and into the stomach through what is known as (geeky word alert!) the cardiac sphincter (no, ancient Egyptians didn't build this). Digestion continues in the stomach, where the pH stays between 1.5 and 3.0 for the perfect environment for the food to be digested using stomach acid and other digestive juices. The stomach is where the proteins are primarily broken down by HCl and pepsinogen. If stomach pH is greater than 3.0, the protein sits in the stomach and eventually causes problems.

HCl plays two major functions in the stomach. First, it helps to disinfect the stomach to guard against foreign invaders (like bacteria and parasites) so that they don't penetrate any further into the body. Second, it activates pepsin (a digestive enzyme in the stomach that breaks down protein) to properly deal with the meat, eggs, and other proteins in your diet.

HIGH-PROTEIN DIETS

There are several reasons we don't think high-protein diets are a good idea for most people who are pursuing nutritional ketosis. As we shared in Chapter 5 and mention again in Chapter 11 on blood sugar, when you consume more protein than your body can use, the body converts the protein to glucose (remember that big long G word—*gluconeogenesis*), which prevents your body from producing therapeutic levels of ketones and disrupts your blood sugar. Also, digesting protein is very hard on the body. Part of the reason for this, which you read more about later in this chapter, is that upward of 90 percent of the population has stomach acid levels that are too low, and stomach acid is necessary for stimulating pepsin that aids in the digestion of proteins. Without HCl, your body can't produce adequate pepsin, which leads to poorly digested proteins that irritate the intestinal wall. An irritated intestinal wall increases gut permeability and can eventually lead to the development of various autoimmune conditions and an imbalance in your gut microbiome. This is exactly why Christine developed Hashimoto's thyroiditis, endometriosis, and psoriasis.

Fun fact: We get a whole new set of taste buds and stomach lining every 21 days. See, you really can break a habit in that amount of time. Or at least give Brussels sprouts another try every three weeks.

NERD ALERT: Get your thinking caps on because the geeky words are back again. Here we go!

Once the food has been broken down in the stomach, the bolus is converted into *chyme* (pronounced like *lime* with a *k*), which matches the acidity of the stomach pH. The chyme travels from the stomach to the upper part of the small intestine—the duodenum—through the pyloric sphincter. (We know that might be a lot of new words to grasp but hang with us.) If the pH of the chyme is where it needs to be (around 2.0), then it passes from the stomach to the duodenum. The duodenum is triggered to secrete mucus and two key digestive hormones you need to know about because they're the magic of this digestive process: secretin and cholecystokinin (CCK).

Secretin stimulates the pancreas to release bicarbonate and pancreatic juices. A normal-functioning pancreas releases about eight cups of pancreatic juices into the duodenum each day. Bicarbonate is released in response to the pH of the chyme entering the duodenum. It's the bicarbonate that helps make the chyme more alkaline so that it can pass into the rest of the small intestine without harming it. Pancreatic juices help continue the digestive process of the proteins and carbohydrates you consume in the duodenum as well.

Cholecystokinin (CCK) is what stimulates the gallbladder to release bile. Bile serves two amazing purposes in the process of digestion: It aids in the digestion of fat, and it's where the liver dumps unwanted toxins that become trapped like quicksand and are removed from the body so they can't harm it. At this point, the chyme is ready to leave the duodenum, and digestion is almost complete. The carbohydrates have been broken down to glucose molecules, proteins have been broken down into their various amino acid profiles and polypeptides (many amino acids strung together), and fats have been broken down into the fatty acids your body needs.

Now is when things start to get really fun! Once the chyme exits the duodenum and travels to the rest of the small intestine, the villi and microvilli (tiny elongated projections close together on the lining or surface of the small intestine that increase the surface area for better absorption of nutrients) begin to absorb nutrients into the bloodstream. These nutrients are then sent throughout the body to be used for all the purposes we discuss throughout *Real Food Keto.* Every organ of the body is connected to nerves that lead to the intestines in what is known as the enteric nervous system (ENS).

Once the chyme goes into the large intestine through the ileocecal valve, all that's left is indigestible fiber, bile, water, and cells. The large intestine recycles the water, nourishes the colon with reusable waste matter, and captures any lingering nutrients that might have gotten lost (the ones that went down a dead-end road). With the help of the bowel and gut microbiome, the large intestine turns these remaining nutrients into vitamin K, vitamin B1, vitamin B2, vitamin B12, and butyric acid. We explain later in the book the very important reasons why these specific vitamins and fatty acids are produced at the end of the digestive process. Stay tuned.

Finally, the end of the road for digestion is defecation, which is such a horrible-sounding word. But you don't want all that crap (literally!) sticking around in your body. All that's left is waste product that serves no good purpose in the body. Expelling feces out of the body removes toxins, metabolic waste, and other gunk you really don't want in your body. As Jimmy's *Keto Talk* podcast cohost Dr. Will Cole explains, someone with optimal gut health should poop out two snakes a day. Anything other than that indicates that there's something off in your microbiome, which might impact the digestive process.

One of the main reasons it's so critical to make sure digestion is working properly is that if it isn't, every single function of the body can be negatively impacted. Let us say that again in another way to hammer home this point: If your digestion is off even a little, there's a domino effect on the way the rest of your body operates, no matter how good your diet and exercise routine might be. It's a sobering thought, but it illustrates the significance of digestion in your health.

Now that you know how digestion is *supposed* to work, let's turn our attention to where things can and will go wrong. These issues are unfortunately not uncommon, so don't feel bad if you see yourself in some of the descriptions in the next section. That's one of the areas where an NTP like Christine can assist you with healing your gut.

DIGESTIVE DYSFUNCTION

It's important to know that digestion works north to south, which means food starts at the top of your body and works its way down until it's excreted out your back side. Many people erroneously think digestion starts in the mouth, but, as we shared earlier, digestion actually begins in the brain. Far too many people are disconnected not only from real food sources of nutrition but also from being present in the moment with the food they're eating. When you multitask while eating, your brain has to deal with a bunch of other "stuff" that's going on in your body as it also sends signals to various digestive systems (the salivary glands, for example) to deal with the food as you're feeding it. Simply being more mindful of food and the act of eating would ease many of the digestive issues people are dealing with.

The reality is that many people in our fast-paced society are guilty of eating on the go or while doing other everyday activities. We've done it, and so have you. Sometimes eating on the run is a necessity of life, but it doesn't hurt for us to remind you that it's optimal to relax and slowly and thoroughly chew your food. Because of everything from a busy and stressful job to raising rambunctious kids to money problems, health concerns, and a wide variety of emotional and psychological issues from every direction of life, taking the time to eat leisurely can be extraordinarily difficult. How do you simply chill out in the midst of living life? You must permit yourself to have these moments of relaxation while eating; your body will reward you.

Other stressors that can negatively affect digestion include things that you wouldn't necessarily think about, such as toxic chemical exposure and pollution. Maybe someone is wearing a very strong perfume right before it's time for you to eat your lunch, which can be taxing for your body to deal with. Perhaps you live someplace where the air is filled with a mix of car emissions, fossil fuel waste, and smoke that's so thick it hides the sun. We probably don't need to tell you just how horrible poor air quality is on many aspects of your health. It's fairly common knowledge that suboptimal living conditions are a serious problem, and living in a smog-filled area like the one in the photo takes a toll on your body. Studies have been done to measure the impact pollution is having on gut health, digestive disorders, and other environmental-related health problems.

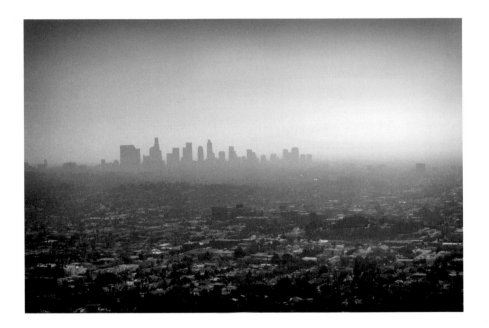

Remember when we shared earlier that salivary amylase is necessary to help digest and moisten the food when it's in the mouth and that carbohydrates are primarily digested with this enzyme? Well, guess what happens when your body is under stress because it's dealing with troublesome lifestyle issues? The brain is too busy to signal to your salivary glands to produce salivary amylase. Say what? That's right, you could be eating the best organic leafy green, nonstarchy vegetables in the world as part of your healthy ketogenic plan, but you can't properly digest them and get the amazing nutrients out of them without salivary amylase.

So what happens instead? These undigestible carbohydrates work their way down your digestive tract but then start to ferment in the intestines, which leads to unwanted and undesirable side effects such as bloating, inflammation, and worse. If you can take some time to chill out, then this should be your motivation for doing it before you eat every single meal. See, it's not just about the food you put in your mouth. It's also about how you prepare your body for that food before it even reaches your taste buds.

When you chew slowly for about thirty seconds, the food is fully broken down to aid in the digestive process as it works its way through the digestive tract. When you eat too quickly, a whole host of problems can occur, including intestinal inflammation, which then can develop into leaky gut (which is when your intestines have more and larger holes in them to allow things that shouldn't be in the bloodstream to pass through). Leaky gut can lead to many other health issues that you may be experiencing right now: irritable bowel syndrome (IBS); seasonal allergies; polycystic ovary syndrome (PCOS); autoimmune diseases such as Hashimoto's thyroiditis, psoriasis, and celiac disease; chronic fatigue; attention deficit hyperactivity disorder (ADHD); skin problems like eczema; small intestinal bacterial overgrowth (SIBO); food allergies; and more. Are you shocked to see so many ways your health can be affected? Another reason (as if you need one more) for being mindful while eating is to let digestion work the way it's supposed to.

NOTE FROM CHRISTINE

I'll be honest with you—I still struggle with taking my time to eat because I used to work as an assistant manager in a retail store, and I had just a short half-hour lunch break. I'd often begin eating my food only to be interrupted by a coworker who had some cash register or customer issue that needed my attention. The situation was especially nerve-wracking during the busy Christmas holiday season when I seemingly never had a break. Consequently, I generally rushed through my meal without chewing my food well; it was a preemptive strategy for being available on a moment's notice. Add the stress of being in a management position, and I had a recipe for a health disaster. Because that was my lifestyle for so many years, I developed a very bad habit of not relaxing and simply being in the moment with the food I eat. So now you know that I'm not perfect at this either. I have to consciously think about being present with my food every single time I eat so I don't slip into those old habits again.

We shared earlier in this chapter that the proper pH of the stomach should be between 1.5 and 3. The stomach acid, HCl, has a pH of 0.8 to 3. It combines with other gastric juices to form an acidic environment for digesting the foods you've consumed. As we've noted many times throughout this book, nine out of ten people don't produce enough stomach acid. Consequently, the stomach pH gets off kilter, and the chyme sticks around in the stomach way longer than it needs to because the pyloric sphincter fails to receive the signal to release the chyme into the duodenum promptly. Each of the macronutrients responds in a wickedly different way to this lack of proper stomach acid:

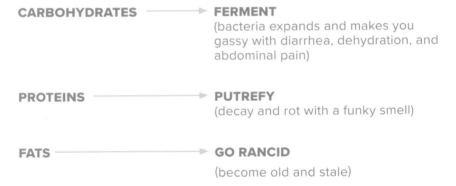

CARBOHYDRATES ——————▶ **FERMENT**
(bacteria expands and makes you gassy with diarrhea, dehydration, and abdominal pain)

PROTEINS ——————▶ **PUTREFY**
(decay and rot with a funky smell)

FATS ——————▶ **GO RANCID**
(become old and stale)

This lack of proper stomach acid that impacts the stomach pH messes things up for the two key digestive hormones we told you about earlier—secretin and CCK. Once the chyme enters the duodenum, if the pH of the chyme is not where it needs to be, then secretin isn't released to trigger the pancreas to produce bicarbonate and pancreatic juices. Also, when the pH of the chyme is out of whack, then CCK isn't released to trigger the gallbladder to produce bile to break down the fats consumed. These undigested fats go rancid in the colon and begin to become congested like Interstate 405 in Los Angeles! People on a congested highway eventually reach their destination when the traffic clears out, but undigested fats lead the body to become fatty acid deficient because they're never absorbed properly for use by the body. So if you're eating a low-carb, high-fat diet but your stomach acid is too low, the consequences might be that you're not getting all the nutrients that you think you are from eating keto. One indicator that you're not breaking down the fats you're eating is that you'll have shiny, greasy-looking stools. Ewww!!!

So what happens to all that undigested food? It goes into the small intestine and begins to change the makeup of the microbiome or gut flora there. The lining of the small intestine becomes much more permeable (gets holes in it), which allows undigested fats and proteins to pass through the intestinal wall directly into the bloodstream. The immune system then responds as if a foreign invader is attempting to cause harm to the body because it's confusing normal body tissue with this undigested food. This is the beginning of an autoimmune disease in which the body starts attacking perfectly healthy tissue. Remember, all of this started because of low stomach acid, and it cascaded from there.

Food is supposed to pass very easily through the ileocecal valve between the large intestine and small intestine, but when the undigested food leaves the small intestine, it can clog the valve. Without an easy way for these poorly digested foods to exit the body, they rot and go bad in the colon, which negatively affects your gut flora by greatly increasing the number of bad bacteria in the small intestine. That can lead to SIBO, which develops into gas, bloating, abdominal pain or cramping, diarrhea, constipation, irritable bowel syndrome (IBS), food intolerances, fibromyalgia, chronic fatigue syndrome, diabetes, neurotransmitter disorders, B12 deficiency, and leaky gut. Other than all that, you'll be okay. Seriously, though, if the gut flora is disrupted and there are not enough good bacteria to take on these enemies to your health, then the epithelial lining of the intestine doesn't regenerate, and you have big problems coming your way—like what we describe for you next.

THINGS THAT CAN HAPPEN IF DIGESTION DOESN'T WORK RIGHT

You might be wondering what kinds of physical issues manifest if digestion becomes compromised. The list of things that can happen if digestion doesn't work right is so daunting that it should make optimizing this part of your health your top priority. All the issues—including GERD, stomach ulcers, bloating, diarrhea, constipation, leaky gut, autoimmune disease, mental illness, detoxification problems, and cardiovascular risks—are preventable when you make a concerted effort to dial in your digestive health.

Let's take a look at the most common health problems associated with poor digestion.

STOMACH ULCERS

A big thing that can happen as a result of too little HCl production is that a person can develop stomach ulcers. As we mentioned earlier in this chapter, one of the functions of HCl is to help disinfect the stomach and kill foreign invaders like parasites and bacteria. If someone isn't producing enough HCl to kill off these invaders, it's possible that person will have an overabundance of *H. pylori,* which is the bacteria that causes some stomach ulcers.

The usual solution is for a person to take antibiotics to deal with the infection, and those antibiotics also compromise the health of the intestines by killing off all or most of the good bacteria along with the bad bacteria.

My mother had several things going on that caused her ulcers; one was an overgrowth of *H. pylori*. Between that and having to take a lot of aspirin for her joint pain, she eventually ended up in the hospital to have surgery to remove her stomach with a gastric bypass. When they did the surgery, the doctors found that the ulcers in her stomach had developed and healed over and over again, which eventually resulted in her pancreas, gallbladder, and stomach fusing together. This was one of the most bizarre things I'd ever seen in my life.

The surgeons had to carefully separate the organs, which made for a long and difficult surgery. They couldn't save her gallbladder, so the surgeons had to remove it along with her stomach. We are incredibly fortunate Mom is still alive today because this was a very serious condition brought on because of the stomach ulcers that developed from poor digestion.

These days, Mom is doing much better, but she has many nutrient deficiencies because her digestive system was all messed up from the damage that led to surgery. To address this, she takes regular vitamin B12 shots and gets blood transfusions often to avoid anemia. Even if she took vitamin and mineral supplements, her body wouldn't be able to absorb or use them because of her compromised digestive system. Let my mom's experience be your motivation for doing everything you can to get your digestion working well now so you don't suffer the same fate that she did.

GUT MICROBIOME

We've talked a lot about gut health throughout this book and for good reason. If your microbiome isn't happy, then your body isn't going to be very happy in general. We have more microbial cells in our body than we do human cells. In fact, microbial cells outnumber our human cells by a factor of 10:1. There are 100 trillion (yes, trillion with a *t*) microbes in us, and they weigh upward of four pounds. When you eat food, you're primarily feeding the gut microbiome. The good bugs are like the Super Friends—Superman, Batman, Robin, Wonder Woman, and Aquaman—who do some incredible work in the body to keep it protected and thriving. However, the bad bugs are like the villains of the Super Friends—Bizarro, Brainiac, Lex Luthor, and Cheetah—and their only job is to disrupt and wreak havoc on what would otherwise be a normal, happy, healthy system. Curses! Foiled again!

Just as we are all bioindividual in our metabolic needs, so too are we unique in our gut health. The composition of gut bugs can vary from person to person so significantly that each person needs a customized plan for regaining their health; the one-size-fits-all approach that far too many health experts have been promoting doesn't work. In fact, your gut microbiome is constantly changing throughout your life, and it's affected by age, what foods you eat, and even where in the world you live.

The term *microbiota* refers to all the microbes that live in the gut, including both the beneficial and the harmful bacteria. Two examples of the beneficial microbes include *lactobacillus* and *bifidobacterium*.[1] Harmful microbes are things like yeast, parasites, viruses, and fungi. Here's an interesting fact: If a baby is born by Cesarean section and doesn't go through the birth canal, then that baby doesn't inherit the beneficial bacteria from the mother. The result is possible compromised gut health and digestive issues as the child gets older.

There are two primary types of microbes living in your gut—transient microbes and native microbes. Transient microbes are like day workers who do their work and then exit the body through the stool. Our supply of these microbes comes mostly from fermented foods like sauerkraut and Greek yogurt as well as from probiotic supplementation from primarily the *Lacto-* and *Bifido-* species. Native microbes are environmental; we get them from the air, soil, and water supply, and they include *Bacteroides, Bacillus,* and *Streptomyces* (not to be confused with *Streptococcus,* which is the infection that leads to sore throat, fever, and swollen lymph nodes). All these native microbes have antifungal, antiparasitic, and antiviral properties and are resistant to your stomach pH and antibiotics.

TOP FIVE THREATS TO YOUR GUT MICROBIOME

Permanent changes to your gut microbiome can happen for a variety of reasons, but these are the top five:

- Stress
- A crappy carbage diet (mostly refined grains, starches, and sugars)
- Contraceptives
- Vaccinations
- Overuse of antibiotics or other prescription drugs

The lack of a strong level of good microbes in the gut is devastating to your health. Here's a list of some of the things that can and will happen if the bad guys outnumber the good guys:

- Chronic ear infections
- Yeast infections
- Diarrhea/Constipation
- Flatulence
- Excess bloating

- Nail fungus
- Hormonal imbalances
- Eczema
- Acne
- Mood disorders

The good microbes help produce three critically important B vitamins—B1 (thiamine), B2 (riboflavin), and B12 (cobalamin)—as well as vitamin K2. Additionally, the good microbes help protect the intestinal wall, absorb nutrients, digest foods, balance intestinal pH, fight foreign or harmful microbes, improve bowel transit time, and improve mood. That last one may seem like a fish out of water on this list, but the connection between the brain and the gut is undeniable (in fact, researchers now refer to the gut as "the second brain"). In fact, 90 percent of the serotonin in the body is produced by the good bacteria in your gut! See, a healthy gut means a healthy mental state as well.

SOURCES OF PREBIOTICS

It's important that you get quality *Real Food Keto* sources of prebiotics in your diet to feed the good microbes in the gut. Prebiotics (not to be confused with probiotics) are soluble and insoluble fibers that serve as the "food" for the microbiome to "eat." Outstanding whole food and ketogenic sources of prebiotics include the following:

- Low-sugar fruits and their skin, such as blueberries, strawberries, and blackberries

- Vegetables, especially dark leafy green ones

- Fresh herbs and spices

- Dark chocolate (80 percent cacao or higher)

NOTE FROM CHRISTINE

My gut health has been compromised because of the overuse of antibiotics. Because I was born prematurely, I was sick so often as a child that my doctor would give me antibiotics every single time my parents took me to see him. In the first year that Jimmy and I were married, I had a series of urinary tract infections (UTIs) that prompted my primary care physician to put me on an intensive round of a very strong antibiotic for three straight months. Of course, I had no idea what this was doing to my gut health because my doctor never said anything about it causing me any harm. Had he simply told me to take a probiotic supplement or to consume fermented food to help replenish the good microbes in my gut, then perhaps I wouldn't have developed the various autoimmune diseases that will be with me for the rest of my life. If I had known of the negative consequences, I never would have been on antibiotics that long and without a plan for offsetting the complications of taking the antibiotics. Let my example educate you in your own health journey.

SOLUBLE FIBER VERSUS INSOLUBLE FIBER

Soluble fiber means the fiber is soluble in water. When the fiber mixes with water, it turns into a gel-like substance and swells. One of the benefits of soluble fiber is that it helps control blood sugar levels. Soluble fibers go by many names, including pectins, gums, and mucilages.

Insoluble fiber doesn't dissolve in water. As it goes through the digestive system, it stays pretty close to its original form. One of the benefits of insoluble fiber is that it helps reduce the risk of hemorrhoids and constipation. (Drinking enough water helps, too!) Insoluble fibers go by several names, including cellulose and lignins.

Supplementing with a probiotic to help replenish your microbiome may be necessary, but make sure you choose one that includes the full spectrum of strains for the most potential benefit. The probiotic should contain transient microbes, native microbes, and a prebiotic in one supplement (make sure the supplement is refrigerated, or you might not be getting as many of those living microbes as you think). It's only necessary to take 3 to 5 billion species of probiotics daily to maintain once you get your gut health under control, but as you begin healing from severely compromised gut health, you might need to take as many as 30 billion species daily. Of course, you could get some of those from fermented foods sources, like kombucha, kefir, sauerkraut, fermented pickles, and kimchi.

LEAKY GUT AND AUTOIMMUNITY

Most people hear the phrase *leaky gut* and have no idea what it is. It sounds like you need to potty-train it or something.

As we previously stated, proteins are only partially digested or not digested at all if we don't have the proper amount of stomach acid. When this happens, the bad bugs survive and start to reproduce like gremlins. The bad bugs follow the undigested proteins into the small intestine and release a dastardly thing known as an *exotoxin,* which begins causing great damage to the mucosal lining that protects the small intestine by increasing the number of holes in the intestinal wall. When there are more holes in the intestinal wall, inflammation levels in the body go up. In short, you have leaky gut when the bad bugs and undigested proteins slip through the holes in the intestinal wall and get into the bloodstream.

Although protein is considered an essential nutrient, when it leaks into the bloodstream through the intestinal wall, the body sees it as a foreign invader that needs to be taken out by the immune system. When the body attacks itself enough times, these perfectly healthy and normal proteins are deemed harmful, and your organs get caught in the crossfire. The type of undigested protein that's most similar to the specific organ under attack determines which organ is the target. For example, did you know the proteins contained in raw tuna mimic the tissues and enzymes that comprise the thyroid gland? Christine used to love eating raw tuna, and now she has Hashimoto's thyroiditis. Coincidence? Maybe, maybe not. The graphic below shows some autoimmune diseases and the organs that are affected by them.

HASHIMOTO'S THYROIDITIS ⟶	THYROID
PSORIASIS ⟶	SKIN
ULCERATIVE COLITIS ⟶	INTESTINES
CELIAC DISEASE ⟶	SMALL INTESTINE
RHEUMATOID ARTHRITIS ⟶	JOINTS
MULTIPLE SCLEROSIS ⟶	MYELIN SHEATH OF NERVES

YOUR APPENDIX AND GUT MICROBES

If you've had your appendix taken out, it's important that you supplement with a good full-spectrum probiotic. The appendix has long been considered an unnecessary organ, but recent research shows that it acts as a haven for good gut microbes. In the appendix, these good gut microbes start to be replenished after a round of antibiotics. If you don't have an appendix, then your gut has a much more difficult time promptly repopulating with healthy gut bacteria to fight against infection and foreign invaders.

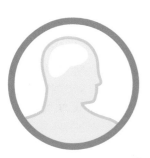

MENTAL HEALTH

The connection between good mental health and digestion might not be as obvious as it is for other systems, but it is an important relationship. Proper stomach pH is necessary to break down or split amino acids to become neurotransmitters, which are the brain chemicals that communicate information throughout the brain and body. These neurotransmitters are what relay signals between nerve cells (neurons). If this process is interrupted for some time because of chronic poor digestion, your brain health is negatively impacted, and you have symptoms of depression, anxiety, and bipolar disorder, just to name a few. Poor digestion prevents the body and brain from absorbing the micronutrients in the foods we eat, and it's these micronutrients that are the precursors for the ever-important neurotransmitters.

One important factor is what happens to serotonin levels. Serotonin, which is known as the "happy hormone," is a monoamine neurotransmitter that's made in the intestines. If digestion isn't working properly, then your body can't produce healthy amounts of serotonin. Trying to function with low serotonin levels in the brain is like trying to get your car to run on fumes. At some point, everything stops working until you get adequate fuel for your vehicle. The same goes for serotonin in the brain. Serotonin directly affects mood, social behavior, appetite, digestion, sleep, memory, and sexual function and desire. Someone with a deficiency in serotonin often suffers from depression.

Unsurprisingly, there's a macronutrient and micronutrient connection to this digestion/mental health issue. (See? Everything is interconnected.) The gallbladder and liver need to be functioning well so that they can digest healthy fats and the fat-soluble vitamins A, D, E, and K. The brain is made up of approximately 70 percent fatty acids, so having enough fat in the diet and good digestive health help ensure you can absorb these fat-soluble vitamins for good brain function. Proper bowel flora is needed to produce vitamin B12, which is required for the production of dopamine, gamma-aminobutyric acid (GABA), norepinephrine, and serotonin—all major elements of proper brain health. Dopamine is what determines your emotional state, your ability to move naturally, and the sensations of pleasure and pain. GABA helps relax and calm you when you're stressed. Norepinephrine (also known as noradrenaline) is released from the sympathetic nervous system in response to stress (the fight-or-flight response) and helps the brain pay attention and respond to events. Remember, it all starts with getting your digestion right.

CARDIOVASCULAR PROBLEMS

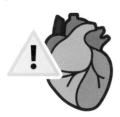

Most people have no clue about the connection between proper digestion and the health of their heart, but the two are intricately involved. First, if you don't properly digest protein, then the heart-healthy amino acids taurine and carnitine can't be made. Second, if you don't produce enough stomach acid, you can't absorb calcium and magnesium, which both help with the contraction and relaxation of the muscles, including the heart muscle. Third, if the liver and gallbladder, both of which are involved in the digestive process, aren't functioning well, then the body can't digest the healthy fats and fat-soluble vitamins that impact cardiovascular health. Finally, proper gut bacteria are necessary to produce vitamins B1, B2, B12, and K2, which all contribute to improvements in heart health. In fact, vitamin K is necessary to prevent calcium from becoming deposited in the coronary arteries.

DETOXIFICATION ISSUES

Even the most perfect whole foods–based ketogenic diet in the world can't overcome the negative effects of the toxins in the body. If the digestive process is less than ideal, then your intestines, which are involved in eliminating toxins, are compromised. Thus, your ability to experience detoxification is impaired. The lymph system gets clogged, and that leads to the liver being clogged, which cuts off any ability for the body to fully get rid of the gunk and junk. Read Chapter 13 for a whole lot more on this important issue. For now, the point is that good digestion is the key to making detoxification work optimally.

ANTACIDS AND DIGESTION

Growing up, we always heard when you have heartburn or acid reflux that you needed to turn to tum-ta-tum-tum-Tums. Some people eat antacids and proton pump inhibitors, such as Prilosec OTC, like candy because people mistakenly think they're suffering from an overproduction of stomach acid. As we've stated previously, upward of 90 percent of Americans produce too *little* hydrochloric acid (HCl). Jonathan Wright, MD, author of the book *Why Stomach Acid Is Good for You,* discovered this issue of underproduction by using Heidelberg Gastrotelemetry equipment to measure the pH of the digestive tract of thousands of patients. The test also showed how much stomach acid was being produced.[2] Furthermore, Dr. George Goodheart, a chiropractor and the creator of the technique of testing muscles called applied kinesiology, found the same thing that Dr. Wright did using kinesiological analysis and functional assessment.[3]

So why isn't heartburn or acid reflux an indication of excessive stomach acid? Great question. The reality is that whether your level of stomach acid is too low or too high, the symptoms are amazingly the same. That's why testing to see where you stand is so critically important. Ask your doctor about running the Heidelberg Gastrotelemetry test (also known as the Heidelberg Gastric Analysis) to see how well you're doing at producing stomach acid.

People have heartburn or acid reflux because the food sits in the stomach too long, and sometimes, when the cardiac sphincter is weak, the food comes back up into the esophagus. Poor nutrition, smoking, alcohol, pregnancy, medications, obesity, and hernia all contribute to a weakening of the cardiac sphincter. The stomach acid is what triggers the cardiac sphincter to close, so when stomach acid isn't sufficient, the signal to close the sphincter isn't sent. Consequently, stomach contents can come back up into the esophagus through the opening. Because the stomach pH is acidic (even when there's too little stomach acid), you feel a burning sensation in the esophagus, and you reach for an antacid. The antacids provide temporary relief because they change the pH of the chyme (remember, that's the term for the digested food going through the digestive tract after it hits the stomach) to a more neutral pH, and the burning stops. However, the unintended consequence of this is that the chyme pH becomes too alkaline, which leads to even lower stomach acid. That makes the food sit in the stomach, and further problems start to develop, as we've already described.

Go to your medicine cabinet right now, remove those antacids, and throw them away. They're doing you a lot more harm than good. They're taking you farther from your goal of improved digestion. Instead, they're making your body's ability to digest food properly next to impossible. In addition, the long-term effects of taking these products (with brand names like Mylanta, Prilosec, Rolaids, Tums, and Zantac) are frightening because they deplete the body of vitally important nutrients, including calcium, phosphorus, zinc, vitamin B12, and vitamin D. They also can lead to constipation, loss of appetite, unusual tiredness, muscle weakness, confusion, and depression. Talk to your doctor, Nutritional Therapy Practitioner, or other healthcare professional about how you can come off of these medications safely.

We hope we've given you new insight into the myriad ways that your digestion impacts your state of health. Let this be motivation for doing everything you can to keep your digestive system running in tip-top shape. If your digestion is happy, then the rest of your body has the best chance at being as healthy as it can be. That's what we all want, right?

CAUSES OF HYPOCHLORHYDRIA

Throughout *Real Food Keto*, you've learned all of the negative consequences that come from having too little stomach acid production, or *hypochlorhydria*, but we haven't gotten into how it happens. That's about to change. In this section, we give you six reasons this deficiency in HCl occurs.

Because nine out of ten Americans deal with the issue of too little stomach acid, a lot of these things are probably very familiar to you and your situation. You're not alone if you have one or more of these problems. This section includes our reminders to you that these things can have consequences that negatively impact your health.

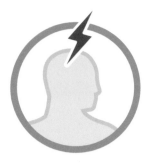

STRESS

Did you know *stressed* spelled backward is *desserts*? Well, that doesn't have anything to do with this subject, really, but these days it seems that everyone is stressed. Although we all deal with stress, not everyone deals with it very effectively. This constant, chronic drip-drip-drip of stress keeps you in a perpetual sympathetic state, which leads to the condition we know as "fight or flight." When this mode kicks in, it takes blood and all the nutrients in it away from the stomach so they can be used in other parts of the body, such as the heart and muscles, to help with the stress response. The result is that the stomach is more vulnerable when you're in this state because the raw materials of blood and the nutrients in the blood that are necessary for producing stomach acid are no longer there. Consequently, stomach acid production drops.

EXCESSIVE CARBOHYDRATE CONSUMPTION

Now is when we talk about desserts, because carbohydrates play a role in low stomach acid production. One of the reasons why we advocate for a low-carb, high-fat, ketogenic diet is because carbohydrate consumption, especially the crappy carbage such as refined sugar, grains, and starches, can wreak havoc on the body in many ways. In the case of stomach acid, these inferior carb sources deplete the body of the nutrients such as vitamin B6 and zinc that are required for making stomach acid. Going keto and using real, whole foods doesn't compromise your system like processed carbs do.

ALLERGIES

Achoo! Yes, allergies can put added stress on the body. And as we've discussed, stress pulls blood and the nutrients in it away from the stomach and toward other areas of the body that are in distress. Virtually any allergic reaction, including seasonal allergies, food allergies, chemical allergies, and more, is a form of stress. There is some debate about whether the allergies lead to low stomach acid or low stomach acid leads to the development of allergies. Either way, it isn't good news for health.

OVERCONSUMPTION OF ALCOHOLIC BEVERAGES

When you consume too many alcoholic beverages, it can actually eat away at and shrink the gastric mucosa, the mucous membrane layer of the stomach. The normal thickness of the mucosal lining is 1 millimeter. The gastric mucosa contains the glands and gastric pits that are crucial to the production of stomach acid. However, when someone consumes alcohol in excess and the thickness of the lining falls below the healthy level, there are fewer glands and pits, which means there's a significant reduction in the amount of stomach acid produced.

CARBONATED BEVERAGES LIKE SODA

All carbonated beverages, both the sugary and the diet versions, contain phosphoric acid, which is a colorless and odorless liquid. Phosphoric acid is what gives these drinks the "bite" that people seem to enjoy. Even if you use the popular SodaStream to make soda or bubbly water at home, the carbonated beverage still contains some phosphoric acid because of the process the water goes through to become carbonated. The downside of repeated consumption of beverages with a lot of phosphoric acid is that it depletes stomach acid production little by little.

NUTRIENT DEFICIENCIES, ESPECIALLY ZINC AND VITAMIN B6

One of the core messages of *Real Food Keto* is the prevention of nutrient deficiencies. So it should not come as a surprise that one of the reasons for hypochlorhydria is a lack of two critical nutrients—the mineral zinc and vitamin B6. Both zinc and vitamin B6 aid in the production of HCl. If you lack either one of these nutrients, then you can't produce adequate amounts of stomach acid.

Now that you know the causes of low stomach acid, we want to share a few of the telltale signs to watch for so you can take appropriate action to remedy this situation. This is invaluable information because 90 percent of the people reading this book have hypochlorhydria. See if you recognize any symptoms that you're experiencing right now.

SIGNS OF HYPOCHLORHYDRIA

Low stomach acid is a little off the radar of most people because they don't recognize the signs that they have it, so we're here to tell you what to watch for. The table lists early signs and advanced signs that may indicate that you're running low in your supply of stomach acid.

EARLY SIGNS	ADVANCED SIGNS
Uncomfortable fullness after meals	Osteoporosis
Undigested food in stool	All allergies
Thinning hair	Cardiac arrhythmia
Candida (yeast overgrowth)	Asthma
Rectal itching	Acne
Thin or peeling nails	Ulcerative colitis
Gas	Autoimmune disease
Abdominal cramping	Depression
	Type 2 diabetes
	Hives
	Eczema

Consuming a ketogenic diet generally leads to a decrease in appetite and an increase in satiety, which allows the body to go many hours without eating while still having the ability to function perfectly fine. One reason why you might not feel hunger while eating keto (or any diet, for that matter) is that low stomach acid production forces the food to sit in the stomach longer than it needs to, which leads to feelings of fullness and even bloating. So, if you feel full while you're eating keto, keep in mind that it may be the satiating effects of the healthy fats and ketones that are fueling you, or it might be the result of too little hydrochloric acid. If you're concerned about this, ask your doctor to run the Heidelberg Gastrotelemetry test to see where you stand with the pH of your stomach.

FOODS THAT AID DIGESTION

Certain foods aid the digestive process. Let's examine those foods that can help you improve your digestion.

1. Apple cider vinegar has a high acid content that helps digest proteins in the stomach by lowering stomach pH to make it more acidic.

2. Beets contain high levels of folate and manganese, which supports gallbladder function.

3. Cabbage juice contains vitamin U, which helps to heal ulcers in the stomach and duodenum. The juice has a high sulfur content, which is helpful in killing parasites that steal nutrients in the digestive process.

4. Garlic is good for killing parasites.

5. Radishes contain sulfur, which helps improve bile flow and therefore helps remove deposits and stones from the gallbladder.

6. Fennel contains healthy amounts of vitamin C, potassium, fiber, and trace minerals, which are great for overall digestive support.

7. Jerusalem artichokes are a great source of fiber-based inulin, which helps promote healthy bacteria in the intestinal tract.

8. Dandelion root helps improve bile production and flow to contract the gallbladder so it can release stored bile. It also helps with liver congestion, bile duct inflammation, gallstones, and jaundice, and it's a good source of inulin, which promotes the growth of good bacteria.

9. Ginger promotes the elimination of intestinal gas by relaxing and soothing the intestinal tract, and it's good for stimulating digestion.

10. Lemon water is alkaline until it enters the stomach, where it turns acidic and helps stimulate stomach acid production.

11. Chard, kale, and spinach are great sources of fiber, which aids in digestion. Kale, yeah!

12. Bone broth is a great gut-healing and joint health–improving agent.

FOOD SOURCES THAT CONTAIN ZINC

Because zinc plays such a critical role in having adequate levels of HCl, which makes digestion happen, here's a list of the *Real Food Keto*–approved food sources of this critical mineral:

- Oysters
- Grass-fed beef
- Turkey
- Full-fat cheeses
- Swiss chard
- Pumpkin seeds
- Lamb
- Cocoa powder
- Cashews
- Kefir (fermented milk) or yogurt
- Mushrooms
- Spinach
- Chicken

NO GALLBLADDER? NO PROBLEM!

If you have had your gallbladder surgically removed, or if your gallbladder isn't functioning well, you need to be mindful of the foods that aid in the digestion of fats. The gallbladder produces the bile to digest fats, so when your gallbladder doesn't work properly (or has been removed), you need to assist your digestive system with processing fats. Remember, eating fat helps keep the bile flowing so that your liver and gallbladder work properly. Here's the list of foods to eat if you don't have a gallbladder:

- Beets
- Radishes
- Artichokes
- Lemons
- Dandelion root

SUPPLEMENTS GOOD FOR DIGESTION

Sometimes it's necessary to add certain supplements to your dietary plan to aid in achieving your goal of having good digestion. Christine regularly takes HCl, pancreatic enzymes, B6, and zinc. These supplements boost or help the production of hydrochloric acid in the stomach to aid in digestion. Consult with a practitioner like a naturopath, functional medicine practitioner, or NTP to make sure you don't get too much HCl, which can do more harm than good. Pancreatic enzymes are necessary to break down all the macronutrients, especially fat, which is especially helpful for those who no longer have a gallbladder. As for zinc, most people are zinc-deficient and require supplementation. Be careful, though, as taking too much zinc on an empty stomach and with low stomach acid can lead to nausea.

NOTE FROM CHRISTINE

I started taking HCl supplements knowing I had low stomach acid production. After just a few doses, my stomach started hurting, and it hurt for four days. It turns out that the stomach ulcers I had back in 2006 had not healed because my digestion was still off. So taking the HCl supplementation was not a good idea for me until my stomach healed. I started taking other supplements that aided in healing my stomach; then, once healed, I could start back on HCl supplementation.

Not all supplements are created equal, so try to access quality pharmaceutical-grade products from an NTP or another nutritional healthcare provider who can procure supplements from companies such as Biotics Research (www.bioticsresearch.com). Also, before experimenting with various supplements, it's advisable that you speak with an experienced healthcare provider to determine which supplements you need.

TIPS TO IMPROVE DIGESTION

Before we wrap up this chapter, we have some last-minute tips on how you can improve your digestion. These suggestions will help you put your body in the best possible position for digestion to work correctly. Try these tips on for size:

- Don't rush through your meals. Chew your food for approximately thirty seconds, which helps break down the food so the stomach can digest it more easily. Try to eat in a relaxed state while sitting down and without doing any other activities at the same time. Eat *slowly*.

- Make sure you get enough fats in your meals to stoke bile production. Eating a low-fat or no-fat diet causes bile to become stagnant and viscous, which can lead to gallstones forming. This might be the reason Christine ended up having to have her gallbladder removed. Because she ate a low-fat diet in her early twenties, she wasn't keeping her bile moving. In the wake of having had the gallbladder surgery, she makes sure to take supplements that help support bile production, and she eats foods that support bile production and flow.

- Take some apple cider vinegar to stimulate your stomach to produce HCl and also supplement with digestive enzymes to help digest the proteins you eat. Taking digestive enzymes helps process the fats you eat if you've had your gallbladder removed or if your gallbladder isn't functioning optimally. However, make sure to consult with an NTP or another healthcare provider before starting these digestive enzymes or HCl supplementation.

- If you know you're deficient in zinc, take a zinc supplement or eat more foods containing zinc to help aid HCl production.

- Have your stomach pH tested. Ask your doctor to run the Heidelberg Gastrotelemetry test. If you find that your stomach pH is low, consult with an NTP or your healthcare provider about the possibility of taking HCl supplements. (Make sure to talk to a professional because taking too much HCl can harm your stomach.)

- Don't drink carbonated beverages with meals. These can affect the pH of your stomach and interfere with your body's ability to absorb and use certain vitamins and minerals. If you drink carbonated beverages, drink them between meals and limit them as much as possible.

If you have gut health issues, slowly incorporate fermented foods into your diet. Adding too much fermented food at once can cause issues like gas and bloating.

- Add a small amount of fermented food to each meal. It can be as little as a tablespoon of any fermented food. Eating fermented foods has many benefits, like strengthening metabolism, boosting immunity, balancing blood sugar, and supporting digestion (of course!). See page 114 for a list of fermented foods you can incorporate into your meals. Also, see the Resources section in the back of this book for a great place to find recipes for fermented foods.

Whew, that was a lot to, er, digest. But we hope you learned a lot about the importance of digestion. The topic of Chapter 11 is of equal importance in your pursuit of improved health. Find out next why blood sugar balance is critical if you want your body to function like it's supposed to.

REAL FOOD KETO TAKEAWAYS FROM CHAPTER 10

- Not feeling hungry is the hallmark of a ketogenic diet, but it also could mean low stomach acid production.
- Proper digestion is a north-to-south process, and the body gleans nutrients from food from start to finish.
- Carbs are digested in the mouth, proteins in the stomach, and fats in the duodenum.
- The food you eat is called the bolus after you swallow it, and then it turns into chyme in the stomach.
- HCl disinfects the stomach to guard against foreign invaders and activates the digestive enzyme pepsin to deal with the protein you consume.
- The stressors of life in our fast-paced society can lead to digestive dysfunction.
- Chewing your food slowly for about thirty seconds can help aid in the digestive process.
- If there's a lack of stomach acid, carbs ferment, proteins putrefy, and fats go rancid.

- Poor digestion leads to stomach ulcers, compromised gut health, autoimmunity from leaky gut, mental health issues, cardiovascular problems, detoxification complications, and more.
- The causes of low stomach acid (hypochlorhydria) include stress, a high-carb diet, allergies, alcohol, soda, and nutrient deficiencies.
- Don't ignore the early signs of low stomach acid. Address them so they don't turn into the more severe advanced signs.
- Eat more of the foods that are high in zinc for better stomach acid production and to help with digestion. If you don't have a gallbladder, focus on foods that aid fat digestion.
- Supplementing with extra HCl, pancreatic enzymes, and zinc may be necessary to heal your digestion.

CHAPTER 11

Blood Sugar Balancing Act

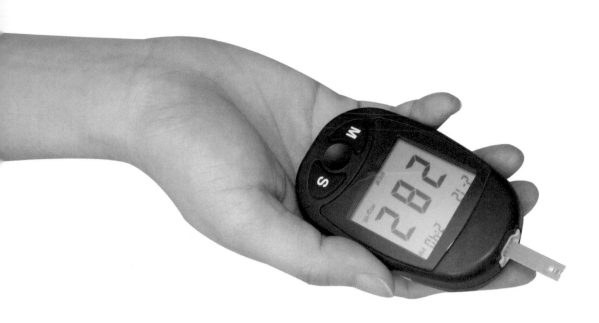

One of the major benefits of a low-carb, high-fat, ketogenic nutritional approach is the positive effect it can have on blood sugar. When blood sugar and corresponding insulin levels are out of whack, the result can be a series of health problems.

Most people hear "blood sugar" and automatically dismiss it if they don't have diabetes. But here's the thing—you don't suddenly wake up one morning and have type 2 diabetes. (Type 1 diabetes is different; it's an autoimmune disease wherein the pancreas stops pumping out insulin.) It happens over time as blood glucose levels go up and down like a roller coaster, with your body constantly working hard to keep this blood sugar balancing act from making you less and less healthy. We can directly attribute the rise in cases of type 2 diabetes, metabolic syndrome, and insulin resistance to the heavy load of refined sugars, grains, and starches in the standard American diet.

We want to challenge you to do something you've probably never done before unless you already have diabetes—start testing your blood sugar levels. You might be saying, "What? But I don't have diabetes." You don't need to have diabetes to find value in testing your blood sugar levels. Jimmy first started testing and sharing his results online many years ago even though he didn't have diabetes. Knowing your blood sugar levels helps you dial in your nutrition so that you can nourish your body in the best way possible for your unique needs.

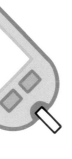

Here's what you need to do: Get a glucometer from your local pharmacy or an online vendor (such as BestKetoneTest.com). This blood sugar testing kit usually comes with a testing meter, disposable strips, and a lancet for pricking your finger and testing your blood. Yes, some people are squeamish about testing their blood, but it provides such a wealth of information about how well you're managing your blood sugar and your overall health that it's worth the momentary discomfort (and it's not as bad as people think it is). Testing once or twice a year at your doctor's office during your routine checkup simply is *not* enough. The technology for testing more frequently exists, and it's inexpensive to see where you stand. Taking this next step in your health journey will open your eyes to the effects food and lifestyle are having on you.

As previously noted, virtually every packaged food product in our food supply is loaded with added sugars and corn derivatives. One of the most egregious ingredients is a double whammy on both blood sugar and insulin levels: high-fructose corn syrup (HFCS). This stuff is in many things Americans are eating, and many people have no idea how incredibly damaging it is to the liver, pancreas, and entire body. The Corn Refiners Association has attempted to respond to the negative backlash by renaming it corn sugar—but don't be fooled! Sugar is sugar is sugar, and the body can't handle the negative effects it causes.

MORE INFO ABOUT HFCS AND CORN PRODUCTS

One of our favorite resources to point people to for information about the problems with HFCS and corn products is *The Omnivore's Dilemma* by journalist and health activist Michael Pollan.[1] He notes that many nonedible products contain HFCS and/or corn substances, including toothpaste, trash bags, cosmetics, disposable diapers, cleaning products, charcoal briquettes, matches, batteries, magazine covers, vegetable waxes, pesticides, adhesives, and the coatings on cardboard, linoleum, and fiberglass. It's virtually impossible to avoid exposure to corn in this day and age. The potential detrimental effects on blood sugar levels simply cannot be ignored.

Let's examine how blood sugar is supposed to work. Later we'll get into blood sugar imbalances and how they affect the body.

We're going to throw a lot of terms at you in this chapter that you might not be familiar with, so here's a quick glossary that defines some terms you might not understand yet. These terms can be difficult to distinguish because they look and sound so similar, but knowing the differences between them and grasping their importance is critical to understanding the information in this chapter.

Glucose: The simple sugar circulating in the bloodstream that's used as energy

Glycogen: The stored form of glucose in the liver and muscles

Ketones: The substance made from the breakdown of fats for energy

Glycolysis: The process of breaking down glucose into usable energy

Gluconeogenesis: The process of converting protein and some fats to glucose for energy

Glycogenesis: The creation of glycogen from glucose to be stored in the liver and muscles

Glycogenolysis: The breakdown of glycogen back into glucose to be used for fuel

Check out the lengthier Glossary at the end of the book to see definitions for other terms we use throughout the book.

HOW BLOOD SUGAR IS SUPPOSED TO WORK

Before you can fully understand the problems associated with blood sugar levels being out of balance, you need to understand how blood sugar is supposed to work in a healthy person. Normal blood glucose levels are between 70 and 100 mg/dL (3.9 and 5.5 mmol/L), and being on a ketogenic diet should make staying within this range quite manageable. Three primary organs are involved in keeping blood sugar under control—the liver, pancreas, and adrenal glands. Although many people know that the pancreas is what helps produce the hormone insulin to respond to blood sugar going up, there are other hormones involved, too, such as glucagon, cortisol, and epinephrine. Let's first look more closely at the role of the pancreas.

BLOOD SUGAR AND INSULIN RESISTANCE ▬▬▬

If you're dealing with insulin resistance, which we've discussed a lot in this book, your normal range for blood sugar may be a little higher than for someone who is more insulin sensitive. As Jimmy and his coauthor Adam Nally, DO, wrote in their book *The Keto Cure*,[2] the normal range for blood glucose in people with insulin resistance is 70 to 120 mg/dL (3.9 to 6.7 mmol/L), which accounts for the glucose-sparing effect that happens with higher blood sugar levels in the morning. This effect is transient and freaks out a lot of people who eat keto, but relax; it's normal. Your glucose readings for the rest of the day are down in the healthy range. Healing insulin resistance can take eighteen to twenty-four months or longer, so be patient with yourself. Keep an eye on your A1c, and aim for less than 5.5 mmol/L and optimally less than 5.0 mmol/L.

The pancreas is both an endocrine gland (it secretes hormones and other substances directly into the blood) and an exocrine gland (it secretes substances to the surface of the skin, like sweat, saliva, and mucus). The pancreas functions as an exocrine gland by releasing digestive enzymes and sodium bicarbonate to contribute to digestion. For blood sugar regulation, the pancreas functions as an endocrine gland by releasing insulin and glucagon.

Insulin is the master hormone released by the beta cells of the pancreas. The insulin signals the liver to push glucose (sugar) into the cells for storage to create glycogen (this process is known as *glycogenesis*). Any excess glucose beyond what the body can store is converted to stored body fat. In other words, insulin is the driver pushing the sugar into the cells, and this is the reason a high-carb diet makes you gain weight (from the added stored body fat). It's also why people refer to insulin as a fat-storing hormone.

The alpha cells of the pancreas release the hormone glucagon. The glucagon signals the liver to turn the stored glycogen back to glucose through *glycogenolysis* so it can be used as fuel. Glucagon also tells the liver to make glucose from the protein you consume through a process known as *gluconeogenesis*. (We know we're throwing a lot of big long *G* words at you, but we'll explain more about the key differences between them in a moment, and you can refer to the glossary on the previous page in the meantime. We're just laying the groundwork for how blood sugar is supposed to work.)

Then the action shifts to the largest solid organ of the body—the liver. The liver plays very specific roles in blood sugar regulation, and all are critical to understanding how this process works. It's the liver that responds to the signals given by the pancreas that indicate whether blood sugar levels are outside the normal range. In other words, the liver doesn't allow blood sugar to go too high or too low. When blood sugar is too high, the liver receives signals to pump out insulin to bring the level down. When blood sugar is too low, the liver receives signals to pump out glucagon to bring the level up. If the health of your liver is compromised in any way, your body has difficulty controlling blood sugar and keeping it within a healthy range.

The liver stores extra glucose in the form of glycogen (through glycogenesis) to be ready to provide the body with emergency fuel at a moment's notice, if necessary. The body can easily convert glycogen stores back to glucose when the need arises. If glucose is still in demand, the liver can turn some of the protein you consume into glucose through gluconeogenesis. And because the focus of this book is the ketogenic approach to eating, you should know that the liver also can create an alternative fuel source known as ketone bodies, which are created from the whole food–based fats consumed in the context of a low-carb, moderate-protein nutritional intake.

Let's shift our attention to the adrenal glands, which are located right on top of the kidneys. They produce three hormones that are crucial in managing blood sugar levels: cortisol, epinephrine (adrenaline), and norepinephrine (noradrenalin).

Most people think of cortisol as the stress hormone, but it's much more than that. Cortisol is released by the adrenal cortex when blood sugar levels are too low because of insufficient glucagon. The adrenal glands create glucose from proteins in the skeletal tissue to send back to the liver to convert it to glucose through gluconeogenesis, which then normalizes blood sugar levels. The adrenal glands also help fill glycogen stores when glycogenesis is lagging and stimulate the breakdown of triglycerides and release stored body fat, which is known as lipolysis.

Epinephrine is what signals the liver to convert glycogen back to glucose. When you have an adrenaline rush and you need quick energy to flee danger, epinephrine kicks in to increase blood flow to the heart, muscles, and liver, to raise your heart rate, and to dilate your airway. It also helps in the process of gluconeogenesis by signaling to the liver to break down protein and some fats into glucose.

The third hormone from the adrenal glands, norepinephrine, takes blood away from the deep organs and puts it into the muscles and heart so that the body can react to emergency situations effectively. The three hormones work diligently to keep blood sugar from going haywire.

Now that you know how blood sugar is supposed to work in a healthy metabolism, let's pull back the curtain on all the things that can go wrong when your blood sugar goes whackadoodle on you.

A quick reminder from earlier in the book: the three ketone bodies are acetone (measured in the breath), beta-hydroxybutyrate or BHB (measured in the blood), and acetoacetate (measured in the urine).

BLOOD SUGAR IMBALANCES AND THE EFFECTS ON THE BODY

Let's face it—people love their sugary, carbohydrate-based foods. Cakes, pies, candy, soda, and other similar items dominate the "food" supply, and these things are highly addictive. When Jimmy gave up drinking sixteen cans of soda and eating whole boxes of snack cakes in 2004, it was like watching a meth addict detox from his drug of choice. We know that the same biochemical pathways in the brain that make people addicted to drugs also lead them to become addicted to (and have withdrawal symptoms from) sugar and carbohydrates. Even though sugar and carbohydrates aren't illegal drugs, we can't ignore the serious health effects on the body from blood sugar levels going up and down all day long. This section describes fifteen of the most prevalent problems that consistently elevated blood sugar levels can lead to.

NUTRIENT DEFICIENCIES

Because high blood sugar levels prevent nutrients from being absorbed through the small intestine (which is where the nutrients get dispersed into the rest of the body), your body might become deficient in key nutrients such as vitamin D, vitamin C, calcium, magnesium, and chromium. Some people might argue that our ancestors consumed sugary foods and seemingly did just fine. That's true because they ate the *whole-food* versions, like sugarcane, which included all the various vitamins, minerals, enzymes, and other nutrients that the body metabolizes well. These days, those nutrients are stripped from the sugar that we consume, and our blood sugar levels respond negatively.[3]

FLUCTUATING ENERGY LEVELS

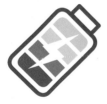

If you work in an office building with lots of other people, then you likely see a steady stream of zombies lurching toward the snack machine a few hours after you get to work or after lunch. Those people likely eat a high-sugar breakfast or lunch and need a boost of energy because their blood sugar spikes and then crashes. This is the ruthless roller-coaster ride that so many people go on every single day, and they never figure out why they feel so sluggish.

WEAKENING OF THE ORGANS AND BLOOD VESSELS

When we look back over Christine's health history, we can see that this is one of the major reasons why her eyesight progressively worsened year after year until she started eating a real food–based ketogenic diet. The blood vessels of her eyes were damaged by chronically high and fluctuating blood sugar levels. The vessels were hardening, so blood flow to them was far less than optimal. This is why so many diabetics have vision issues that, in some cases, eventually lead to blindness.

Poor blood flow to the organs and various parts of the body is a side effect of elevated blood sugar levels, and it explains why many people with diabetes need to have limbs amputated. Blood flow to those body parts becomes so restricted that the limbs, in essence, die through a process known as *glycation* (yes, another *G* word that's extremely important to understand). When blood glucose is elevated, especially as a result of sugar consumption, it quickly reacts with proteins to make them sticky and unusable by the body's cells for structure and communication. These glycated proteins (also known as advanced glycation end products, or AGEs) begin to harden, which is why a hardening of the arteries, joints, organ tissues, and cell membranes happens, too. When the arteries harden, blood flow becomes constricted, which can lead to a heart attack or other cardiovascular issue. See, it's not the fat in your diet that makes that happen; it's the sugary carbs.

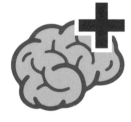

COMPROMISED BRAIN HEALTH

It's not just the blood flow to your limbs that's affected. Elevated blood sugar levels also directly impact the blood vessels in the brain by restricting blood flow. This can lead to a decline in cognitive function, dementia, Alzheimer's disease (which is also known as type 3 diabetes), depression, and other mood and mental health disorders.

HORMONAL IMBALANCES

Elevated cortisol levels lead to high blood sugar levels, which can alter the normal production of hormones. High blood sugar levels also cause imbalances in the pituitary gland, which is responsible for producing a lot of hormones that trigger the glands of the endocrine system to produce other hormones. An example is thyroid-stimulating hormone (TSH), which triggers the thyroid to produce thyroxine (T4), which gets converted to triiodothyronine (T3). T3 is what regulates the body's metabolism, and we see lower levels of T3 when blood sugar levels and cortisol levels are elevated. You'll learn more about TSH and other hormones in Chapter 12.

DETERIORATION OF THE ADRENAL GLANDS

When blood sugar levels remain high, the adrenal glands, which help regulate blood sugar, wear out. The adrenal glands are the glands that produce cortisol, which is one of the hormones that helps us deal with stress. Consistently high blood sugar levels lead to chronically elevated cortisol, which puts us in a constant state of stress. Because the adrenal glands place a priority on dealing with stress (blood sugar regulation being one indicator of stress) over all other functions, they work overtime when the body is in a constant state of stress, which wears them out. When the adrenal glands are worn out, blood sugar is elevated, which in turn raises cortisol and causes a deficit in sex hormones. For example, a reduction in estrogen production is common, which leads to hot flashes in menopausal women.

OVERTIME FOR THE LIVER

The liver is responsible for performing more than 500 functions in the body, one of which is blood sugar regulation. When blood sugar levels are consistently high, the liver might have difficulty converting glycogen back to glucose (glycogenolysis) and converting fats and proteins to glucose (gluconeogenesis). If the liver gets tired from trying to regulate blood sugar all the time, the other functions are compromised. A key function that might suffer is detoxification.

UNRESPONSIVENESS OF THE BETA CELLS OF THE PANCREAS

Riding the blood sugar roller coaster eventually tires the pancreas so that it's unable to produce enough insulin to deal with the blood sugar spikes. It's the beta cells of the pancreas that produce insulin. Consistently high blood sugar levels mean an increase in insulin production. When this happens, the insulin receptor on cells becomes unresponsive to the insulin production, so the pancreas has to pump out more insulin to have the same effect. As a result, the beta cells of the pancreas begin to wear out and eventually quit working.

NONREACTIVE HYPOGLYCEMIA

Nonreactive hypoglycemia happens mainly in type 1 and type 2 diabetics when blood sugar drops below 60 mg/dL for any reason, not just consuming food. The cause could be stress, illness (especially one that affects the liver, heart, or kidneys), pregnancy, or medications.

REACTIVE HYPOGLYCEMIA

Hypoglycemia occurs when blood sugar levels drop below baseline postprandial (after eating) and when blood sugars are 60 mg/dL or 90 mg/dL and lower with symptoms. A person can experience fatigue, trouble sleeping, mood disorders like depression, infertility, and weight gain. Often people suffering from hypoglycemia crave sweets, become irritable if they skip a meal, get jittery or shaky, have blurred vision or memory problems, or feel light-headed.

HYPERGLYCEMIA

Hyperglycemia is when an excessive amount of sugar in the blood (most likely from a high carbohydrate intake) raises blood sugar levels way too high. When you eat a meal, the most you want to see your blood sugar rise is about 10 to 20 points above baseline (the level before you eat). Hyperglycemia occurs when fasting blood sugar levels reach 130 mg/dL.

INSULIN RESISTANCE (PREDIABETES)

When the body becomes unresponsive to insulin, a person can have many problems, such as difficulty losing weight, fatigue, trouble remembering things, wounds that heal slowly, joint pain or other joint-related problems, thyroid problems, infertility, and mood disorders like depression. People with insulin resistance often crave sweets, which is why someone might want dessert after a meal.

Insulin resistance is a big cause of hormonal imbalances that manifest in many different ways. In women, they can manifest as polycystic ovarian syndrome (PCOS), irregular periods, acne, mood swings, infertility, and hair loss. In men, insulin resistance can manifest as a reduction in progesterone levels (progesterone helps protect the prostate) and an increase in aromatization, which is the conversion of testosterone to estrogen.

METABOLIC SYNDROME

Similar to insulin resistance, metabolic syndrome is where cells have become so unresponsive to insulin that a whole host of cardiometabolic health markers are negatively affected, such as high triglycerides, low HDL cholesterol, high blood pressure, elevated blood sugar, and excess belly fat. A person has insulin resistance at this point, but it isn't classified as diabetes.

TYPE 2 DIABETES

In type 2 diabetes, there's a loss of most of the beta cell function of the pancreas as a result of a need for high insulin output due to a high-carbohydrate diet or stress. Someone with type 2 diabetes has at least one blood sugar reading higher than 200 mg/dL in a twenty-four-hour period because the cells of the body have become unresponsive to insulin.

TYPE 1 DIABETES

The development of type 1 diabetes is the result of a virus or an autoimmune condition, but it can even happen if someone with type 2 diabetes doesn't get blood sugar levels under control. In type 1 diabetes, all beta cell function is gone, so the pancreas is no longer able to make insulin. A person with type 1 diabetes has to take insulin for the rest of his or her life. Eating keto allows them to take less insulin than if they consume a higher-carbohydrate diet. (The insulin would be used merely to cover the ill effects of their dietary choices.)

THE DIABETES CRISIS

Diabetes has become a major public health crisis, according to the latest U.S. Centers for Disease Control statistics.[4] One out of every five dollars spent on healthcare in the United States goes toward managing either type 1 or type 2 diabetes. It is estimated that nearly 31 million people in the U.S. alone—almost one in ten—have diabetes. According to the World Health Organization, that number worldwide is 422 million as of 2014.[5] The greatest increase in diabetes has been taking place in lower-income countries where carbohydrates are a mainstay of the diet. Diabetes is the seventh leading cause of death in the United States, with more than a quarter-million casualties in 2015 alone.

The illustration below shows the slow progression over decades of insulin resistance that eventually leads to type 2 diabetes—and, if nothing changes, eventually type 1 diabetes. The numbers on the illustration show how fasting insulin levels keep getting higher and higher until beta cell function is nearly or completely burned out.

FASTING TWO-HOUR SERUM INSULIN LEVELS IN INSULIN RESISTANCE STAGING
THIS CAN BE REVERSED IN 18–24 MONTHS WITH A KETOGENIC LIFESTYLE

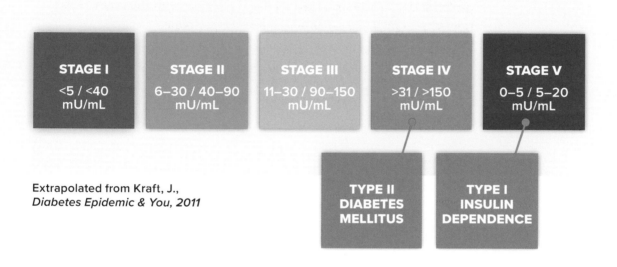

STAGE I	STAGE II	STAGE III	STAGE IV	STAGE V
<5 / <40 mU/mL	6–30 / 40–90 mU/mL	11–30 / 90–150 mU/mL	>31 / >150 mU/mL	0–5 / 5–20 mU/mL

TYPE II DIABETES MELLITUS

TYPE I INSULIN DEPENDENCE

Extrapolated from Kraft, J.,
Diabetes Epidemic & You, 2011

GLUCAGON RESISTANCE

Earlier in the chapter, we discussed how the hormone glucagon helps raise blood sugar to ensure it doesn't go too low into the range of hypoglycemia. Glucagon is what helps raise blood sugar levels between meals and even after the insulin response to food lowers blood sugar. Glucagon resistance is a condition that's just now getting some attention in health circles. Glucagon resistance happens when the alpha cells of the pancreas get worn out and can no longer produce adequate amounts of glucagon. We theorize that Jimmy has this condition because when he eats a meal—even a ketogenic meal—he has a hypoglycemic response, which indicates glucagon is not helping to bring his blood sugar back into normal range. Jimmy has discussed this topic on his show *The KetoHackingMD* podcast (www.ketohackingmd.com).

IMPACT OF BLOOD SUGAR LEVELS ON SPECIFIC SYSTEMS OF THE BODY

Most people think that controlling blood sugar is something only people with diabetes need to be concerned about. However, as we explain in this section, blood sugar affects all of us in ways that you may or may not have thought about before. Maintaining normal blood sugar levels isn't just about controlling diabetes. It's about controlling your health. Uncontrolled blood sugar leads to a whole cascade of undesirable responses in the body. So let's take a look at just a few of the specific systems in the body that are directly impacted by your blood sugar.

BLOOD SUGAR AND ENDOCRINE FUNCTION

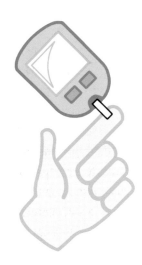

A diet high in sugar and processed carbohydrates is the main culprit in endocrine function getting messed up. Normal blood sugar regulation is needed for the endocrine system to work properly. If blood sugar is out of sorts, the hormone balance in the body will most likely be out of balance as well. This is because elevated blood sugar stresses the liver, which is responsible for deactivating hormones that are in excess or no longer functional. These hormones have to be broken down, conjugated, and removed from the body. Elevated cortisol levels because of high sugar and processed carbohydrate intake decrease the effectiveness of the liver pathways that perform the conjugation.

The pancreas also is affected by blood sugar fluctuation. When cortisol levels are elevated, insulin receptors on cells don't respond adequately to insulin. This puts a strain on the pancreas to secrete more insulin to transport glucose into the cells, which leads to high insulin levels and all the adverse effects that come along with it. Because adrenal function is favored over reproduction, metabolic rate, and other endocrine function, if the adrenal glands need more nutrients or hormonal precursors to function, they "steal" those nutrients and hormonal precursors from the other organs in the endocrine system. If more cortisol is still needed, the gonads may release pregnenolone to help make more cortisol, but this depletes sex hormone reserves.

NOTE FROM CHRISTINE

Proper adrenal function is an issue I've dealt with over the years, and I'm still working to heal my adrenal glands. The adrenal glands produce estrogen before a girl goes into puberty, then the ovaries kick in and start producing the estrogen. Once a woman starts to go through menopause, the job of creating estrogen goes back to the adrenal glands. As I mentioned in my story in the Introduction, I had to have a total hysterectomy when I was forty-four. Consequently, I went into what is called surgical menopause; without ovaries to produce estrogen, my body gave the job back to my adrenal glands. A week after my hysterectomy, I started having horrible hot flashes, and a lot of them . . . twenty-five-plus a day! I was having hot flashes because my adrenals were worn out from so many years of eating a bad diet before I started keto. The chronic stress I was under (I'm like my mother in that I worry a lot, and I have a bit of OCD) also contributed to the problem. Having an autoimmune condition doesn't help, either, because of the effects autoimmune conditions can have on blood sugar. It takes many years for stressed-out adrenal glands to heal, but I'm getting there.

BLOOD SUGAR AND IMMUNE FUNCTION

Too often we are stressed out. Stress has many effects on the body. An organ that's significantly affected by stress is the adrenal glands. These are known as an "emergency" organ, meaning they play a big part in dealing with stress, whether short-lived or prolonged. When the adrenals fire and release cortisol, the body goes into fight-or-flight mode. Cortisol, which is a hormone produced by the adrenal glands, plays a big part in how the immune system behaves. So when the adrenal glands respond to stress by releasing cortisol, your immune system is affected. If your cortisol levels are too high, the result is a depression of lymphocytes (white blood cells) and diminished salivary immunoglobulin A, or SIgA, levels (antibodies that help fight infection and play a role in allergic reactions). When your cortisol levels are too low, your immune system can become too active, which increases inflammation in the body and can lead to autoimmunity.

The immune system is depressed when blood sugar levels are consistently high because the high blood sugar levels reduce white blood cell activity. This is because minerals that are important for healthy immune function get depleted when someone eats a diet high in sugar and processed carbohydrates. Zinc is a prime example of a mineral that is easily depleted, and zinc is critical to a healthy immune system.

BLOOD SUGAR AND CARDIOVASCULAR HEALTH

Your cardiovascular health can be affected by consistently high blood sugar or blood sugar imbalances because the blood sugar imbalances lead to too much cortisol production. As we previously mentioned, the adrenal glands are an "emergency" organ. Consistently high blood sugar puts our bodies in a state of emergency, causing the adrenal glands to release tons of cortisol. Consistently high cortisol levels can lead to insulin resistance, which affects how well the body can absorb and use the minerals we take in that are so necessary for heart health.

Remember the prostaglandins we talked about in Chapter 4? Well, excess insulin production blocks the prostaglandin 1 (PG1) pathway, which helps control inflammation in the body and helps prevent heart disease. Excess insulin also is very abrasive to the arteries. When irritation occurs, cholesterol is released to go to the site of the irritation and patch it up. If this happens often enough, the artery can become clogged, which increases the chances of heart attack and heart disease in general.

BLOOD SUGAR AND DETOXIFICATION

Even detoxification of the body can be negatively affected if both blood sugar levels and cortisol levels are elevated for long periods because both stress the liver. Blood sugar imbalances also deplete the body of the B vitamins. Vitamin B2 plays a big part in phase 1 detoxification. Vitamin B6 is necessary for all liver enzyme functions and neurotransmitter synthesis (epinephrine and serotonin).

Blood sugar levels that remain consistently high cause a buildup of free radicals. They also put the body in a general catabolic state, which robs the body of nutrients it needs to detoxify properly.

HOW TO TELL THE DIFFERENCE BETWEEN A SUGAR BURNER AND A FAT BURNER

We explained earlier in this chapter that the body is always burning sugar and fat at the same time. Whether you're a sugar burner or a fat burner is determined by the thing the body primarily uses as fuel. A sugar burner uses more glucose for fuel, and a fat burner uses more fat for fuel. You're probably thinking, "That's great and all, but I want to be able to tell if my body is burning more sugar or more fat. How do I do that?" Well, we have some information that we think will help. The following table lists the differences between sugar burners and fat burners.

A SUGAR BURNER...	A FAT BURNER...
Can't effectively access stored fat for energy	Burns stored body fat for energy throughout the day
Can't effectively access dietary fat for energy	Can effectively oxidize fat for energy
Depends on a quick-burning source of energy	Has plenty of energy on hand
Burns through glycogen fairly quickly during exercise	Can rely more on fat for energy during exercise, sparing glycogen for when it's needed
Gets hungry really quickly after meals	Has sustained energy between meals

FOODS TO AID IN BLOOD SUGAR REGULATION

- **Almonds** contain high levels of manganese, which aids in blood sugar regulation. Almonds also contain arginine, which plays an important role in promoting the secretion of insulin.

- **Asparagus** contains high levels of potassium, which is needed for the conversion of blood glucose to glycogen.

- **Chili peppers** contain high levels of vitamin A, which plays a role in adrenal hormone production and activity.

- **Cinnamon** helps manage blood sugar because it acts as an insulin substitute by increasing the uptake of glucose by cells and stimulates glycogen synthesis.

- **Collard greens** and **kale** contain high levels of vitamin A, which aids in adrenal hormone production and activity. **Onions** contain high levels of chromium, which functions in a critical enzyme system called the *glucose tolerance factor,* which is involved in blood sugar regulation. Having adequate levels of chromium in the diet can help ward off insulin resistance.

- **Dandelion root** contains high levels of vitamin A, which plays a role in adrenal hormone production and activity. It also contains good amounts of vitamin B6 (pyridoxine), which is involved in creating body proteins and chemical transmitters and helps maintain hormone balance. Another vitamin it contains is B1 (thiamine), which helps with carbohydrate metabolism, energy production, and nerve cell function.

- **Eggs**, known as nature's perfect food, contain high levels of vitamin B3 (niacin), which aids in carbohydrate metabolism and adrenal hormone creation. When you get eggs from your own backyard chickens, they're even better!

- **Fish** also contains high levels of vitamin B3 (niacin) for carbohydrate metabolism and adrenal hormone production. Fish is a good source of vitamin B5 (pantothenic acid), which is important in the production of adrenal hormones as well as for the utilization of fats, carbohydrates, and potassium. Potassium is crucial for the conversion of blood sugar to glycogen.

- **Kombucha** is a fermented tea that contains vitamin B6 (pyridoxine), which helps maintain hormonal balance in the body. Kombucha also contains vitamin B1 (thiamine), which helps in carbohydrate metabolism, energy production, and nerve cell function.

- **Liver** contains high levels of chromium and good amounts of vitamin B3 (niacin), which helps in carbohydrate metabolism and adrenal hormone creation. Liver also contains vitamin B5 (pantothenic acid), which aids in the absorption of fats and carbohydrates.

- **Olive oil** contains high levels of vanadium, which aids in blood sugar metabolism.

- **Oysters** contain high levels of chromium.

- **Parsley** contains high levels of vanadium, which helps in blood sugar metabolism, as well as vitamin A, which helps in adrenal hormone production and activity.

- **Pecans** contain high levels of manganese, which aids in the management of blood sugar.

- **Raw milk** can provide some nutrients that are otherwise stripped out of pasteurized milk (pasteurization is the heating process that kills harmful bacteria but also the beneficial nutrients); however, raw milk isn't legal in every state. We live in South Carolina, and we're fortunate because we have access to raw milk. If you live in a state that allows you to purchase raw milk, it's a great source of vitamin B5 (pantothenic acid), which aids in the production of adrenal hormones and helps in the utilization of fats and carbohydrates. Find sources of raw milk at www.realmilk.com/real-milk-finder.

- **Turmeric** contains curcumin, which aids the liver in keeping blood sugar in check and improves the pancreas' ability to make insulin. Turmeric also slows the metabolism of carbohydrates after meals.

TIPS FOR GOOD BLOOD SUGAR REGULATION

A true food allergy is related only to foods that are protein based. Sensitivities to any type of food can occur.

Now that you know more than you thought you would ever know about blood sugar regulation and the importance of keeping your blood sugar steady, here are some things you can do to help keep your blood sugar under control. First, limit the amount of sugar and processed carbohydrates in your diet. Also, if you're eating a low-carb, moderate-protein, high-fat (ketogenic) diet, stay away from starchy vegetables and stick with nonstarchy vegetables and leafy greens. Some people can have an occasional sweet potato and not be kicked out of ketosis, but you have to test your blood sugar to see how certain foods affect your blood sugar to know for sure. (See page 49 for information on how to do a series of blood sugar tests to find out how a particular food affects your blood sugar.) Remember, you don't have to eat carbohydrates to produce glucose. Eat the foods listed earlier in this chapter that are good for blood sugar regulation and keep a good variety in your diet to help prevent food allergies or sensitivities from developing.

To help you figure out how much sugar is in a particular food, you can look up the carbohydrate content of that food, or, if you get something with a label on it, you can look at the carbohydrate total there. Carbohydrates, which all get turned to sugar in the body, are listed in grams. Take the number of carbohydrates in that food and divide by 4. The number you come up with is the number of teaspoons of sugar in that food. For example, a 12-ounce can of Pepsi has 41 grams of carbohydrates. When you divide that 41 grams by 4, you get more than 10 teaspoons of sugar in one small can!

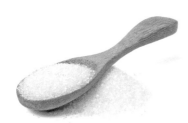

That's a *lot* of sugar in one little can! Now, guess how much sugar is floating around in the blood of someone with normal blood sugar levels. Would you believe it's just one single teaspoon? Yep, just one, and a sugary soda delivers more than ten times the amount of sugar that you would normally have in your bloodstream. It's a sobering thought, right? Jimmy used to drink sixteen cans of Coca-Cola a day, so that was more than 160 teaspoons of sugar each day just from soda! EEEK!

If diet alone doesn't fully resolve the issue, you can take supplements to aid in lowering blood sugar. Three good ones are chromium, berberine, and cinnamon. For example, you can add cinnamon to food or beverages to get more into your diet.

In today's world, it can be hard to reduce stress levels, but that's another thing you can try to help regulate your blood sugar. Meditation, yoga, or any activity you like can help reduce stress. As we previously mentioned, stress causes the adrenals to produce cortisol, which has a negative impact on blood sugar. Making sure you take time every day to get in a parasympathetic state will go a long way in helping to control blood sugar.

Adequate sleep is very important for blood sugar regulation. If we don't get enough sleep, then our blood sugar levels will probably be elevated the next day. Have you ever noticed that you have certain cravings the day after you get a poor night's sleep? That's not a coincidence; it's a result of blood sugar imbalances.

We need seven to nine hours of quality sleep each night. Some people doing a ketogenic lifestyle report that they find they need less sleep than they did before they changed their diets. We believe this is due to the better nutritional profile of eating a real, whole foods–based diet. To ensure good-quality sleep, don't eat too soon before going to bed. When you eat too close to bedtime, you might find you have a hard time getting to sleep because your body is spending so much energy on digesting the food you just ate. (Christine struggles with this.) Also, limit your exposure to blue light before going to bed. If we use our mobile devices at night, we make sure that the Night Shift feature is activated while we're using them. This feature blocks blue light by turning the screen an orangish color. You also can buy blue blocker glasses to wear.

You can find them online by typing *blue blocker glasses* in a search engine. If you wear prescription glasses, you can ask your optometrist about blue blocker prescription lenses. We also try to minimize household lights at night. Bright lights can mess up circadian rhythms. Getting out in the sunlight each day when you first wake up helps keep your circadian rhythm normal so you will start to produce melatonin at the proper times.

SLEEP STAGES

There are four stages of sleep, and we need to go through each of them to get the best benefits from resting. The first three stages vary from 5 to 15 minutes each. We start out awake, resting with our eyes closed. Having our eyes closed blocks out external stimuli that can keep us from getting to sleep. Then the first stage of sleep, which is known as *transitional sleep,* happens. We don't dream during this stage, and it's considered light sleep.

Stage 2 is known as *typical sleep*. This stage is also considered light sleep. People who take "power naps" or "cat naps" go through these first two stages. When it's time to get up, you want to awake from stage 2.

The next stage is the beginning of *deep sleep,* which is where physical healing and repair happen, and the brain filters data from the day. Muscles and tissues are repaired, growth and development are stimulated, the immune system gets a boost, and we build energy for the next day. It's harder to be woken from this stage of sleep. If you awake from this stage, you tend to feel groggy and sluggish.

Stage 4 is known as *R.E.M.*, or Rapid Eye Movement. Dreams occur during this stage of sleep. Mental and emotional healing and clearing happen, and our brains make connections emotionally and consolidate information that will be stored in long-term memory. You usually enter R.E.M. sleep around 90 minutes after going to sleep. Each R.E.M. stage can last up to one hour, and the length of the R.E.M. cycles grows longer as the night goes on. These different stages of sleep vary in duration depending on age.

Certain medications also have negative effects on blood sugar. For example, Jimmy's mom, Judiann, has had to take high-dose steroids for quite a while to treat myasthenia gravis, an autoimmune condition that affects the communication between nerves and muscles. The steroids have made it hard for her to lose weight even though she eats a ketogenic diet. The good news is that even though she hasn't lost as much weight as she wants to, she has seen other health benefits from the ketogenic lifestyle. For the longest time, Judiann hadn't been able to sleep in her bed because of pain and trouble breathing, but now that's changed and she sleeps in bed again. She also has experienced a reduction in the swelling in her body from excess fluid. She was diagnosed with type 2 diabetes in 2016 and went on the ketogenic diet in 2017.

In just a few short months, her A1c dropped from 7.5 to 5.5 and she came off all of her diabetes medications simply from eating the way we describe in *Real Food Keto.* Always consult with your doctor or another healthcare professional before making a change in your diet; that way he or she can monitor any medications you take.

Now that you better understand blood sugar and why it's so important to get it under control, Chapter 12 shifts our attention to something a little more complex but incredibly important in the health equation: the endocrine system. If you're applying the principles of nutritional therapy to your ketogenic diet as we recommend in this book, then knowing the ins and outs of the endocrine system and the hormonal connection to every aspect of your health is critical.

REAL FOOD KETO TAKEAWAYS FROM CHAPTER 11

- One of the biggest benefits of a ketogenic diet is the positive effect it has on balancing blood sugar.
- The liver, pancreas, and adrenal glands work in harmony to keep blood sugar under control.
- The hormones insulin, glucagon, cortisol, and epinephrine work together like instruments in a symphony to keep blood sugar within the normal range.
- The plethora of negative effects of blood sugar dysregulation cannot be ignored.
- There are five progressive stages of insulin resistance, which leads to type 2 diabetes—and eventually type 1 diabetes if nothing changes.
- Blood sugar imbalances affect the endocrine system, immune function, cardiovascular health, and detoxification.
- There are clear differences between being a sugar burner and being a fat burner.
- Certain foods that fit within a whole foods–based ketogenic lifestyle aid in controlling blood sugar levels.
- If you want to know about the effect of a food on your blood sugar levels, divide the total carbohydrates by 4; the result is the number of teaspoons of sugar in that food.

CHAPTER 12

Endocrine System— The Hormonal Connection

You're probably wondering why you need to know what the endocrine system is all about. When you've finished reading this chapter, it will be abundantly clear why understanding this system is a critical part of knowing how and why your body works the way it does and how it contributes to your pursuit of health. In short, the endocrine system is a set of glands that perform an array of functions in the body, including controlling and regulating metabolism, promoting growth and development of the body and tissues, facilitating sexual function and reproduction, aiding in sleep, stabilizing mood, and so much more.

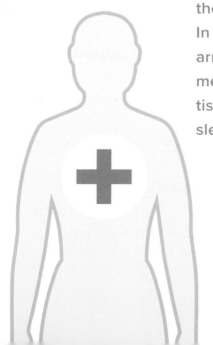

Because we're all bioindividual, each of us has specific needs. That's why there's no easy fix for any particular endocrine problem; it's very case dependent. But, as we've shared throughout this book, the basics of what you need to do to put your body in the best possible position for optimal health haven't changed: eat real food, control carbohydrate intake, moderate protein consumption, eat whole food–based fats to satiety, get your digestion in order, control blood sugar levels, maintain good levels of vitamins and minerals, and drink plenty of water for proper hydration. When any one of these is less than ideal, the way your endocrine system works is compromised.

The illustration of the endocrine system on the next page shows all the things it helps regulate in the body. As you can see, it's a pretty big deal.

What about having extra fat on your body? That can't possibly be healthy for you, right? Well, having a slight amount of excess fat can help cushion and shield your organs and joints from shocks. This is a great example of why it's not healthy to be stick thin. It's perfectly healthy to have a little weight on you.

A CLOSER LOOK AT THE ENDOCRINE GLANDS

The endocrine glands play so many amazing roles in the body that you really should know about all eleven of them—where they are, which hormones and fluids they secrete, and exactly what they do. Ready for a crash course on the entire endocrine system? Here goes!

ENDOCRINE SYSTEM

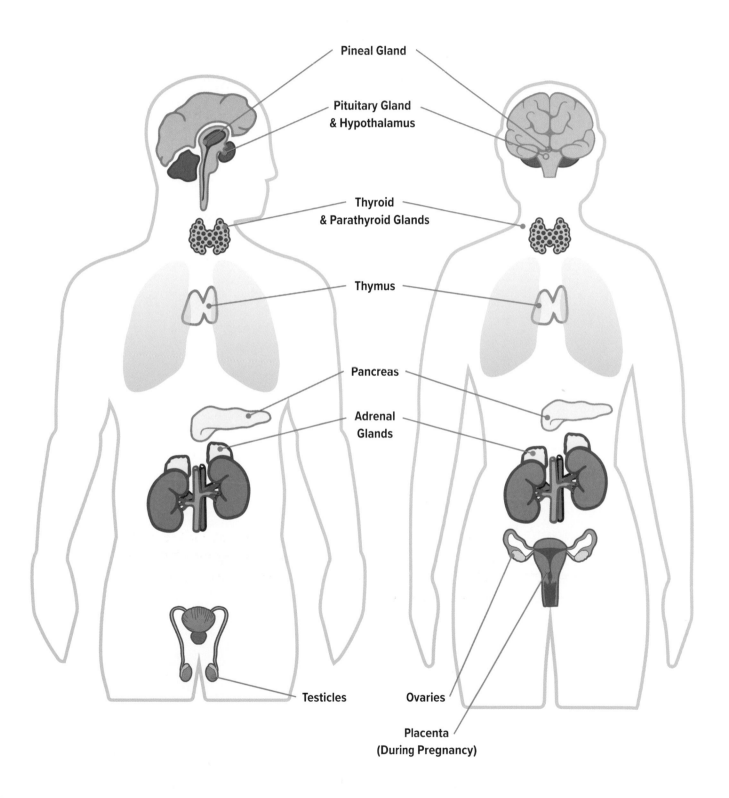

Pineal Gland

Pituitary Gland & Hypothalamus

Thyroid & Parathyroid Glands

Thymus

Pancreas

Adrenal Glands

Testicles

Ovaries

Placenta (During Pregnancy)

The hypothalamus is part of the brain, and it's the control and relay center of the endocrine system. It links the nervous system to the endocrine system through the pituitary gland and releases seven or eight hormones that control the pituitary gland. The hormones the hypothalamus releases include the following:

- *Thyrotropin-releasing hormone (TRH)* is a hormone that stimulates the release of thyrotropin (thyroid-stimulating hormone, or TSH) and prolactin from the pituitary gland.

- *Gonadotropin-releasing hormone (GnRH)* signals the pituitary gland to create two hormones: luteinizing hormone (LH) and follicle-stimulating hormone (FSH).

- *Growth hormone-releasing hormone (GHRH)* stimulates the pituitary gland to produce and release growth hormone into the bloodstream. Once growth hormone is released, it affects just about every tissue of the body to control metabolism and growth.

- *Corticotropin-releasing hormone (CRH)* stimulates the pituitary gland to produce adrenocorticotropic hormone (ACTH).

- *Somatostatin* regulates the secretion of hormones coming from the pituitary gland, including growth hormone and thyroid-stimulating hormone. It also inhibits the secretion of pancreatic hormones, which include glucagon and insulin.

- *Dopamine* functions as a neurotransmitter, which is a chemical released by neurons or nerve cells to send signals to other nerve cells. The brain has many distinct dopamine pathways; one of these pathways plays a big role in reward-motivated behavior.

The pituitary gland, also part of the brain, has been described as the "master gland" because it secretes certain key hormones that control other endocrine glands. The pituitary gland secretes these hormones:

- *Oxytocin* controls key aspects of the reproductive system and some aspects of human behavior.

- *Antidiuretic hormone (ADH)* tells your kidneys how much water to conserve and constantly regulates and balances the amount of water in your blood.

- *Prolactin (PRL)* helps women produce milk after childbirth; it's important to both male and female reproductive health.

- *Human growth hormone (HGH)* encourages growth in children and adolescents; helps regulate body composition, bodily fluids, and muscle and bone growth; helps regulate sugar and fat metabolism; and may help with heart function.

- *Thyroid-stimulating hormone (TSH)* or *thyrotropin* or *thyrotropic hormone (hTSH)* stimulates the thyroid gland to produce thyroxine (T4), which gets converted to triiodothyronine (T3). T3 directly affects the metabolism of just about every tissue in the body.

- *Adrenocorticotropic hormone (ACTH)* regulates levels of the steroid hormone cortisol, which is released by the adrenal glands.

- *Luteinizing hormone (LH)* triggers ovulation in women and stimulates the production of testosterone. It's chemically identical to interstitial cell-stimulating hormone (ICSH) in men.

- *Follicle-stimulating hormone (FSH)* plays different roles depending on gender. In women, this hormone stimulates the growth of follicles in the ovaries before the release of an egg from one follicle at ovulation, and it increases estradiol production. In men, FSH stimulates sperm production (a process known as *spermatogenesis*).

- *Melanin-stimulating hormone (MSH)* stimulates the release of melanin (a dark brown to black pigment in the hair, skin, and iris of the eye in people and animals that is responsible for the tanning of skin exposed to sunlight). It's located in the hypothalamus, and it suppresses appetite and contributes to sexual arousal.

- *Gonadotropins* include any of a group of hormones secreted by the pituitary gland that stimulate the activity of the gonads. Two primary examples are luteinizing hormone (LH) and follicle-stimulating hormone (FSH).

- *Interstitial cell-stimulating hormone (ICSH)* stimulates the production of testosterone by the testes in men and works alongside follicle-stimulating hormone (FSH). It's chemically identical to luteinizing hormone (LH) in women.

- *Intermedin* or *melanocyte-stimulating hormone (MSH)* regulates skin color.

The pineal gland in the brain is commonly referred to as the "third eye" because the Third Eye chakra in the Hindu belief system is located in the center of the forehead, near the pineal gland. It produces melatonin, which helps regulate the circadian rhythm.

The thyroid gland is located in the front of the neck just below the Adam's apple, and it's considered one of the major glands in the regulation of metabolism. It produces T4, which gets converted to T3 with the help of selenium. T3 controls basal metabolic rate. The thyroid also produces calcitonin, which is responsible for the uptake of calcium to the bones.

A WORD ON THE THYROID

Because the thyroid plays such an important role in controlling metabolism, I want to go into just a little more detail about it. T4 and T3, two of the hormones produced by the thyroid, have many functions in the body. The big one is controlling basal metabolic rate. But the thyroid hormones do so much more. They help control growth and development and the activity of the nervous system. You might not be aware that the thyroid hormones help stimulate the synthesis of protein and increase the use of glucose for adenosine triphosphate (ATP) production, which is the cells' usable form of energy. They also increase the chemical breakdown of fats (lipolysis), which we cover briefly in Chapter 11, and help reduce blood cholesterol levels by improving the excretion of cholesterol.

The thyroid is a very sensitive organ. Things like heavy metals, aspirin, food allergies, and endocrine imbalances can interfere with how well the thyroid functions. In addition, certain foods can block the conversion of T4 to T3. Those foods are known as *goitrogenic foods* and include cabbage, soy (which we try to stay away from on a ketogenic diet), broccoli, kale, millet (often called a grain, but it's actually a seed), cauliflower, rutabaga, turnips, and Brussels sprouts. You don't have to shun these foods—just eat them in smaller amounts.

The thyroid depends on iodine and tyrosine for good health, so seaweed (kombu, kelp, hiziki, wakame, arame), herbs like dulce and spirulina, haddock, cod, shrimp, yogurt, strawberries, and full-fat cheeses are great foods for supporting the thyroid. Selenium is necessary to convert T4 to its active form, T3; some selenium-containing foods are yellowfin tuna, halibut, sardines, grass-fed beef, beef liver, chicken, turkey, free-range eggs, chard, spinach, Brazil nuts, and sunflower seeds.

There are many disorders of the thyroid, and treating these disorders can be difficult. I have hypothyroidism (low thyroid function) and Hashimoto's thyroiditis. I suspected that I had the latter after dealing with several symptoms for a couple of years. For example, I tended to be cold, especially in my hands; my hair fell out in larger amounts than normal after I took a shower; I was gaining a little bit of weight; and I was tired a lot. At one of my annual physicals, I talked with my doctor about these symptoms, and he ran a thyroid panel. However (and this is important), he didn't run a *complete* thyroid panel; he just ran TSH, T3, and T4. When those numbers came back within normal ranges, he told me that nothing was wrong. Needless to say, I was discouraged.

I knew the symptoms I was experiencing weren't just in my head. So, after hearing different medical experts in the low-carb, high-fat, ketogenic world recommend a full thyroid panel, Jimmy and I decided I should have one run. We used a website called privatemdlabs. com. Use of this website is not legal in some states, but ours (South Carolina) happens to be one in which it is allowed. A full thyroid panel that includes the antibodies costs about $250. It's a little pricey, but if you're concerned that you might be having thyroid issues and you're not getting answers from your doctor, then you need this test. Even if the TSH, T3, and T4 numbers all come back from a typical thyroid panel within normal ranges (like mine did), you can still have thyroid issues.

When my full thyroid panel test results came back, they showed that my thyroid peroxidase antibodies were elevated. So I took the results to my doctor and asked him to prescribe Armour Thyroid. I don't often ask my doctor to do things like that, and I'm fortunate that he's always been willing to try anything I ask him to try. With the Armour Thyroid and a ketogenic diet, I have kept my antibodies down, and my symptoms are managed pretty well now.

Besides hypothyroidism and Hashimoto's thyroiditis, a person can develop other thyroid conditions, like hyperthyroidism (high thyroid function), goiter (an abnormal enlargement of the thyroid gland), nodules or cysts (growths or lumps on the thyroid), and Graves' disease (in which the thyroid gland produces too much thyroid hormone). Iodine deficiency is a common cause of these issues. Hashimoto's thyroiditis and Graves' disease are autoimmune conditions whereby the immune system attacks normal thyroid tissue.

NOTE: If you have either Hashimoto's thyroiditis or Graves' disease, supplementing with iodine is not a good idea because it can make things worse. Always consult with a healthcare provider before supplementing with iodine.

The parathyroid gland is located in the neck behind the thyroid and produces parathormone (PTH), which is associated with the growth of muscle and bone and the distribution of calcium and phosphate in the body.

The thymus lies across the trachea and bronchi in the upper thorax and produces thymosin. Thymosin activates the immune system by activating the T-cells and T-lymphocytes, which are white blood cells associated with antibody production.

The pancreas lies behind the stomach and produces insulin through the beta cells, which is responsible for the conversion of glucose to glycogen, the cellular uptake of glucose, and the conversion of excess glucose into fat. The pancreas also produces glucagon through the alpha cells, which is responsible for the conversion of glycogen to glucose.

The adrenal glands are on top of the kidneys and produce adrenaline, which prepares the body for fight-or-flight mode; noradrenaline, which has similar effects to adrenaline; and the corticosteroids, which include cortisol, cortisone, and corticosterone.

ADRENAL FATIGUE

James L. Wilson, ND, DC, PhD, notes in his book, *Adrenal Fatigue: The 21st Century Stress Syndrome,* that adrenal fatigue is something most people have dealt with or will deal with in their lifetime.[1] An estimated eight out of ten American adults suffer from some level of adrenal fatigue due to the high stress of modern living. Work, diet, environmental factors, and physical illness are the main sources of this stress.

Adrenal fatigue often goes undiagnosed because doctors fail to see the underlying cause of the symptoms and instead give patients unnecessary medication or chalk it up to aging. The sad reality is that mainstream medicine is ill-equipped to deal with adrenal fatigue until it becomes severe, as in the case of Addison's disease or Cushing's disease, both of which can be tested for and treated with a drug.

Interestingly, adrenal fatigue and breathing infections such as asthma, bronchitis, and pneumonia are interconnected. If a person gets an infection in the lungs, that infection makes them more likely to develop adrenal fatigue. Then the adrenal fatigue makes it more likely that the person will develop a breathing issue. It's a ruthless cycle that's difficult to break once it starts. The stress of being sick makes the adrenal glands work very hard, especially if the person has poorly developed lungs because of a genetic tendency or premature birth. As Christine shared in the Introduction, she was born premature, and her lungs never fully developed. As a result, she often had respiratory issues as a child and into adulthood, and we hypothesize that this is why she deals with adrenal fatigue today.

Another important thing to note about the adrenal glands is that while a woman goes through menopause, the adrenal glands may need extra support. Why? Before a girl hits puberty, the job of producing estrogen belongs to the adrenal glands. Beyond puberty, the job of producing estrogen is handed over to the ovaries. Then, when menopause begins, the ovaries return the job to the adrenal glands. If a woman has been consuming a high-carb diet or her body has been under stress for most of her life, by the time her adrenal glands have to start producing estrogen again, they're worn out and may not be able to produce sufficient amounts of estrogen. This is why some women experience bad hot flashes during this time.

The adrenal glands can heal, but it takes time, especially because, even if we follow a ketogenic diet, we still have to deal with everyday stressors from work, family, health issues, and environmental toxins. All these things can slow the healing process.

The ovaries are in the lower abdomen in women. They're responsible for producing estrogen, which is necessary for the breakdown of the uterine wall. They also produce progesterone, which builds up and maintains the uterine wall for embedding the fertilized egg. Progesterone is associated with body hair, breast enlargement, and the physical changes that occur during puberty.

The testes are located outside the pelvic cavity in men and produce testosterone, which is responsible for the development and function of the sex organs and is associated with body hair, muscle development, and voice changes.

The prostate is about the size of a walnut and sits between the bladder and the penis in men. It produces prostate-specific antigen (PSA), which helps keep the sperm in liquid form. Although women don't have a prostate, there are two small anatomical structures called Skene's glands (or paraurethral glands) that are sometimes referred to as the "female prostate."

THYROID ———————————→ **IODINE**
(seaweed, cod) and
TYROSINE (cheese, pork)

PROSTATE ———————————→ **ZINC**
(oysters, beef, lamb)

PITUITARY GLAND ———————————→ **MANGANESE**
(nuts, leafy green vegetables)

PANCREAS ———————————→ **CHROMIUM**
(broccoli, grass-fed beef)

GONADS ———————————→ **SELENIUM**
(testes or ovaries)
(Brazil nuts, meat)

HYPOTHALAMUS ———————————→ **CHROMIUM**
(brewer's yeast, pastured eggs)

ADRENAL GLANDS ———————————→ **COPPER**
(beef liver, dark chocolate)

PINEAL GLAND ———————————→ **IODINE**
(raw yogurt, raw milk) and
BORON (almonds, walnuts)

PARATHYROID ———————————→ **CALCIUM**
(cheese, other dairy, sardines, leafy green vegetables)

THYMUS ———————————→ **ZINC**
(spinach, pumpkin seeds, nuts)

THE HORMONES PRODUCED BY THE ENDOCRINE SYSTEM

Many people haven't heard of the endocrine system, but when you mention the word *hormones,* they think of testosterone, estrogen, and perhaps even insulin, the master hormone we've discussed in this book. But what are hormones, and why do the endocrine glands produce them? Hormones serve as regulatory substances that travel through the fluids in the tissues to help the body maintain normal cellular and tissue health. For example, insulin and glucagon work in tandem to regulate blood sugar levels so that you don't become hyperglycemic (high blood sugar) or hypoglycemic (low blood sugar).

There are two major classifications of hormones: *fat (lipid)-soluble* and *water-soluble.* Do those terms sound familiar? Well, in Chapter 9, we tell you that vitamins A, D, E, and K are fat-soluble, and that the rest of the vitamins are water-soluble. Hormones are either fat-soluble or water-soluble, too.

Fat-soluble hormones dissolve in fat (that is, they are *lipophilic*). They consist of steroid hormones, which come from cholesterol (see, this is why you don't want to lower your cholesterol!), and thyroid hormones, which come from iodine atoms and tyrosine. These fat-soluble hormones easily pass through the target cell membrane to act directly on the cell because they bind directly to the receptors inside the cell.

FAT-SOLUBLE HORMONES

Aldosterone is a hormone produced by the adrenal glands. If our bodies can't produce aldosterone, the likely result is electrolyte imbalances, because aldosterone helps prevent the body from dumping salt through urination.

Cortisol is a hormone produced by the adrenal cortex. It helps control blood sugar in emergency situations or when the liver isn't working at its best.

Dehydroepiandrosterone is a weak hormone produced by the adrenal glands that helps with antiaging properties. It also aids in athletic performance and prevents osteoporosis.

Estradiol is a major estrogen produced in the ovaries.

Estriol is a weak estrogen and a minor female sex hormone.

Progesterone is a hormone that stimulates the uterus to prepare for pregnancy.

Testosterone is mainly produced in men by the testes. It stimulates the development of male secondary sexual characteristics. It also can be produced by the ovaries and adrenal cortex.

Triiodothyronine (T3) and **thyroxine** (T4) are tyrosine-based thyroid hormones whose primary responsibility is the regulation of metabolism. T3 is more potent than T4.

Water-soluble *(hydrophilic)* hormones dissolve in water and are developed from amino acids. Unlike fat-soluble hormones, water-soluble hormones can't pass through the target cell membrane (because it's made of fat), but they do affect the target cell by binding to receptors on the surface of that cell. The water-soluble hormones include amines, peptides, and eicosanoids.

AMINES
- Dopamine[2]
- Histamine
- Phenylethylamine
- Serotonin
- Tryptamine
- Tyramine

PEPTIDES
- Angiotensin
- Endothelin
- Glucagon
- Glutathione
- Insulin[3]
- Oxytocin
- Somatostatin

EICOSANOIDS

- *Leukotrienes* are a family of lipid mediators that play a key role in the pathogenesis of inflammation. They're synthesized in the leukocytes from arachidonic acid (AA) via the actions of 5-lipoxygenase (5-LO). Leukotrienes are divided into two classes: LTB4 and cysteinyl LTs (CysLTs).[6]

- *Prostaglandins* are one of many types of hormone-like substances that participate in a wide range of body functions, such as contraction and relaxation of smooth muscle, dilation and constriction of blood vessels, control of blood pressure, and modulation of inflammation.[4]

- *Thromboxane* is a substance made by platelets that causes blood clotting and constriction of blood vessels. It also encourages platelet aggregation. There are two thromboxanes: A2 and B2.[5]

PROBLEMS THAT UPSET THE ENDOCRINE SYSTEM

The endocrine system is a complex web of relationships. If one aspect of the endocrine system gets out of balance, a cascading effect occurs that will disrupt the entire endocrine system.

You know term *bioindividuality* that we have used throughout this book? Well, each person has different endocrine issues. It's important to look at all the individual parts of the endocrine system as well as view the endocrine system as a whole.

One important thing to realize is that hormonal imbalances cannot be addressed until blood sugar is under control. This means getting blood sugar back within normal ranges (or as close to it as possible) and controlling blood sugar swings (hypoglycemia and hyperglycemia). Blood sugar stability is just one of the foundations that need to be addressed in order to ensure that the endocrine system is working at its best.

Here are some other things that need to be working right for the endocrine system to be able to do its job effectively.

DIGESTION

We hammer on this point again and again throughout this book, but proper stomach acid production is necessary for the body to absorb the nutrients you consume. Our bodies and the endocrine system can make the hormones we need to function well from the food we consume only if there's enough stomach acid to digest and break down proteins. We also need adequate digestive enzymes and bile production to break down fats and other food components. Always be mindful of this; it's one of the major takeaways from *Real Food Keto*.

FATTY ACIDS

Taking in proper amounts of essential fatty acids (EFAs), along with the other healthy fats we describe in this book, is necessary to help the endocrine system work at its best because these fats are critical to the endocrine system's performance. The body can't make hormones without adequate fat in the diet because fat comprises cell membranes. The endocrine factories are inside the cells, and phospholipids (lipids containing a phosphate group) control what comes into and goes out of the cell. Also, because cell membranes are made of fat, fat is required to ensure that cellular-hormonal communication takes place.

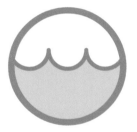

WATER

When you drink enough water, your body can effectively transport hormones to where they need to go. Proper hydration improves the viscosity of the blood and interstitial fluids so that they don't become too thick. Additionally, adequate water intake combined with exercise helps keep the lymphatic system running.

THE NEGATIVE EFFECTS OF AN UNHEALTHY ENDOCRINE SYSTEM

Perhaps you're getting a clearer picture of why the endocrine system is at the heart of everything we've been sharing in *Real Food Keto*. If any one thing in your diet or lifestyle is outside the ideal range for being healthy, then you face the consequences: your endocrine glands working less well than they are supposed to. It's a delicate balancing act that far too many people ignore; instead, they blame genetics, feign ignorance, and adopt a "you only live once" kind of attitude. Well, we want you to start caring, and we want you to know exactly how not taking proper care of your body is simply not an option. The following sections explain the various negative effects that are a direct result of the endocrine system being out of whack.

WEIGHT GAIN

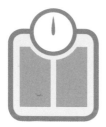

In a person who has adrenal gland problems brought on by prolonged stress, the stress hormone cortisol is released and begins storing fat around the vital organs in the midsection (a state known as abdominal obesity). Someone with thyroid issues also tends to carry extra weight because the thyroid controls the metabolism in the cells. Women who have problems with their ovaries gain weight in their hips and the lower part of their stomach. Those suffering from liver problems carry weight in their upper body and have thin legs.

BLOOD SUGAR

Here is where being on a low-carb, high-fat, ketogenic diet shines. If blood sugar is going up and down throughout the day because of poor nutritional and lifestyle choices, then endocrine function and hormonal balance suffer. The pancreas, liver, and adrenal glands work together to help keep blood sugar levels normalized. When one of them (particularly the adrenals or liver) gets worn out due to poor blood sugar control, then all endocrine functions become compromised, which results in the entire endocrine system getting out of sorts and not running as efficiently as it should.

ADRENAL GLANDS

The function of the liver in the endocrine system is to deactivate hormones where there are sufficient amounts and to remove them from the body. If the adrenal glands are pumping out too much cortisol as a result of a poor diet or stress, then the liver pathway that's necessary for breaking down these hormones loses its effectiveness, resulting in hormonal imbalances. Additionally, high cortisol levels can push the insulin receptors on cells toward insulin resistance, causing you to start experiencing all the negative effects that come from chronically elevated insulin. Finally, when the body is under stress, the adrenal glands place top priority on responding to that stress while sacrificing responses to reproduction, metabolic rate, and other endocrine functions; consequently, the adrenal glands "steal" nutrients and other hormonal precursors that the rest of the endocrine system needs to function optimally. The result is endocrine system disruption, and it ain't good.

THE PERILS OF THE CORTISOL TSUNAMI

People generally know that high cortisol levels brought on by stress are not healthy, but most people have no clue why. Let us explain. The release of cortisol is a completely natural reaction by the body. However, it becomes a problem when too much cortisol is released over a sustained period, causing it to overstay its welcome, wreaking havoc on the entire endocrine system by preventing the glands from releasing enough hormones to do what the body needs to do with them.

Before long, adrenal exhaustion sets in, blood sugar goes whackadoodle, the body becomes more insulin resistant, and obesity and insulin-related health issues set in with a vengeance. One function of the adrenal glands is to produce a steroid hormone called pregnenolone, which is a precursor to sex hormones like progesterone, estrogen, and testosterone, and other hormones like aldosterone and cortisol. Why should you care? When a person is under chronic stress, more cortisol is needed so

the cortisol pathway "steals" pregnenolone from sex hormone pathways and causes an imbalance in the sex hormones that can lead to a man becoming estrogen dominant (with symptoms such as man boobs, low libido, and loss of muscle mass) and a woman becoming testosterone dominant (with symptoms like a deeper voice, facial hair, and thinning hair). As if all that were not bad enough, elevated cortisol levels affect the thyroid. High cortisol decreases the production of T3, the active thyroid hormone, and T3 plays a role in nearly every organ of the body by acting as a modulator of cell function. If T3 production is low because of high cortisol from stress or a bad diet, then oxygen use and basal metabolic rate, cellular metabolism, body growth and development, the activity of the nervous system, and cholesterol excretion (which reduces blood cholesterol levels) are inhibited.

Now do you see why reducing cortisol is so important? The domino effect is difficult to stop.

MINERALS

If hormone production from the endocrine system isn't working properly, then managing mineral levels in the body to get the benefits that they provide is next to impossible. Parathyroid hormone helps regulate calcium levels. The thyroid hormone prevents the loss of calcium in the bones and decreases calcium levels in the blood (critical for preventing cardiovascular disease, among other things). Adrenal hormones keep electrolytes like sodium and potassium in the proper ratios in the body so that calcium functions correctly. Finally, estrogen prevents bone loss, progesterone builds new bone, and testosterone serves as a precursor to both estrogen and progesterone.

TIPS FOR SUPPORTING ENDOCRINE FUNCTION

We've shared some pretty sobering information in this chapter about a subject you probably never gave much thought to before, but there's hope in the midst of the gloom and doom—which is why you're reading this book, right? We have lots of easy-to-implement tips to help you support your endocrine function, and you'll start seeing improvements in your overall health as a result. (We've mentioned some of these things before, so by this point in the book, we might be sounding like a broken record.)

Get your digestion working properly by making sure you're producing enough stomach acid. Ask your doctor to run a Heidelberg Gastrotelemetry test to check the pH of your stomach. It's an easy test that provides you with the information you need to make sure you're producing enough stomach acid. Also, try to avoid drinking carbonated beverages with your meals; the phosphoric acid inhibits stomach acid production and directly affects how well the body absorbs and uses calcium. Remember, you can take HCl supplements and digestive enzymes to help with digestion, but you should consult with an NTP or another healthcare provider for assistance.

Next, consume enough healthy fats because they're absolutely necessary for proper hormone production. Make sure you're getting a healthy balance of the essential fatty acids—omega-3s and omega-6s—as well as saturated fats and even some omega-9 fats. Fat is necessary, especially to the fat-soluble hormones discussed earlier in this chapter, such as steroid hormones and thyroid hormones.

To help control your blood sugar, you should know which diet is best: a real foods–based low-carb, moderate-protein, high-fat, ketogenic diet! There are fantastic supplements you can take to normalize blood sugar levels, including berberine, chromium, and cinnamon, to name a few. When blood sugar is stable, the adrenal glands can do their job of making the hormones your body needs. Additionally, a good multivitamin with methylated folate (like the KetoEssentials Multivitamin from www.ketoliving.com) will shore up any potential deficiencies that could affect the endocrine system.

As for the foods you consume, make them whole foods as much as possible, and choose a wide variety of colors to maximize your exposure to the full complement of available nutrients. Only eat foods when they're in season (in most locales, strawberries don't grow in January, for example, so stop buying them at that time of year), and you'll help prevent food allergies or sensitivities from popping up.

Last but not least, drink enough water to stay properly hydrated and help your endocrine system function well. Remember, don't gulp down large quantities of water at once, because that forces your body to dump electrolytes. Sip it throughout the day by having a water bottle with you all the time. (Try keeping a water bottle by your side to remind you to drink.) Staying hydrated keeps your blood and interstitial fluids flowing well so that hormones can be transported effectively throughout your body. And now you know that that's a good thing!

Okay, enough about the endocrine system. We have one more chapter to share with you about a topic that's been completely misrepresented by well-meaning health influencers. Detoxification doesn't require juicing, drinking fruit smoothies, undertaking a fiber cleanse, or any of that stuff that our minds might associate with that word. The reality is something far different from those stereotypes.

REAL FOOD KETO TAKEAWAYS FROM CHAPTER 12

- The eleven endocrine glands produce the hormones that control every single aspect of how the body functions.

- Proper mineral intake is required for each endocrine gland to do what it's supposed to do.

- The endocrine glands produce fat-soluble hormones and water-soluble hormones.

- An unhealthy endocrine system can lead to weight gain, blood sugar dysregulation, adrenal gland imbalances, and more.

- Improving stomach acid production, eating healthy fats and a variety of real foods, controlling blood sugar, and drinking enough water can help to improve the health of the endocrine system.

CHAPTER 13

Detoxification to Eliminate What's Harming You

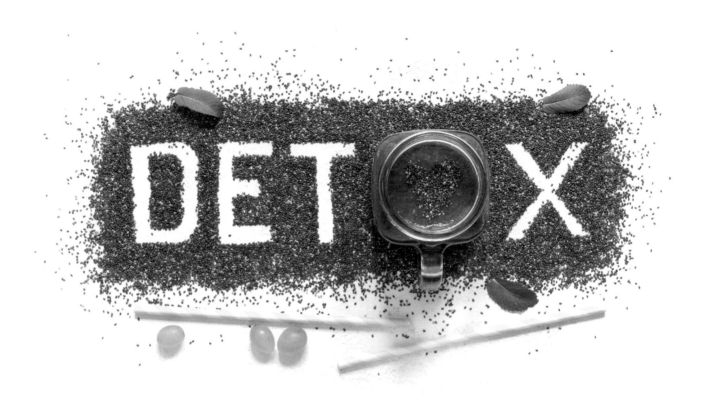

When you say the word *detox* or *detoxification,* the reactions you get are usually at one end or the other of the spectrum. Either you get someone who enthusiastically embraces it and dives right in, trying everything, or you get someone who rolls their eyes at all the marketing gimmicks that promise robust health or weight loss in some pill, shake, or juice. Let us be very clear: That's not the type of detoxification we're referring to in this book.

No matter where you stand on the subject of detoxification, the reality is that your body is detoxifying 24 hours a day, 7 days a week, 365 days a year, from the beginning of your life until the good Lord decides to take you home. But there are times when the process happens at an accelerated rate, which is what this chapter is about. Simply put, detoxification is the removal of waste and toxins from the body. Unfortunately, there are both good and bad ways of doing it. Having extra weight on the body might be a sign of toxins hiding in body fat, which protects the body from being harmed by them. There are various ways to get rid of that extra body fat that may or may not help you detoxify.

The priority of detoxification is to clear the elimination pathways so the body's natural detoxification process can occur and provide the benefits of getting rid of these toxins that harm you. In this modern age, toxins are literally all around us in our food, household products, and environment, so it's next to impossible to be completely toxin free. But there are ways to greatly reduce toxins so that your body can function well enough to make you healthy. Let's take a look at the history of various detoxification methods. You'll quickly see that this isn't some new fad.

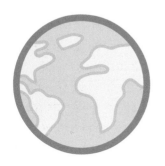

DETOXIFICATION THERAPIES

The history of detoxification is almost as old as the history of the world. Many of the therapeutic methods for doing a detox have been a dominant part of both health and religious culture. Let's explore a little more about the various types of detoxification traditions that are still in use today.

CULTURAL TRADITIONS

Detoxification has been practiced by many cultures throughout history.

AYURVEDA

The Ayurvedic (literally means "science of life") teaching, which originated in India more than 3,000 years ago, states that the reason we get sick is toxins in the body. It teaches that if disease is treated before the toxins have been removed from the body, the toxins will just be pushed deeper into the tissues of the body, and the problem will come again in the same form or in a different disease down the road.

There are two types of Ayurvedic treatments: elimination of toxins (called panchakarma) and the neutralization of toxins (called palliation). Ayurvedic teaching also states that if a person represses their emotions and doesn't deal with them in a healthy way, the emotions will cause an imbalance in the body that will lead to disease-causing toxins. Panchakarma involves physical elimination techniques that help to cleanse the body, mind, and emotions, including therapeutic vomiting to clear mucus in the lungs, laxatives to remove excess bile, medicated oil enemas for cleansing the colon, clearing nasal passages of excess phlegm, and bloodletting to clear toxins from and purify the blood. Palliation, on the other hand, includes fasting to stimulate digestion, exercising, sunbathing, and getting fresh air.

HIPPOCRATIC

The ancient Greeks developed the first principles of the scientific method for practicing medicine. Early techniques focused on bringing balance back to the Four Humors—blood, phlegm, yellow bile, and black bile. The techniques include enemas for cleansing the digestive tract, vomiting to clear the body of toxins that have accumulated, bloodletting to bring balance back to the Four Humors, massage to remove waste products from the muscles, bathing to purify and cleanse the body, fasting to balance bodily fluids, and counterirritation using an action to create mild inflammation in a localized area to alleviate pain in another part of the body.

NATIVE AMERICAN

Native American medicine involves various purification rituals. Smudging is when smoke from a protective herb like sage is waved around a person to eliminate negative energy that's causing sickness. Sweeping involves herbs being swept over a person's body to clean out bad spirits and invite good spirits to come in. Sweat lodges (similar to steam saunas) increase sweating to release physical, emotional, and spiritual toxins from the body. Some groups practice the Navajo sweat-emetic rite in which people sweat and vomit around a fire in a hut as they replenish their bodies with liquid herbs, and others fast to purify the body before ceremonial dances.

NATURAL HYGIENE

Natural Hygiene, which is also known as orthopathy, is a school of medical thought founded in the nineteenth century. This detoxification teaching involves four things to keep health optimal: diet, environment, activities, and psychology. Water fasting and plenty of rest also are considered parts of a healthy lifestyle. Fasting is considered one of the best ways for the body to heal itself naturally.

TRADITIONAL HERBAL MEDICINE

This detoxification philosophy, also known as botanical medicine or herbalism, first showed up in written texts as early as 2800 B.C. This philosophy teaches that the elimination pathways in the body need to keep functioning properly or an acute illness will lead to chronic disease. Thus, it encourages the use of mild herbal laxatives to help keep the bowels moving effectively, medicinal herbs to stimulate the liver (which helps in the detoxification process), mild diuretics to help move fluid and acid waste out of the body, lymphatics to drain excess lymph fluid, expectorants to clear congested airways, blood cleansers to clear various detoxification channels, diaphoresis to force perspiration, and heating therapy to bring on a therapeutic fever.

TRADITIONAL CHINESE MEDICINE

Acupuncture is the major detoxification technique of traditional Chinese medicine and has been practiced for more than 2,000 years. The primary goal of acupuncture is to restore and balance the flow of energy in and through the body.

RELIGIOUS TRADITIONS

Detoxification also is a component of a number of religions.

JUDAISM

The Jewish tradition of Shabbat (also known as the Sabbath) includes regular periods of fasting that involve abstaining from work, food, and drink from sunset on Friday until sunset on Saturday. The spiritual detoxification process also involves attending prayer services, engaging in fellowship with family and friends, reading the Torah, and resting. Many people are familiar with the two-day Jewish new-year celebration ritual known as Rosh Hashanah, which is the beginning of a ten-day period of repentance. The period concludes with Yom Kippur, which is a twenty-five-hour period of fasting and prayer. No eating, drinking, or working is allowed during this time of spiritual cleansing.

CHRISTIANITY

The Sabbath, Lent, and Advent often involve fasting. Similar to Judaism, Christianity teaches to rest on the seventh day because it is holy; no work is to be done. This comes from the Old Testament in Genesis 1 where God created the world in six days and rested on the seventh day. Lent is a six-week period of fasting, reflection, and repentance that begins on Ash Wednesday. During Lent, people prepare to celebrate the resurrection of Jesus Christ. Fasting can take many different forms during this time; it's not restricted to food. Advent is the four-week period before the celebration of Christmas. Orthodox Christianity calls for a forty-day fast from meat and dairy during this time.

If you're curious about fasting and want to learn more about it, Jimmy collaborated with a Toronto-based nephrologist named Jason Fung, MD, on a book called *The Complete Guide to Fasting.*[1] Make sure to consult with your physician or other healthcare provider before beginning a fasting regimen.

ISLAM

The tradition of Ramadan calls for fasting for twenty-nine or thirty days based on the crescent moon. From sunrise to sunset during this month, adult Muslims are not allowed to eat, drink, smoke, or have sex. It's supposed to be a time for reflection, repentance, and purification. Ramadan ends when the lunar cycle reaches the new moon phase. Another Muslim celebration is Ashura, which involves two days of fasting leading up to the celebration.

HINDUISM

Two celebrations that Hindus observe are Maha Shivaratri and Rama Navami. Maha Shivaratri is a festival of the new moon that starts with a twenty-four-hour fast. During this festival, people offer gifts to the god Shiva and break the fast at sunrise. Rama Navami is a festival that celebrates the birth of the god Rama; celebrants fast for different periods of time during the eight days leading up to the festival.

FASTING

Fasting has experienced a huge resurgence in popularity as a major health modality in recent years. When most people hear about fasting, they think of religious tradition or preparation for going into surgery. But fasting has some truly incredible healing and detoxification effects that hardly anyone ever thinks about. You're not starving yourself if you're making a proactive choice to go without eating for some time.

The body has a way of getting rid of old or damaged cells and making new ones, which is known as *autophagy.* It is a normal physiological process that helps maintain homeostasis or normal functioning by protein degradation and turnover of the destroyed cell organelles for new cell formation. During cellular stress, the process of autophagy is upscaled and increased. Fasting allows the number of toxins entering the body to be reduced so that there is not more damage to cells going on, and the body can clean out the old and damaged cells. This process helps the body to detoxify more efficiently.

Fasting also gives the gallbladder and liver a break from having to digest and break down foods and regulate blood sugar so much. This allows these organs to focus on the detoxification process.

Fasting might be as simple as skipping breakfast and pushing the first meal of the day to noon. If your last meal was at six o'clock the night before, then you fasted for eighteen hours. This is called *intermittent fasting*. Some people choose to eat every other day to fast, and that's called *alternate-day fasting*. Finally, for those people who are especially metabolically challenged and find it hard to lose weight and improve their health even with a healthy real food–based ketogenic diet, extended periods of fasting of a few days to a week might be necessary to get things moving again in the pursuit of health. Please consult with a physician before starting any fasting protocol, and keep learning about the science of this ever-evolving topic of fasting.

SHINTO

Believers perform a ritual rinsing of the mouth and washing of the hands before entering a shrine. The acts represent internal and external cleansing. They do this because purity is very important in this religion. One of the rituals involves a priest reciting prayers while passing a purification stick over the worshipper's head as a means of drawing out pollution from the worshipper.

BUDDHISM

Buddhism uses the detoxification method of meditation to help free the mind of emotions like passion, anger, jealousy, ignorance, and pride. Chanting also is used to help focus the mind and protect it from negative influences.

WHAT IS DETOXIFICATION, AND WHY IS IT NECESSARY?

Now that you understand the history of various detoxification methods that have been around for most of human civilization, let's take a look at what detoxification is and why you need to make it a priority in your health journey.

What is a *toxin*? The basic definition of a toxin is any substance that causes irritation or harm to the body, which even can include positive things that your body needs, such as water, vitamins, and minerals. Although these things are essential to our well-being, as we shared earlier in this book, they can be toxic when consumed in larger quantities than the body requires.

There are other toxins that we instinctively know are harmful, and they're everywhere today. It's extremely difficult to get away from them because we're exposed to them via air pollution, water pollution, chemicals in cleaning supplies, chemicals in hair and other beauty products, food additives, radiation, pesticides and herbicides, pharmaceutical and over-the-counter drugs, and even stress. That list merely scratches the surface of all the toxins we're exposed to daily. Just because these toxins are ubiquitous doesn't mean that we should give up on detoxifying. It's still worth pursuing for the sake of your health.

TOP FOODS CONTAINING HIGH LEVELS OF PESTICIDES

The following is a list of foods that contain the highest amounts of pesticides. Yes, we know—ewwww! Some of these foods aren't part of a ketogenic diet because they're too high in sugar, but others are acceptable when you're eating keto. The pesticide problem is why we decided several years ago to start growing a vegetable garden, which has since expanded to two gardens and a greenhouse. The effort of growing your own produce is worth it so you don't have to worry what toxins you're getting from foods like those listed here:

1. Strawberries
2. Bell peppers
3. Spinach
4. Cherries
5. Peaches
6. Cantaloupe
7. Celery
8. Apples
9. Apricots
10. Green beans
11. Grapes
12. Cucumbers

HOW DETOXIFICATION WORKS

Detoxification is a function that occurs primarily in the liver. There are two detoxification pathways, called Phase 1 detoxification (Oxidation) and Phase 2 detoxification (Conjugation).

Vitamins B2 (riboflavin) and B3 (niacin), magnesium, and an enzyme known as cytochrome P450 (which is produced by the adrenal glands) are necessary for Phase 1 detoxification. If a person has poor adrenal function, then Phase 1 detoxification is compromised. In Phase 1 detoxification, a toxic substance transforms into a less toxic or less harmful substance through oxidation, reduction, and hydrolysis. The by-product of this process is free radicals. If there are too many free radicals, the liver can be damaged. Antioxidants like vitamins C and E can help the body deal with the free radicals that are produced during Phase 1 detoxification.

Some toxins, however, are converted to a more harmful substance that Phase 2 detoxification needs to deal with. Methionine, cysteine, glutathione, sulfate, and glycine are necessary for aiding Phase 2 detoxification. In Phase 2 detoxification, the liver adds another substance to the toxin (cysteine, glycine, or a sulfur molecule). Adding these things makes the toxin or drug water-soluble so it can be excreted from the body. Have you ever had coffee and, after not having drunk much at all, you start to become jittery? That jitteriness is a sign that Phase 1 detoxification is compromised. If Phase 1 is compromised, then Phase 2 will be as well.

THE SYSTEMS INVOLVED IN DETOXIFICATION

Several systems are involved in detoxification. They include the cardiovascular system, lymphatic system, digestive system, urinary system, respiratory system, and skin. Did you know that the skin is the body's largest detoxification organ? Oh, yeah, there are so many nuggets of solid gold information in here that you'll be the center of attention at the office water cooler! Here is how each of these systems plays a part in the detoxification process.

THE DIGESTIVE SYSTEM

Several organs of the digestive system play a huge role in detoxification: the gallbladder, intestines, and liver. The intestines are a physical barrier that protects the rest of the body from substances that shouldn't be present. The good bacteria in the intestines help with removing toxic substances, which is one reason we need to make sure digestion is working correctly. Remember how we told you in Chapter 10 that our good gut bacteria can be harmed if digestion isn't working correctly? Well, if those good little buggers aren't there in proper amounts, then our intestines can't help our bodies detoxify properly.

In Chapter 11, we mention that the liver is responsible for more than 500 functions in the body. Cleansing the blood of toxins is one of those functions. Once the liver has cleansed the blood of toxins, the toxins move on to the gallbladder, and the toxins are removed from the body through the rest of the digestive tract before being excreted in feces.

You might have heard that it's not a good idea to eat too close to bedtime. We've heard many reasons for this, but the most common reason is that it can stall weight loss or cause weight gain. Although that explanation isn't completely accurate, there is a grain of truth behind it. You see, detoxification is a parasympathetic process, meaning the body has to be in a relaxed state for detoxification to happen. You tend to be in a parasympathetic state while you're sleeping, so your body has the best chance to detoxify and heal at night. Eating too close to when you go to sleep delays the detoxification process because the body always prioritizes digestion over detoxification. When you eat close to bedtime, your body is busy because it's focused on digesting the food you ate rather than getting immediately to the detoxification processes that help heal your body.

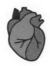

THE CARDIOVASCULAR SYSTEM

All the organs in the body are linked to the cardiovascular system by the blood. Because of the role it plays in our bodies, the blood is sensitive to toxin exposure. The blood delivers oxygen and nutrients to every part of the body while at the same time taking away waste. It works with the lymphatic system to help clear areas of the body that aid in detoxification and support the immune system. Once the blood has been exposed to toxins, it carries those toxins throughout the body, which affects every single organ.

THE LYMPHATIC SYSTEM

Similar to the blood, the lymph is a very important fluid that helps with the detoxification process. The lymph nodes—which are in the neck, the groin, the mammary area, and right behind the knees—filter toxins and foreign invaders the lymph has brought to them. This helps to prevent the liver from getting clogged and overloaded. After the lymph filters through the lymph nodes, it's returned to the bloodstream through the thoracic duct, which is in the chest. The lymphatic system has no pump like the cardiovascular system does (the heart), so the lymph moves much more slowly than the blood. This is why exercise is so important. You've probably heard that exercise is critical for weight loss, but we think exercise plays a bigger role in keeping the lymph moving so that it can better transport toxins to where they need to go to be filtered out of the body. Dry brushing and bouncing exercises also help drain the lymphatic fluid. (Read more about these therapies later in this chapter in the "Detoxification Therapies" section.)

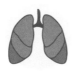

THE RESPIRATORY SYSTEM

Even the respiratory system aids in detoxification. When we exhale, we're removing carbon dioxide from our bodies. The respiratory system also is a major player in keeping the pH of the body where it should be.

THE URINARY SYSTEM

Toxins are removed from the body in two ways. The first is through the intestinal tract when you eliminate feces. The second is through the urinary system—specifically the kidneys. The kidneys help filter the blood by removing waste found in water and bile. This is why, especially when you're dehydrated, your urine looks yellow; the color is a result of the bile pigments.

THE SKIN

As previously stated, the skin is the body's largest detoxifying organ. The skin has sweat glands in it to help remove waste from our bodies when we exercise. Both exercise and sweat therapy are very effective methods for detoxification.

THINGS THAT CAN IMPACT THE EFFECTIVENESS OF DETOXIFICATION

As with everything else we've been sharing in this part of the book, all of the systems in the body are so intricately interconnected that you have to look at how they interact with one another. If just one thing is less than optimal, issues can pop up in another area. This section explores things that can hinder the effectiveness of the detoxification process.

DETOXIFICATION AND DIGESTION/ELIMINATION

Before you try a detoxification therapy, you need to make sure that digestion and elimination are working optimally. Even if you eat the healthiest diet, your digestive system could still be clogged. If the digestive system is clogged, then your body won't efficiently get rid of the toxins it needs to. You might experience bad side effects, including becoming very sick if the toxins aren't effectively removed from your body. You have to make sure your stomach is producing enough acid to digest the foods you consume.

Certain amino acids are necessary for proper functioning of the specific detoxification pathways in the liver. If you're not properly digesting proteins, those detoxification pathways in the liver won't work right, no matter how clean you eat. You can't properly digest those proteins if your stomach acid is low. Also, you need to make sure your vitamin and mineral status is good. Production of stomach acid depends on zinc and vitamin B6. If you're deficient in some vitamins and minerals, your ability to digest and absorb nutrients and convert them into amino acids will be compromised.

Another important factor in detoxification is proper bile production. Bile helps you break down the fats you consume so your body can use the proteins you eat. The bile is where the liver dumps the toxins to be trapped. If the bile becomes thick and sludgy, the toxins can't move fluidly to exit the body.

Finally, the intestines should be working properly before you attempt to detox. Compromised intestines might not be able to eliminate toxins from other parts of the body because the organs and intestines will be unable to communicate with each other.

DETOXIFICATION AND BLOOD SUGAR REGULATION

One of the problems with elevated cortisol levels is that they reduce the liver's ability to detoxify because high cortisol levels and blood sugar imbalances stress the liver. The liver is responsible for deactivating hormones that are at excess levels or are no longer functional. These hormones have to be removed from the body, and when cortisol is high for prolonged periods, the liver's pathways that perform the conjugations decrease in effectiveness.

High blood sugar levels also deplete the B vitamins needed to help with detoxification. Vitamin B6 is necessary for every liver enzyme function and for the production of neurotransmitters like epinephrine and serotonin. Remember our earlier discussion about Phase 1 detoxification and Phase 2 detoxification? Well, vitamin B2 is needed to help make Phase 1 detoxification work as it should.

DETOXIFICATION AND MINERALS

Detoxification can create an acidic environment in the blood. If we don't have access to proper amounts of minerals in our bodies, the pH of the blood can get out of whack. When we're exposed to toxins, our bodies can become depleted of minerals that help make the enzymes necessary for the detoxification process to work correctly. You might remember that earlier we mentioned heavy metals as being toxins. Certain minerals help keep these heavy metals from collecting in body tissue. If you go to a healthcare provider who informs you that you have heavy metal toxicity and recommends chelation therapy, make sure that the therapy includes replenishing your body with the various vitamins and minerals that chelation therapy removes.

DETOXIFICATION AND HYDRATION

Proper hydration keeps blood and lymph moving as it should so that toxins can go to the right places to be removed from the body. Keeping yourself hydrated helps ensure that your body can flush out the toxins. Consuming enough water also keeps your bowels moving regularly and causes you to urinate more frequently so that toxins are eliminated. In addition, being adequately hydrated ensures that your body can sweat like it needs to when you exercise.

DETOXIFICATION AND FATS

At the beginning of this chapter, we mentioned that the fat in our bodies holds on to difficult-to-remove toxins. These toxins can include heavy metals or chemicals. The liver transforms the fats we eat into usable forms. If we don't consume enough dietary fat, the liver becomes stressed, which affects how well our bodies can go through the detoxification process. When we don't consume enough fat, the bile becomes viscous and sludgy, and the toxins aren't transported out of the body effectively.

Fats also help make healthy cell membranes. The health of the cell membranes determines how effectively toxins can be removed from the cells. When the membranes aren't healthy because we haven't eaten enough fat, toxins can't be effectively removed from the cells.

DETOXIFICATION THERAPIES

Now that you know the basics of detoxification and how it benefits the body, we want to go over some therapies you can use to help with detoxification. Detoxification can actually make your health worse if all elimination pathways are not clear, so before using these detoxification techniques, it's very important that you consult with your NTP or another healthcare provider. The following sections describe the therapies and the purpose of each.

DRY BRUSH MASSAGE

The skin is the largest eliminative organ. It is estimated that one-third of all body impurities are excreted through the skin. Chemical analysis of sweat shows that it has almost the same constituents as urine, including large amounts of uric acid (the main metabolic waste product in urine). If the skin becomes clogged and the pores are choked with millions of dead cells, uric acid and other impurities must remain in the body or attempt to find an alternative route of elimination.

Dry brushing involves taking a long-handled natural-bristle brush with a head that's about the size of your hand (or slightly larger) and brushing vigorously in circular patterns on various parts of your body, including the soles of your feet, legs, hands, arms, back, abdomen, chest, neck, and face. It can seem kind of weird at first, but the benefits of dry brushing greatly outweigh any criticisms someone might have. Some of the major benefits include removing dead skin to open the pores, stimulating better blood circulation and oxygenation, making the skin more receptive to minerals and other health-promoting nutrients, and stimulating hormone- and oil-producing glands.

BOUNCING EXERCISES

We know what you're thinking: "Bouncing? Really? What's that supposed to do?" Stick with us here, because it does a whole lot more than you think.

Remember when we shared that the lymphatic system doesn't have a pump to keep the lymphatic fluid moving (like the cardiovascular system has the heart to circulate the blood)? Well, bouncing exercises help make up for the absence of a pump. Bouncing exercises get the lymph moving so the toxins can effectively travel to where they need to go. Examples include jumping rope, doing jumping jacks, doing a trampoline workout, lightly jogging, and even lightly bouncing on an exercise ball. Jimmy has a vibration plate that he stands on to simulate the effects of bouncing.

SWEATING THERAPIES

Another beneficial detoxification therapy is sweating. Exercise that elevates the heart rate is an obvious way to sweat, but using steam or an infrared sauna works as well. Jimmy loves getting in his infrared sauna to aid the detoxification process; other benefits include improved sleep and pain management. You also can induce sweating by consuming certain herbs and spices, including ajwain, Angelica, black pepper, burdock root, cayenne pepper, cinnamon, elder, elecampane, garlic, and ginger.[2]

CONSTITUTIONAL HYDROTHERAPY (HOT AND COLD TOWEL THERAPY)

The purpose of this therapy is to enhance circulation, detoxification, and immune function over a half-hour period. Enhancing or improving circulation helps toxins be easily transported out of the body. Also, improving immune function can help our bodies better deal with toxins that might be in the body.

In constitutional hydrotherapy, your chest is covered with hot towels before you're wrapped with a sheet and blankets for five minutes. Then the hot towels are replaced with cold towels, and you're rewrapped with a sheet and blanket for ten minutes. This alternating hot and cold towel therapy is repeated on your back. It sounds strange, but this detoxification technique could be just what you need to feel well again.

WATER ENEMA

Many people have heard of doing a water enema, but very few are willing to try this detoxification method because it sounds uncomfortable. However, those who love it live by this cleansing of the colon, which helps stimulate the liver to dump bile to reduce headaches, fatigue, and mood issues.

Simply put, a water enema is the injection of fluid into the lower bowel through the rectum. It's commonly used to relieve constipation and stimulate stool evacuation. Various enema fluids can be used, including water, saline, and mineral oil. This is a delicate procedure that you might want to ask your natural healthcare provider to assist you with.

COFFEE ENEMA

We know this sounds kind of weird, but coffee enemas are a great way to help with detoxification. During a coffee enema, the coffee is absorbed into the bloodstream and sent to the liver, where glutathione production increases. Glutathione is an antioxidant enzyme that is important for helping to drive out toxins from the body.

OIL PULLING

Oil pulling is known as Karach's therapy in honor of Ukrainian physician Dr. Fedor Karach. This detoxification method helps remove germs and bacteria from the gums and removes toxins and microbes from the body through the mucous membranes and tongue. It involves swishing either organic sunflower oil, sesame oil, or cold-pressed coconut oil in the mouth for fifteen to twenty minutes without swallowing.[3] Swishing for that long is a lot of work, but people who swear by oil pulling enjoy it.

TIPS FOR HELPING WITH THE DETOXIFICATION PROCESS

Now that you understand why detoxification is so incredibly important and have learned about some therapies you can use to aid with detoxification, we have a few tips for you. Please consult with an NTP or another healthcare provider to make sure all your elimination pathways are open. If you have blocked pathways and you try to detoxify, you'll have an unpleasant experience because you'll become sick when the toxins are unable to leave the body. Also, remember not to eat anything too close to bedtime, because the majority of restorative detoxification and healing happens while we sleep. If your body is having to digest food, then it cannot also be detoxing. You have to pick one function or the other, and we highly recommend that you choose detoxification over digestion at bedtime.

Use natural household and personal products as much as possible to limit your exposure to chemicals. We've been using essential oils for several years instead of air fresheners, perfumes, and colognes. We also use shampoos and conditioners with essential oils and choose only organic cleaning products for our home. These little things add up to prevent toxins from sneaking into our bodies.

You may not have given it much thought, but your smartphone emits toxins in the form of electromagnetic field (EMF) exposure. Turn off your Wi-Fi at night and use the devices on speaker mode so they're not in direct contact with your ear. Having iPhones and other modern-day gizmos and gadgets is part of life now, but you should use them with caution to prevent any harmful effects.

Before we conclude this part, it bears repeating that consuming a low carb, moderate-protein, high-fat, ketogenic diet gives your liver a chance to detoxify because it won't be distracted by having to deal with regulating blood sugar levels. The low-sugar aspect of eating keto means that nutrients aren't pulled from other parts of the body to help with detoxification.

Now you know that detoxification is not only real but also a serious aspect of your health journey. Don't neglect to do the little things in your pursuit of optimal health; even the little things matter.

Before we move on to the recipes and other odds and ends of *Real Food Keto,* Christine has one more thing to share with you: a call to action to stop sitting on the sidelines and start helping others to begin their health journeys in earnest.

REAL FOOD KETO TAKEAWAYS FROM CHAPTER 13

- Juicing, pills, and shakes consumed as part of a regimen commonly referred to as a *detox* or *cleanse* are not what real detoxification is about.

- A deep cultural and religious tradition has surrounded detoxification for many millennia.

- Toxins are everywhere in our daily lives, and we must make an effort to detoxify from them.

- Having good liver health and open detoxification pathways is the key to eliminating harmful toxins.

- Every major system in the body is involved in the detoxification process.

- If digestion, blood sugar, hydration, fats, and mineral balance in the body are off, proper detoxification can't happen.

- Dry brushing, bouncing exercises, sweating, hydrotherapy, enemas, and oil pulling help stimulate the detoxification pathways.

- Use natural household and personal products, such as essential oils, as much as possible in your daily life.

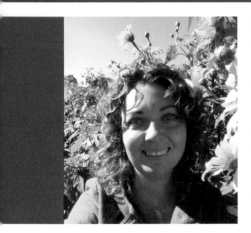

KATIE DILLON, NUTRITIONAL THERAPY PRACTITIONER, INTEGRATIVE HEALTH COACH, DIP. SOC. SCI.

www.empowerednutrition.com.au

I have always had an interest in nutrition, but the idea of studying intimidated me. I was making good money doing what I was doing. Why would I change? When my son was born with eczema, I tried the medical route of moisturizers and steroid creams, and nothing worked. I didn't like using the steroid cream, and it didn't feel right to be trying to fix a symptom without knowing what was causing the problem. I started doing research, which led me to look at diet. Once I cleaned up both of our diets (he was breastfeeding), my son's eczema cleared up, and his sleep improved—as did mine. This sparked my interest in doing more with nutrition. I decided to enroll with the Nutritional Therapy Association, and now I'm working with people with a variety of problems, helping them to improve their health and return to a state where their bodies are able to heal themselves. This is extremely rewarding and very exciting.

I am currently working with a young boy with severe epilepsy, which is uncontrolled by his medication. He also has global developmental delay and cerebral palsy as the result of a traumatic brain injury. We are working at transitioning him to a ketogenic diet to manage his seizures. I'm working with his neurologist to make the transition slowly to ensure the dietary changes do not have an adverse effect on his medication. It's early days, but already we're seeing improvements in many of his symptoms. I'm so excited to see these changes and to see what's to come for him in the future.

A Call to Action:
Your Response to Reading
Real Food Keto

This book has been one of the most gratifying experiences of my entire life because I know the information that was provided to you in these pages is life-changing. When I decided to become a Nutritional Therapy Practitioner in 2017, I had no idea what it would entail. But, as you can see from the depth of knowledge that we have shared throughout *Real Food Keto,* especially in this last part, it's a very advanced nutritional health course that empowers you to take your passion for real food to the next level.

That is why I'm inviting you to check out the Nutritional Therapy Association (NTA) at www.nutritionaltherapy.com and to consider becoming a Nutritional Therapy Practitioner (NTP) or Nutritional Therapy Consultant (NTC) like thousands of others already have. Although it isn't explicitly a ketogenic program, the discussion of healthy fats, the alternative viewpoint on cholesterol, and the importance of controlling blood sugar levels make it the perfect educational choice for anyone who follows keto and wants to teach others about it.

I had always wanted to further my education, but I didn't really know what I wanted to do. I have been interested in health and nutrition ever since Jimmy started his journey and began doing his work. So, when the opportunity to go through the Nutritional Therapy Practitioner program came up, I jumped at the chance. Although most NTPs and NTCs are in the United States, there are programs all over the world for you to begin your education. The class instructors and group leaders are wonderful, and I'll forever be grateful to Brook and Christie for doing a fantastic job at making this experience as stress-free as possible. They were always encouraging and available to answer questions throughout the course.

Perhaps you think you don't have time to invest in this kind of training, but the course lasts only nine months. Yes, it's quite intensive, and it does require a little bit of travel for weekend workshops, but you can do most of the coursework from the comfort of your home and at your own pace. There are deadlines for the coursework, but you control when it gets done. If you have any questions about becoming an NTP or NTC, feel free to reach out to me directly at rebootingyournutrition@gmail.com. Becoming an NTP was one of the best decisions I ever made, and I am so happy to be able to impart this knowledge to you through this book.

So now the ball is in your court. What are you going to do with the knowledge you have gained from reading this book? You could settle for applying it in your own life and perhaps sharing some of it with close family members. But don't your friends, coworkers, and other people in your sphere of influence deserve to hear some of this incredible health-promoting stuff, too? Of course they do! Teaming up with the NTA can help you make that happen. Visit www.nutritionaltherapy.com and see for yourself what this organization is all about. This group is one of the most loving, supportive nutritional health groups you will find anywhere, and the people in this organization have positively influenced my life in more ways than I can name. It changed my life . . . now it's time for it to change yours, too!

part 4
RECIPES

Now that you understand how to apply nutritional therapy to your real foods–based, low-carb, high-fat, ketogenic diet, it's time to apply what we have shared as you get in the kitchen. All of this talk about nutrition and its effect on health is moot if you can't make your way around a refrigerator and stove.

For this part of the book, we asked our good friend and international bestselling ketogenic recipe author, Maria Emmerich, to share some *Real Food Keto* recipes so you can start implementing everything you've learned in this book right away. However, we couldn't resist the chance to share a couple of our own all-time favorite dishes: Fauxtatoes au Gratin (page 304) and Cauliflower Patties (page 306). We handed our recipes over to Maria, and she graciously agreed to test them and give them her "Maria flair."

Before we get to the keto yumminess that awaits you in the coming pages, we have some tips, tricks, and recommendations for you.

SUGAR SUBSTITUTES

In this book, you have read that staying away from sugar is very important because of all the negative effects that sugar has on the body. That doesn't mean that you have to stay completely away from certain fruits like strawberries, blueberries, blackberries, and raspberries (which are lower in sugar than some other fruits) or sweets made entirely with a sugar substitute. However, keep in mind some people's cravings are stoked by the taste of sweetness, and some people can experience blood sugar issues after eating sweet foods. This is where you have to tinker and test to try different things to see how they fit into your ketogenic lifestyle.

We like to use stevia and erythritol when we cook or bake because both are natural sweeteners that don't seem to have any negative effects on blood sugar. One sweetener in particular that we like to use is called Swerve. (Maria often lists this product as an ingredient in her desserts and other recipes that call for a sweetener.) It's a combination of stevia and erythritol, which makes it perfect for use in the recipes in this book. Swerve has been available in granular and powdered forms for some time, and the company has added a baking mix and brown sugar substitute to the product line. You can find Swerve in many grocery stores and online at www.swervesweet.com.

There are a number of artificial sweeteners we recommend you stay away from:

- Maltitol (Maltisorb, Maltisweet)

- Xylitol (Birch Sugar, Meso-Xylitol)

- Aspartame (Equal, NutraSweet, NatraTaste Blue)

- Sucralose (Splenda)

- Acesulfame potassium or ACE K (Sunette, Equal Spoonful, Sweet One, Sweet 'n Safe)

- Saccharin (Sweet 'n Low, Sweet Twin)

- Sorbitol

Even if you can tolerate low-sugar fruits and sugar substitutes, make sure you don't eat too much of them because that could cause blood sugar issues, insulin spikes, and weight loss stalls or even weight gain. We have included a chart Maria developed that shows equivalencies of Swerve to other keto-friendly sugar substitutes if you would prefer to use one of those.

NOTE FROM MARIA ABOUT SWEETENERS

If you're trying keto for the first time, the recipes in this book should have just the right amount of sweetness. But as you continue on with the ketogenic lifestyle, you might find that food naturally begins to taste sweeter, and you may want to reduce the amount of sweetener used in a recipe. Whenever a recipe requires a powdered sweetener, Swerve, which is available in granular and powdered forms, is the go-to choice. I always use the powdered (confectioners') form of Swerve because it gives you a smoother finished product and better overall results. That said, you can always pulverize a granular form of erythritol, such as Wholesome! All-Natural Zero, in a blender or coffee grinder to get the powdered texture.

If a specific sweetener or type of sweetener (such as powdered or liquid) is called for, *do not* substitute any other sweetener; these recipes rely on these particular forms of sweeteners. For example, in recipes where the sweetener has to melt, some sweeteners won't work, so it's important to use exactly what's called for.

If a sweetener in an ingredients list is followed by "or equivalent," such as "¼ cup Swerve confectioners'-style sweetener or equivalent amount of liquid or powdered sweetener," you are free to use any keto-friendly sweetener, liquid or powdered. For example, you could use liquid stevia, stevia glycerite, monk fruit, or Zsweet.

I use Swerve, my favorite keto-friendly sweetener, in many of the recipes in this book. But if you prefer to use another keto-friendly sweetener, here are the conversion ratios:

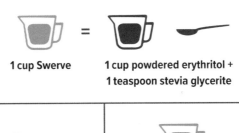

1 cup Swerve = 1 cup powdered erythritol + 1 teaspoon stevia glycerite

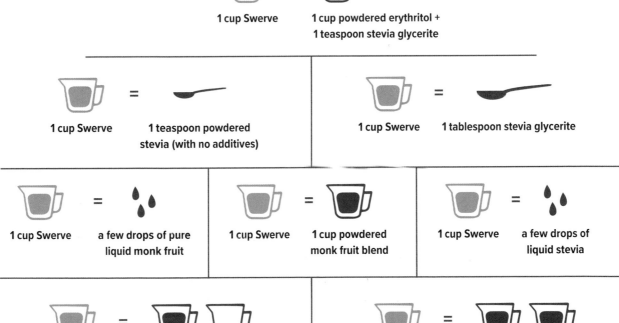

1 cup Swerve = 1 teaspoon powdered stevia (with no additives)

1 cup Swerve = 1 tablespoon stevia glycerite

1 cup Swerve = a few drops of pure liquid monk fruit

1 cup Swerve = 1 cup powdered monk fruit blend

1 cup Swerve = a few drops of liquid stevia

1 cup Swerve = 1 ⅓ cups powdered erythritol

1 cup Swerve = 2 cups yacón syrup

FATS: TO HEAT OR NOT TO HEAT?

In Chapter 4 we cover the important subject of fats. Some fats you can use to cook with and some become very unstable when you cook with them. Read labels very carefully to determine whether a fat is safe to cook with. Stay away from all fats and oils that have the following terms:

- Refined
- Hydrogenated
- Partially hydrogenated
- Cold-processed

Also, don't confuse *cold-PROCESSED* with *cold-PRESSED*. Cold-pressed oils are okay to use.

Look for oils labeled with the following:

- Organic
- First-cold pressed
- Cold-pressed
- Expeller-pressed
- Unrefined
- Extra virgin

The following chart tells you which fats are safe to use for cooking and which fats to keep away from heat.

The oils in the right column of the chart are not to be exposed to heat. You can use these for salad dressings or in a sauce to go over meat or cooked veggies (with the sauce added to the veggies after they have been removed from the heat and are ready to serve).

FATS BEST FOR COOKING AT HIGH HEAT

- Beef and lamb tallow
- Chicken, duck, or goose fat
- Organic and virgin coconut oil
- Butter and ghee
- Lard
- Organic and virgin palm oil (palm kernel oil is also okay)

FATS FOR COOKING AT LOW HEAT (TO STIR-FRY, SLOW COOK, OR SAUTÉ)

- Olive oil (best if yellow or green, unfiltered, and cloudy)
- Avocado oil
- Macadamia nut oil
- Sesame oil

FATS TO KEEP AWAY FROM HEAT

- Flax oil
- Hemp oil
- Pine nut oil
- Pumpkin oil
- Safflower oil
- Sunflower oil
- Grapeseed oil

A WORD ABOUT SNACKING

Fat keeps you from getting hungry between meals so you don't have to snack. If you do get hungry between meals, then it's possible you didn't consume enough fat in your last meal. You shouldn't feel the need eat between meals if you're consuming enough fat.

However, we're not saying you shouldn't snack at all. There will be times, especially during the initial fat-adaptation period, when you might need to eat a little something between meals. Also, in times of stress, we sometimes feel the need to have a little nibble even when it's not time for breakfast, lunch, or dinner. We find this to be especially true when we travel. The rise in cortisol from the stress messes with our blood sugar levels and creates the desire to have a little extra high-fat snack to hold us over until our next meal. This is perfectly fine. Maria has included several snack recipes that are good for such occasions.

GENERAL FOOD SHOPPING TIPS

Throughout this book, we stress the importance of buying organic whenever possible. Buying organic means that the produce or food you get hasn't been treated with pesticides, synthetic fertilizers, sewage sludge, genetically modified organisms, or ionizing radiation. Organic meat, poultry, dairy products, and eggs mean that the animals weren't given any antibiotics or growth hormones. If you choose to buy a packaged food like spaghetti sauce, salsa, salad dressings, mayonnaise, and more, consider things like added and hidden sugars, vegetable oils, natural and artificial flavors, and synthetic vitamins. Read the labels very carefully to see if any of these ingredients are in the product, and don't buy any products that include these ingredients. Our rule of thumb is if you can't pronounce an ingredient on the food label or if it has more than five ingredients in it, don't buy that packaged food.

We know that it won't always be easy to buy organic ingredients because of financial limitations and spotty availability in certain areas. Whatever your circumstances, just make the best choices you can for your situation.

SHOPPING GUIDE

With fermented foods, make sure you select products from the refrigerated section of the grocery store. Otherwise, the good bacteria in these fermented foods have lost their benefits.

You may be wondering which brands are best to purchase when buying ingredients for the recipes in this section. You can either make your own or buy them already prepared. Following is a list of brands that we normally get for items included in the recipes. For other products we recommend, see the Resources section at the end of the book.

Blanched almond flour: Bob's Red Mill Super Fine Almond Flour or Blue Diamond Almonds Almond Flour

Bone broth: Bare Bones Broth or Ali Anderson's Abundant Broth

Cashew milk: So Delicious Cashew Milk Unsweetened

Collagen peptides: Vital Proteins Collagen Peptides Unflavored

Dill pickles: Bubbies Dill Pickles

Egg white protein powder: Jay Robb Egg White Protein

Extracts (rum, almond, maple, apple, raspberry, strawberry, vanilla): McCormick Extracts

Fish sauce: Red Boat Fish Sauce

Make sure to purchase pure extracts rather than imitation flavor extracts.

Grass-fed powdered gelatin: Vital Proteins Beef Gelatin

Hemp milk: Living Harvest Hemp Milk Unsweetened Vanilla

Kimchi: Bubbies Kimchi

Liquid stevia: Pyure Organic Liquid Stevia or SweetLeaf Liquid Stevia

Mayonnaise: Primal Kitchen or Chosen Foods Coconut Oil Mayo

Salsa: Italian Rose Fresh Salsa

Sauerkraut: Bubbies Sauerkraut

Stevia glycerite: Swerve or Pyure Organic Stevia

When you buy a product like tomato sauce, always purchase one that's packaged in a glass jar.

Tomato sauce: Member's Mark (Sam's Club) Organic Marinara Sauce

Unsweetened almond milk: Blue Diamond Almonds Almond Breeze

Unsweetened chocolate: Pascha Organic 100% Cacao Unsweetened Dark Chocolate Baking Chips or Baker's Unsweetened Chocolate

RECIPES

BREAKFAST

SALADS & SIDES

MAINS

DESSERTS & DRINKS

BASICS

STRAWBERRIES AND CREAM
SMOOTHIE

Yield: 2 servings   *Prep time:* 4 minutes

Using frozen strawberries in this smoothie makes it thick and frosty, almost like strawberry ice cream.

1 cup frozen strawberries

½ cup unsweetened vanilla-flavored almond milk, homemade (page 345) or store-bought

½ cup heavy cream

¼ cup Swerve confectioners'-style sweetener or equivalent amount of liquid or powdered sweetener (see page 271)

1 scoop collagen peptides (vanilla or unflavored)

Place all of the ingredients in a blender and blend until very smooth. Divide between two 8-ounce glasses and serve. Store leftover smoothie in an airtight container in the refrigerator for up to 4 days.

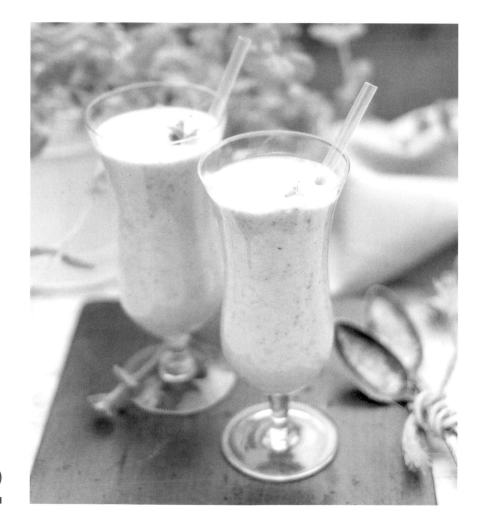

NUTRITIONAL INFO (per serving)

CALORIES	FAT	PROTEIN	CARBS	FIBER
254	23g	7g	7g	1g

PUMPKIN SMOOTHIE

Yield: 2 servings   *Prep time:* 4 minutes

1 cup unsweetened vanilla-flavored almond milk, homemade (page 345) or store-bought

½ cup canned pumpkin puree

2 ounces cream cheese (¼ cup)

2 tablespoons Swerve confectioners'-style sweetener or equivalent amount of liquid or powdered sweetener (see page 271)

1 scoop collagen peptides (vanilla or unflavored)

1 cup crushed ice

Ground cinnamon and nutmeg, for garnish (optional)

Place all of the ingredients in a blender and blend until very smooth. Taste and adjust the sweetness to your liking. Divide between two 8-ounce glasses, garnish with cinnamon and nutmeg, if desired, and serve. Store leftover smoothie in an airtight container in the refrigerator for up to 4 days.

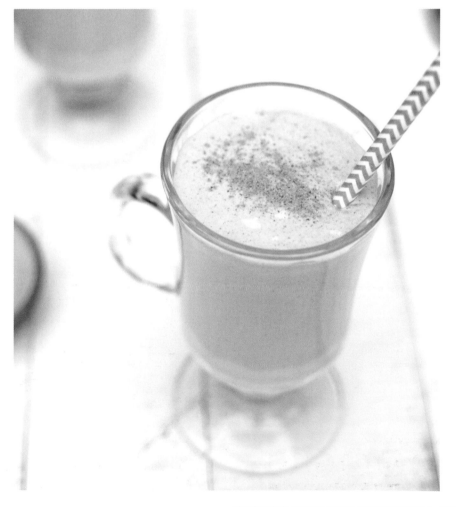

NUTRITIONAL INFO (per serving)

CALORIES 149 | FAT 10g | PROTEIN 8g | CARBS 4g | FIBER 1g

PECAN PIE WAFFLES

Yield: 2 servings   *Prep time:* 5 minutes (not including time to boil eggs)   *Cook time:* 6 minutes

2 large eggs

2 hard-boiled eggs

3 tablespoons unsweetened almond milk, homemade (page 345) or store-bought

2 tablespoons Swerve confectioners'-style sweetener or equivalent amount of liquid or powdered sweetener (see page 271)

1 tablespoon coconut flour

1 teaspoon pumpkin pie spice

½ teaspoon baking powder

⅛ teaspoon fine sea salt

2 tablespoons melted coconut oil or unsalted butter

1 tablespoon almond extract

Melted coconut oil or coconut oil spray, for greasing the waffle iron

DRIZZLE:
2 tablespoons melted coconut oil or unsalted butter

2 tablespoons creamy pecan butter or almond butter (unsweetened and unsalted)

A few drops of stevia glycerite (optional)

Toasted pecans, for garnish

SPECIAL EQUIPMENT:
Waffle iron

1. Preheat a waffle iron to high heat. Place the raw eggs, hard-boiled eggs, milk, sweetener, coconut flour, pumpkin pie spice, baking powder, and salt in a blender or food processor and blend until smooth and very thick. Add the melted coconut oil and almond extract and pulse to combine.

2. Grease the hot waffle iron with coconut oil. Place 3 tablespoons of the batter in the center of the iron and close the lid. Cook for 3 to 4 minutes, until the waffle is golden brown and crisp. Remove from the waffle iron and repeat with the remaining batter.

3. Meanwhile, make the drizzle: Mix together the melted coconut oil and pecan butter until smooth. Add the stevia glycerite, then taste and add more sweetener, if desired.

4. Serve the waffles with the drizzle and garnish with pecans. Store in an airtight container in the refrigerator for up to 4 days or in the freezer for up to a month. To reheat, place in a toaster.

NUTRITIONAL INFO (per serving)

CALORIES	FAT	PROTEIN	CARBS	FIBER
597	60g	15g	6g	3g

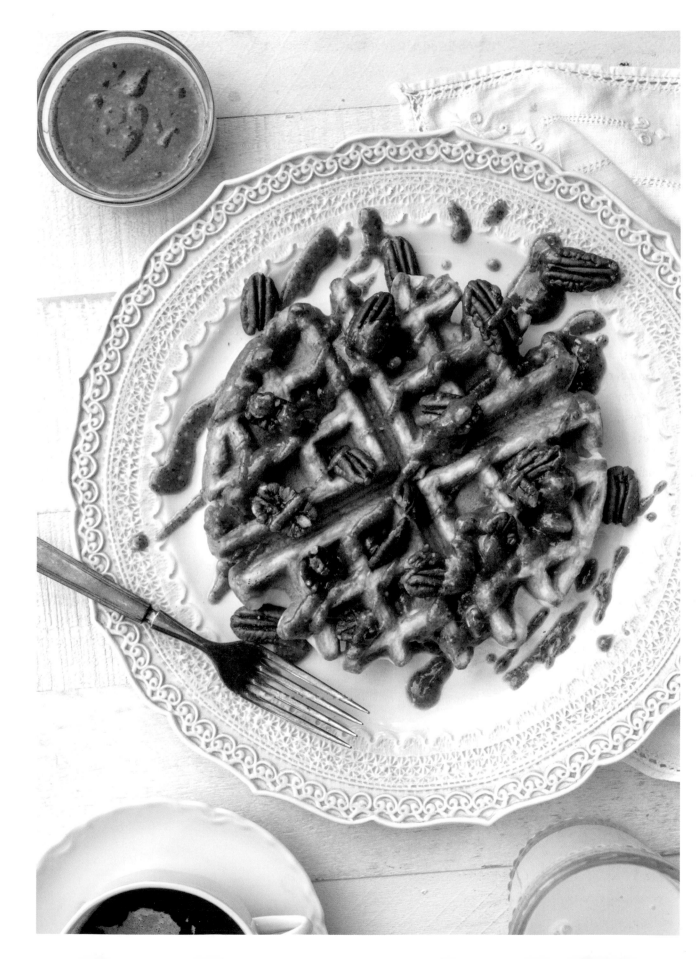

BAKED EGGS
WITH CORNED BEEF AND SAUERKRAUT HASH

Yield: 6 servings   *Prep time:* 10 minutes (not including time to make dressing)   *Cook time:* 22 minutes

Coconut oil or lard, for the baking dish

4 cups shredded green or purple cabbage

1 tablespoon lemon juice

12 ounces thick-sliced corned beef, cut into ¼-inch pieces

¼ cup drained and chopped sauerkraut, homemade (page 294) or store-bought

2 tablespoons chopped fresh dill, or 2 teaspoons dried dill weed, divided

½ teaspoon fine sea salt

½ teaspoon ground black pepper

1 tablespoon ghee or unsalted butter, melted

6 large eggs

¾ cup shredded Swiss cheese (about 3 ounces)

½ cup Thousand Island Dressing (page 349), for serving

1 sprig fresh thyme, for garnish

1. Preheat the oven to 450°F. Grease a 13 by 9-inch baking dish or an 8-inch cast-iron skillet with coconut oil or lard.

2. In a large bowl, toss the shredded cabbage with the lemon juice. Add the corned beef, sauerkraut, 1½ tablespoons of the fresh dill (or 1½ teaspoons dried), salt, and pepper and mix to combine well.

3. Spread the cabbage mixture in the prepared baking dish, then drizzle with the melted ghee. Bake for 20 minutes, until the cabbage is soft. Remove from the oven and, using a large spoon, make 6 evenly spaced depressions in the cabbage mixture. Crack an egg into each depression. Sprinkle the cheese over the cabbage, avoiding the eggs.

4. Continue baking until the egg whites are opaque, the yolks are almost set, and the cheese is melted, about 7 minutes. Remove from the oven, cover with foil, and let stand for 2 minutes. Remove the foil and sprinkle with the remaining dill. Garnish with fresh thyme leaves, if desired. Serve with the dressing.

5. Store in an airtight container in the refrigerator for up to 4 days. To reheat, place in a lightly greased skillet over medium-high heat for 3 minutes or until heated to your liking.

NUTRITIONAL INFO (per serving)

 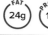

CALORIES	FAT	PROTEIN	CARBS	FIBER
306	24g	17g	5g	1g

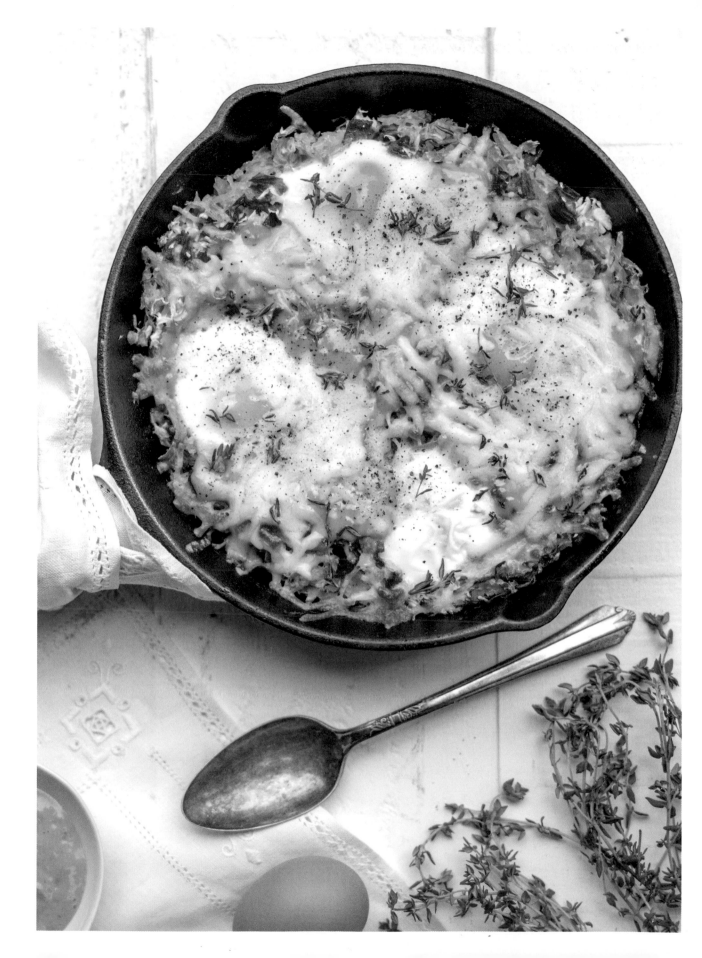

SPRING DUTCH BABY

Yield: 2 servings   *Prep time:* 5 minutes   *Cook time:* 18 minutes

OPTION

2 tablespoons coconut oil

3 large eggs

¾ cup unsweetened cashew milk or almond milk, homemade (page 345) or store-bought (or hemp milk if nut-free)

¼ cup unflavored egg white protein powder

1 teaspoon baking powder

1 teaspoon fine sea salt

2 tablespoons chopped fresh dill or other fresh herbs of choice

8 spears asparagus, trimmed

¼ cup shredded Parmesan cheese

Butter or coconut oil, for serving

1. Preheat the oven to 425°F.

2. Place the coconut oil in an 8-inch cast-iron skillet. Put the skillet in the hot oven.

3. Place the eggs, milk, protein powder, baking powder, salt, and dill in a blender. Blend for about 1 minute, until foamy. Remove the hot skillet from the oven and pour in the batter. Arrange the asparagus on top of the batter (they may fall into the batter, which is fine). Sprinkle with the Parmesan.

4. Bake for 18 to 20 minutes, until the pancake is puffed and golden brown.

5. Remove the pancake from the oven and spread with butter or coconut oil. Cut into wedges and enjoy! Best served fresh.

NUTRITIONAL INFO (per serving)

CALORIES (251) FAT (20g) PROTEIN (16.2g) CARBS (1.4g) FIBER (0g)

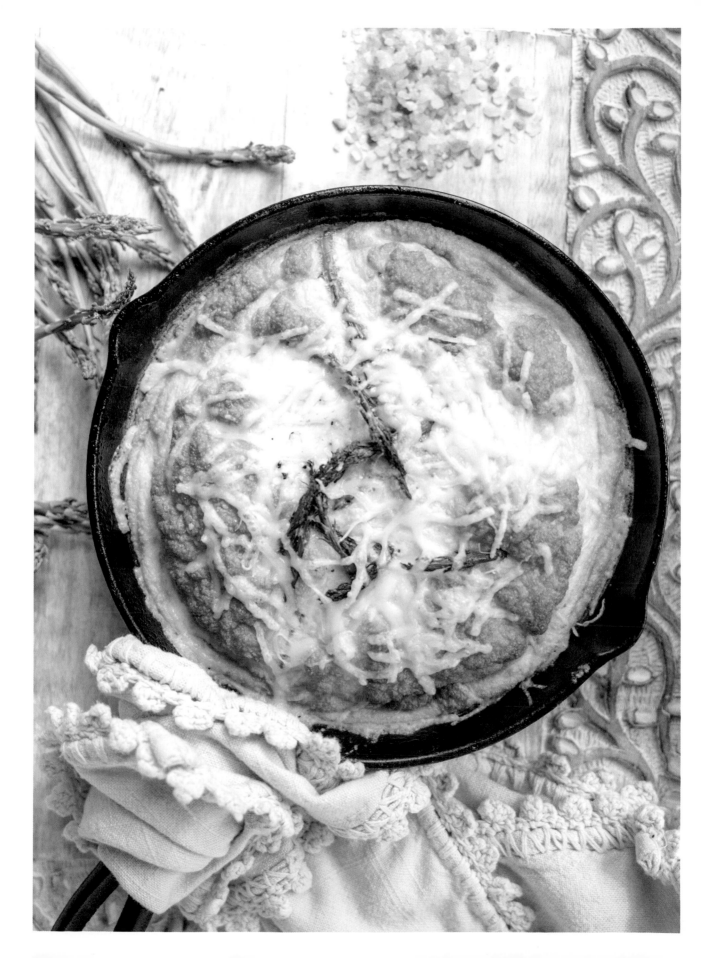

NO-BAKE
MINI BREAKFAST CHEESECAKES

Yield: 8 servings   *Prep time:* 8 minutes, plus 3 hours to chill

Who wouldn't love a mini cheesecake for breakfast? This recipe has a creamy flavor that is reminiscent of French toast.

CRUST:

2 tablespoons blanched almond flour or almond meal

2 tablespoons crushed roasted and salted almonds

2 tablespoons Swerve confectioners'-style sweetener or equivalent amount of liquid or powdered sweetener (see page 271)

2 tablespoons unsalted butter, melted

1 teaspoon ground cinnamon

FILLING:

1 teaspoon grass-fed powdered gelatin

¼ cup Swerve confectioners'-style sweetener or equivalent amount of liquid or powdered sweetener (see page 271)

½ cup unsweetened almond milk, homemade (page 345) or store-bought

1 (8-ounce) package cream cheese, softened

Seeds scraped from 1 vanilla bean (about 6 inches long), or 1 teaspoon vanilla extract

1 teaspoon maple extract (optional)

Whole roasted almonds, for garnish

SPECIAL EQUIPMENT:
8 (2-ounce) dessert cups

1. Make the crust: Using a hand mixer, mix all the crust ingredients until well combined. Place 1 heaping tablespoon in the bottom of a 2-ounce dessert cup. Press down using your fingers to spread the mixture evenly across the bottom and to compress it firmly. Repeat with the remaining crust mixture, filling 8 dessert cups total. Set aside.

2. Make the filling: Mix the gelatin and sweetener in a small saucepan over medium-high heat. Add the milk and heat until hot, about 1 minute. Stir until the gelatin is completely dissolved. Remove from the heat.

3. In a large bowl, beat the cream cheese, vanilla bean seeds, and maple extract, if using, with a hand mixer on medium speed until creamy. With the mixer running, gradually add the gelatin mixture, beating until well combined.

4. Pour about ¼ cup of the filling mixture over the crust in each dessert cup. Place in the refrigerator to chill for about 3 hours. Garnish with whole roasted almonds before serving.

5. Store in an airtight container in the refrigerator for up to 5 days.

NUTRITIONAL INFO (per serving)

CALORIES 172 · FAT 16g · PROTEIN 4g · CARBS 2g · FIBER 1g

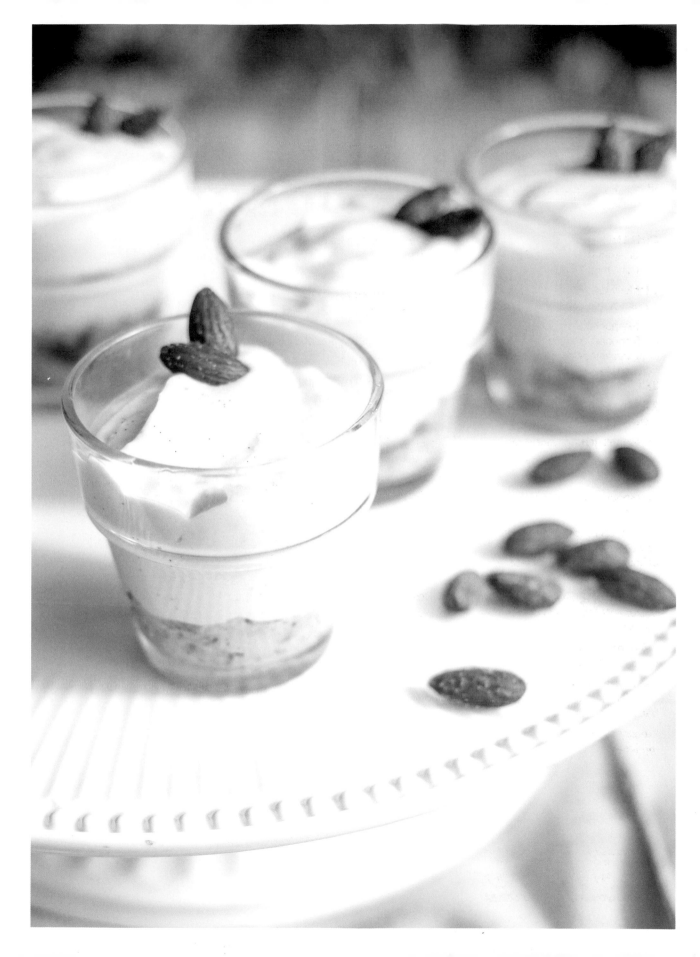

GLAZED CINNAMON FRITTERS

Yield: 4 servings   *Prep time:* 7 minutes   *Cook time:* 16 minutes

OPTION

FRITTERS:

½ cup coconut flour

½ cup egg white protein powder (vanilla or unflavored)

¼ cup Swerve confectioners'-style sweetener or equivalent amount of powdered stevia or erythritol (see page 271)

2 teaspoons baking powder

1 teaspoon ground cinnamon

¼ teaspoon ground nutmeg

¼ teaspoon fine sea salt

2 large eggs

⅔ cup unsweetened almond milk, homemade (page 345) or store-bought (or hemp milk if nut-free)

1 teaspoon vanilla or maple extract

Coconut oil, for frying

GLAZE:

¼ cup coconut oil or unsalted butter, melted

¼ cup Swerve confectioners'-style sweetener or equivalent amount of powdered stevia or erythritol (see page 271)

2 teaspoons ground cinnamon

1 teaspoon maple extract

1. Make the fritters: Place the coconut flour, protein powder, sweetener, baking powder, spices, and salt in a large bowl and whisk to combine. In another bowl, mix the eggs, almond milk, and extract. Add the wet ingredients to the dry and stir well with a hand mixer to combine.

2. Heat about 1 inch of coconut oil to 350°F in a cast-iron skillet. Working in batches, drop 1½-tablespoon balls of the batter into the hot oil and fry until the fritters are golden brown on all sides, about 1 minute per side.

3. Make the glaze: Mix together all the glaze ingredients. Drizzle the glaze over the hot fritters.

4. Store in an airtight container in the refrigerator for up to 5 days or freeze for up to a month. To reheat, place in a lightly greased skillet over medium heat for 2 minutes per side or until heated through.

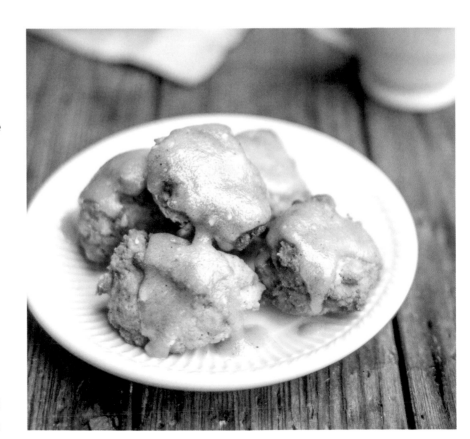

NUTRITIONAL INFO (per serving)

CALORIES 305   FAT 22.4g   PROTEIN 14g   CARBS 12g   FIBER 7.3g

BREAKFAST COBBLER

Yield: 12 servings   *Prep time:* 10 minutes   *Cook time:* 15 minutes

2 (8-ounce) packages cream cheese, softened

1 large egg

¾ cup Swerve confectioners'-style sweetener or equivalent amount of powdered stevia or erythritol (see page 271)

½ teaspoon vanilla extract

¼ teaspoon fine sea salt

3 cups chopped fresh rhubarb

BISCUITS:

4 large egg whites

1 cup blanched almond flour

1 teaspoon baking powder

¼ teaspoon fine sea salt

3 tablespoons very cold unsalted butter, cut into pieces

1. Preheat the oven to 400°F.

2. In a large mixing bowl, use a hand mixer to beat the cream cheese, egg, and sweetener until smooth. Stir in the extract and salt. Fold in the rhubarb. Pour the rhubarb mixture into an 8-inch cast-iron skillet or 8-inch casserole dish.

3. Make the biscuits: Place the egg whites in a mixing bowl or the bowl of a stand mixer and whip with an electric mixer until very fluffy and stiff. In a separate bowl, whisk together the almond flour, baking powder, and salt, then cut in the cold butter, making sure the butter stays in separate clumps. (If the butter isn't chilled, the biscuits won't turn out.) Gently fold the dry mixture into the beaten egg whites.

4. Using your hands, form the dough into 2-inch round biscuits. Place the biscuits on top of the rhubarb mixture in the casserole dish. Bake for 12 to 15 minutes or until golden brown. Serve warm or cold.

5. Store in an airtight container in the refrigerator for up to 5 days. To reheat, place cobbler into a preheated 350°F oven for 5 minutes or until heated through.

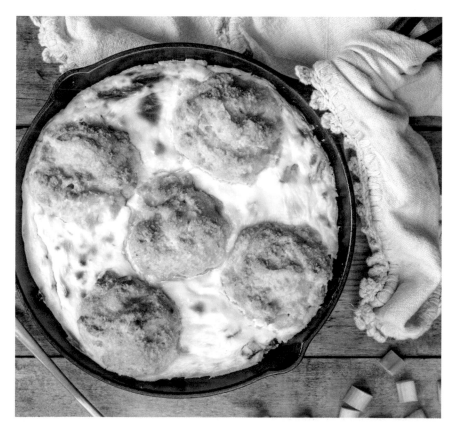

NUTRITIONAL INFO (per serving)

 CALORIES 116  FAT 8g   PROTEIN 7g   CARBS 4.5g FIBER 1g

DENVER OMELET

Yield: 2 servings   *Prep time:* 15 minutes   *Cook time:* 15 minutes

On the TV show Top Chef, *some of the most amazing chefs in the world compete for the title. Some challenges are very difficult, yet some of the simplest challenges are the hardest for these talented chefs. In a recent season, the contestants had to make a perfect Denver omelet, which inspired this recipe.*

1 tablespoon plus 1 teaspoon ghee or unsalted butter, divided

2 tablespoons diced onions

2 tablespoons diced red and green bell peppers

¼ teaspoon fine sea salt, divided

3 large eggs, beaten

2 tablespoons diced ham

2 tablespoons shredded sharp cheddar cheese

Sour cream, for garnish

Sliced green onions, for garnish

1. Melt 1 tablespoon of the ghee in a saucepan over medium-low heat. Add the onions and bell peppers and cook, stirring, until soft. Season with ⅛ teaspoon of the salt.

2. In a mixing bowl, whisk together the eggs, 2 tablespoons of water, and the remaining ⅛ teaspoon of salt. Add the ham and stir well. Set aside.

3. Heat a 12-inch skillet over medium-low heat. Add the remaining teaspoon of ghee and swirl to coat the pan. Pour in the egg mixture. Cover with a lid and cook until the eggs are almost set, about 4 minutes.

4. Remove the lid and sprinkle the cheese over the entire omelet. Place the vegetable filling on top of the cheese.

5. Fold the omelet in half and place on a serving platter. Top with a dollop of sour cream and sprinkle with the sliced green onions. Slice in half and serve.

6. Store in an airtight container in the refrigerator for up to 3 days. Reheat in a sauté pan over medium heat for a minute or two, until warmed through.

NUTRITIONAL INFO (per serving)

CALORIES 361 FAT 31g PROTEIN 16g CARBS 4g FIBER 1g

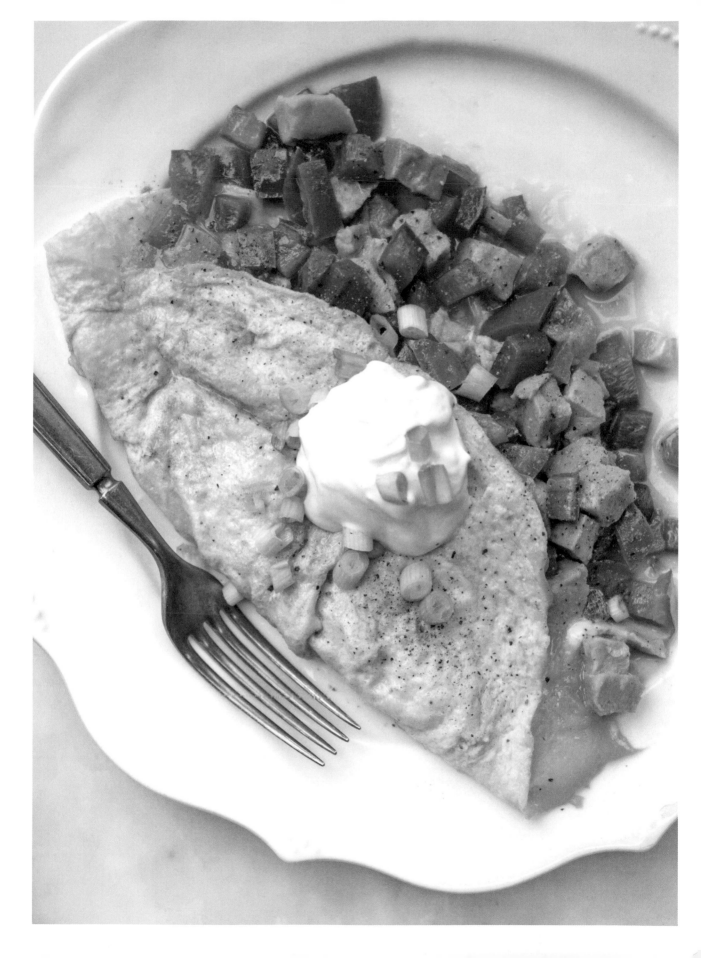

ROAST BEEF SALAD KABOBS

Yield: 4 servings   *Prep time:* 10 minutes (not including time to make dressing)

½ head butter lettuce, cut into 1-inch squares

1 pound roast beef or corned beef, shaved thin

8 (¼-inch-thick) strips dill pickles

1 cup cubed Swiss cheese (about 4 ounces)

A handful of cherry tomatoes, halved

½ cup Thousand Island Dressing (page 349)

SPECIAL EQUIPMENT:
8 (8-inch) skewers

1. Thread several lettuce squares onto a skewer, then fold a roast beef slice into a 1-inch square and thread it onto the skewer. Follow with a dill pickle strip, a cheese cube, and a tomato half. Repeat the layers until the skewer is filled. Repeat with the remaining ingredients and skewers.

2. Place on a serving platter and serve with the dressing for dipping. Store in an airtight container in the refrigerator for up to 4 days.

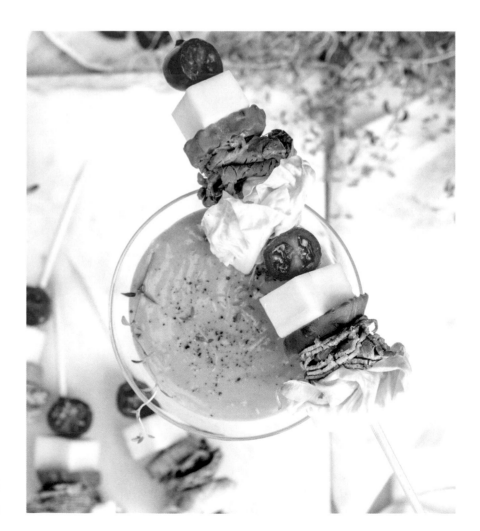

NUTRITIONAL INFO (per serving)

CALORIES	FAT	PROTEIN	CARBS	FIBER
383	26g	32g	5g	1g

COBB SALAD STACKS

Yield: 4 servings   *Prep time:* 15 minutes (not including time to boil eggs or make guacamole and dressing)
Cook time: 4 minutes

4 strips bacon, diced

2 hard-boiled eggs, diced

¼ cup mayonnaise, homemade (page 346) or store-bought

Fine sea salt and ground black pepper, to taste

1 cup Guacamole (page 310)

1 cup chopped romaine lettuce

1 cup diced leftover cooked chicken

½ cup Ranch Dressing (page 347)

¼ cup blue cheese crumbles (about 1 ounce)

1. Cook the bacon in a large skillet over medium-high heat until it is crispy and the fat is rendered, about 4 minutes. Remove the bacon with a slotted spoon and set aside.

2. In a medium-sized bowl, combine the hard-boiled eggs, mayonnaise, salt, and pepper.

3. To assemble, place ¼ cup of the guacamole in the center of a small serving plate and spread into a thick 3- to 4-inch circle. Mound the guacamole with ¼ cup of the romaine, followed by ¼ cup of the diced chicken, one-quarter of the egg salad mixture, one-quarter of the cooked bacon, 2 tablespoons of the ranch dressing, and 1 tablespoon of blue cheese crumbles. Repeat with the remaining ingredients to make a total of four salads.

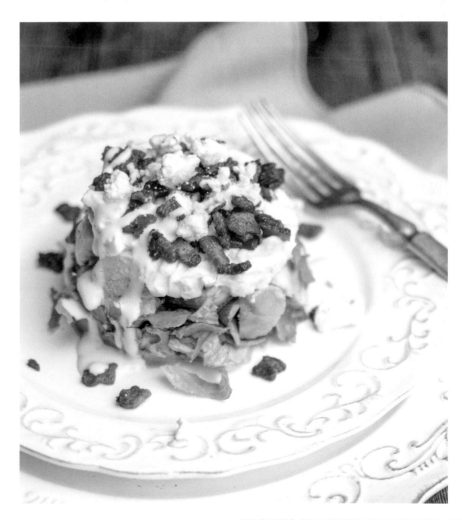

NUTRITIONAL INFO (per serving)

CALORIES	FAT	PROTEIN	CARBS	FIBER
513	49.5g	11.9g	5.1g	2.8g

GREEK CUCUMBER SALAD

Yield: 4 servings   *Prep time:* 5 minutes

OPTION

2 large cucumbers, very thinly sliced

¼ cup thinly sliced red onions

1½ tablespoons fine sea salt

¼ cup coconut vinegar or apple cider vinegar

½ cup sour cream (or coconut cream if dairy-free)

½ cup pitted black olives

1 tablespoon chopped fresh basil, or 1 teaspoon dried basil (optional)

1 tablespoon fresh oregano leaves, or 1 teaspoon dried oregano leaves (optional)

¼ cup feta cheese crumbles (about 1 ounce) (optional; omit for dairy-free)

1. In a colander, toss the cucumbers and onions with the salt and let sit to drain for 10 minutes. Press the liquid out of the vegetables and rinse well with cold water, then drain well.

2. Place the vinegar and sour cream in a medium bowl and stir well.

3. Add the cucumbers, onions, and olives to the vinegar mixture and toss to coat. Stir in the basil and oregano, if desired. Sprinkle with the feta, if desired. Store in an airtight container in the refrigerator for up to 5 days.

NUTRITIONAL INFO (per serving)

 CALORIES 247   FAT 18g   PROTEIN 12g   CARBS 8g   FIBER 1g

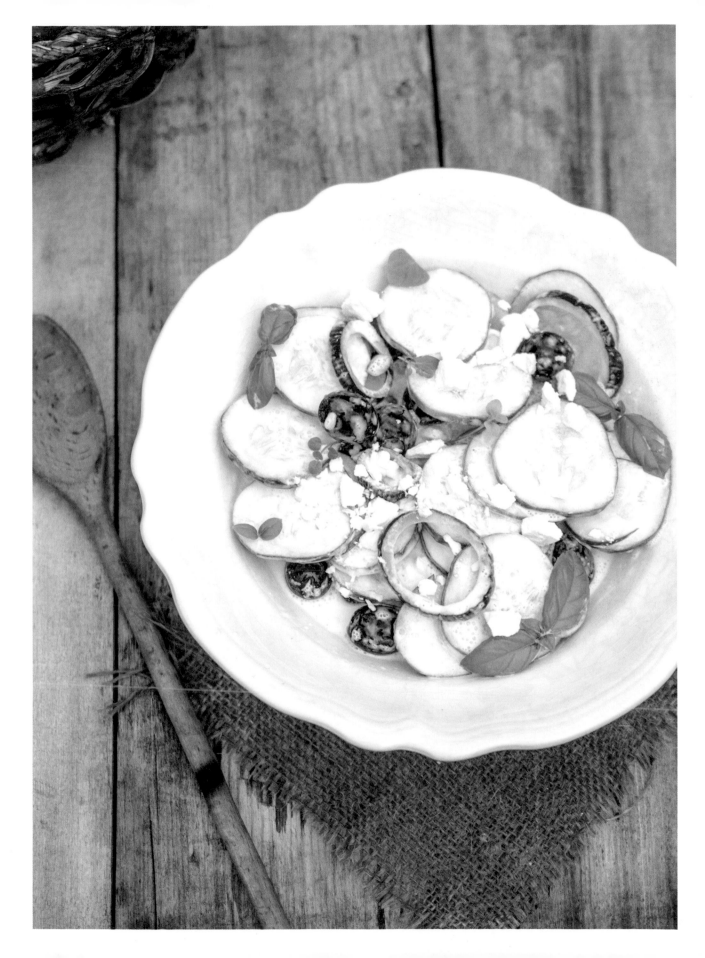

SAUERKRAUT

Yield: 8 cups (½ cup per serving)   *Prep time:* 18 minutes, plus up to 10 days to ferment

If you are new to making sauerkraut, this recipe is an awesome one to start with! Because it makes a small batch, the sauerkraut ferments faster. Here are some helpful tips before you start:

- *Use sea salt or a salt that does not contain iodine or anticaking agents, which can prevent fermentation.*

- *When making fermented foods, it's essential to give the healthy bacteria every chance of surviving by starting off with clean equipment, so always be scrupulously clean! It's very important to clean everything very well before you begin. (Packing jars should be sterilized in boiling water.) Make sure your hands are free from soap residue because you'll be touching the cabbage.*

- *Chlorinated water can prevent fermentation, so if you're using water to top off the jars in Step 6, be sure to use filtered, spring, or distilled water.*

- *If you get gas after eating cabbage, try adding caraway seeds. They help relieve gas by inhibiting its formation. Caraway seeds are very soothing to the digestive tract. The oil in caraway seeds contains antibacterial properties, which allow them to successfully expel infections from the body.*

1 medium head green cabbage (3 pounds)

1½ tablespoons fine sea salt

1 tablespoon caraway seeds (optional)

Nonchlorinated water, such as filtered, spring, or distilled water (to top off the jars, if needed)

SPECIAL EQUIPMENT:
2 wide-mouth, quart-sized canning jars

Something to weight down the kraut while it ferments

1. Remove and discard the wilted outer leaves of the cabbage. Cut the head into quarters and discard the core. Using a large knife, slice the cabbage quarters crosswise into thin ribbons that are 2 to 3 inches long.

2. Place the sliced cabbage in a very large glass mixing bowl and add the salt evenly throughout the cabbage. Use your hands to squeeze and distribute the salt into the cabbage. After a few minutes, the cabbage will become soft and a bit watery. Massage the cabbage for about 10 minutes. Add the caraway seeds, if using, and mix them in well.

3. Stuff the cabbage into two sterile 1-quart wide-mouth mason jars, packing it in tightly. Pour the liquid remaining in the bowl into the jars.

4. Place a clean weight on top of the cabbage to make sure the cabbage remains submerged in the liquid. I place a very clean metal measuring cup into the mouth of the mason jar and weight it down with clean rocks (from our rock polisher).

5. Place a cheesecloth or other clean thin cloth over the mouth of the jar and tie it with a string so air can flow in but the sauerkraut stays clean.

6. Over the next day or two, the cabbage will continue to release liquid. Press the measuring cup into the cabbage every few hours to make sure the cabbage remains submerged. If, after 24 hours, the cabbage has risen above the liquid and hasn't generated enough liquid of its own to cover the cabbage, dissolve 1 teaspoon of salt in 1 cup of water and pour in just enough to submerge the cabbage.

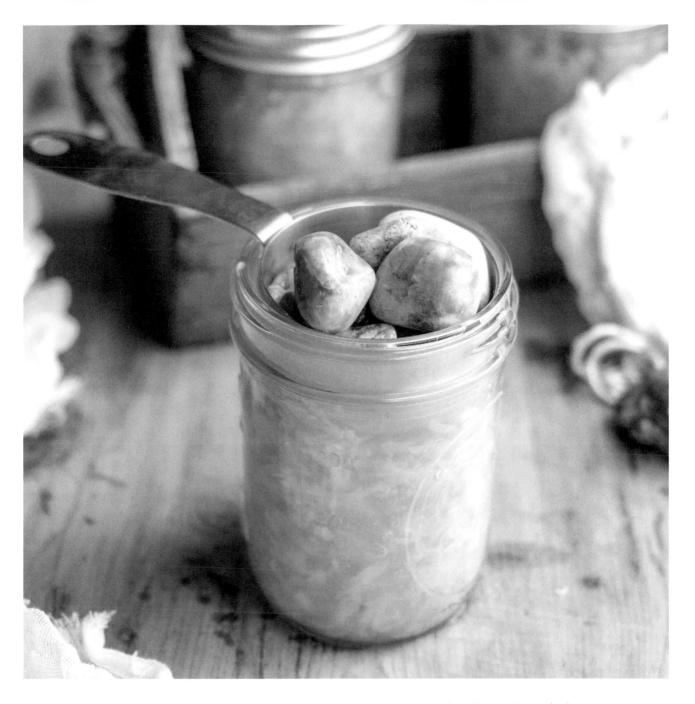

7. Now the fermenting begins. This takes 3 to 10 days. Keep the jars in a cool, dark room (65°F to 75°F), away from sunlight. Check it every day and press the cabbage down if it is floating above the liquid.

8. After 3 days, taste your creation. When it tastes good to you, remove the cheesecloth and the object you used to weight down the cabbage. Seal with an airtight cover and store in the refrigerator. If you prefer a stronger fermented taste, keep fermenting until you have your desired taste. You may notice bubbles and cloudiness in your sauerkraut during fermenting. This is the good bacteria you want for a healthy gut flora.

9. Store in the refrigerator for up to 2 months.

NUTRITIONAL INFO (per serving)

CALORIES	FAT	PROTEIN	CARBS	FIBER
22	0.2g	1g	5g	2g

KIMCHI

Yield: 6 cups (½ cup per serving)   *Prep time:* 25 minutes, plus up to 10 days to ferment

Here are some helpful tips before you start:

- *See the first three tips for making sauerkraut on page 294. The same tips apply here: use the right type of water (nonchlorinated) and the right type of salt (free of iodine or anticaking agents) and be scrupulously clean.*

- *Food-safe gloves are optional but highly recommended to protect your hands from stains or stings when mixing the spicy paste into the veggies.*

- *Fish sauce delivers an umami taste to kimchi. In lieu of fish sauce, you could use salted shrimp paste or a combination of both.*

1 large head Chinese (napa) cabbage (about 2 pounds)

¼ cup fine sea salt

Nonchlorinated water, such as filtered, spring, or distilled water

5 cloves garlic, minced

1 teaspoon grated fresh ginger

1 or 2 drops of stevia glycerite (optional)

2 tablespoons fish sauce

2 tablespoons Korean red pepper flakes, or more to desired heat (see Note)

8 ounces daikon radish, peeled and cut into matchsticks

4 green onions, trimmed and cut into 1-inch pieces

Note:

You can find Korean red pepper flakes at specialty stores or online. They provide a traditional Korean flavor that makes this dish extra special. They have a very bright red color and can range from mild to very hot. The mild version is referred to deolmaewoon gochugaru; the hot version is referred to as maewoon gochugaru.

1. Cut the cabbage lengthwise into quarters and remove the core. Slice each quarter crosswise into 1½-inch-wide strips.

2. Place the cabbage strips in a large glass bowl and cover with the salt. Using very clean hands, massage the salt into the cabbage until it starts to wilt. Add water to cover the cabbage. Put a plate on top and weight it down with something heavy so the cabbage strips are submerged. Let sit for 1 to 2 hours.

3. Transfer the cabbage to a colander and rinse very well with cold water. Drain for 15 minutes. Meanwhile, rinse and dry the bowl in which the cabbage strips were salted.

4. In a small bowl, combine the garlic, ginger, stevia, if using, and fish sauce. Mash until you have a very smooth paste. Add 2 tablespoons of the red pepper flakes, or use more if you like a hotter kimchi.

5. Using your hands, lightly squeeze the water from the cabbage strips and return them to the dry bowl. Add the radish, green onions, and paste.

6. Wearing food-safe gloves or using clean hands, gently work the paste into the vegetables until they're well coated.

7. Stuff the kimchi into two sterile 1-quart wide-mouth mason jars, packing it in tightly. At this point you want to keep it submerged in the liquid. I place a very clean metal measuring cup in the mouth of the mason jar and weight it down with clean rocks (from our rock polisher).

8. Place a cheesecloth or other clean thin cloth over the mouth of the jar and tie it with a string so air can flow in but the kimchi stays clean.

9. During the next day or two, the kimchi will continue to release liquid. Press the measuring cup into the mixture every few hours to make sure the vegetables remain submerged.

10. Now the fermenting begins. This takes 3 to 10 days. Keep the jars in a cool, dark room (65°F to 75°F), away from sunlight. Check it every day and press the kimchi down if it's floating above the liquid.

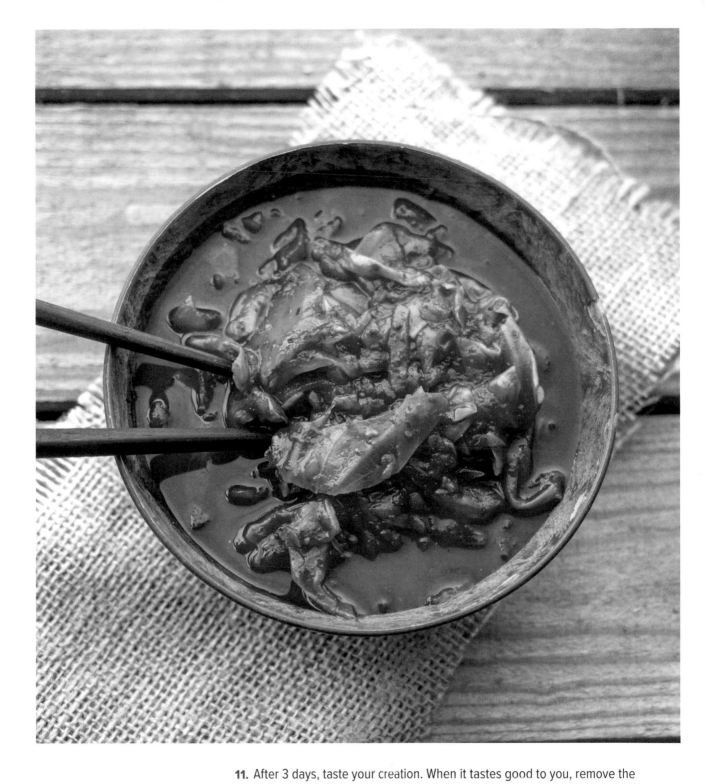

11. After 3 days, taste your creation. When it tastes good to you, remove the cheesecloth and object you used to weight down the cabbage. Seal with an airtight cover and store in the refrigerator. If you prefer a stronger fermented taste, keep fermenting until you have your desired taste. You may notice bubbles and cloudiness in your kimchi during fermenting. This is the good bacteria you want for a healthy gut flora.

12. Store in the refrigerator for up to 2 months.

NUTRITIONAL INFO (per serving)

  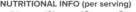

CALORIES	FAT	PROTEIN	CARBS	FIBER
27	0.4g	2g	4g	1g

QUICK ASIAN
FERMENTED CUCUMBERS

Yield: 8 servings   *Prep time:* 5 minutes, plus up to 2 days to ferment

  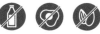

1 pound pickling cucumbers, thinly sliced

¼ cup sliced green onions

1½ tablespoons fine sea salt

1 tablespoon Swerve confectioners'-style sweetener or equivalent amount of liquid or powdered sweetener (see page 271)

1 tablespoon fish sauce

2 teaspoons Korean red pepper flakes (see **Note**, page 296)

2 teaspoons grated fresh ginger

2 cloves garlic, crushed to a paste

1. Place the ingredients in a large bowl. Stir well to combine.

2. Divide the mixture evenly among 4 sterile quart-sized jars, leaving 1 inch of space at the top of each jar. Allow to rest for 1 hour for the juices to release. Eat immediately if you prefer a mild-flavored fermented cucumber, or loosely cover and allow to ferment on the countertop for up to 2 days before chilling in the refrigerator. The flavors will develop over time. Cover and refrigerate until ready to consume. Open the jars every 2 to 3 days to release accumulated gas. Store in the refrigerator for up to 1 week.

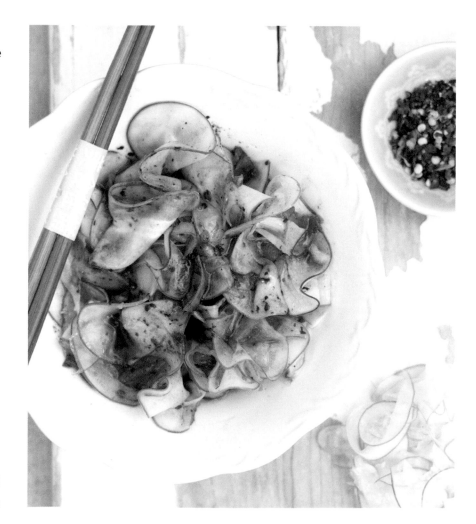

NUTRITIONAL INFO (per serving)

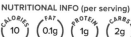

CALORIES	FAT	PROTEIN	CARBS	FIBER
10	0.1g	1g	2g	0.4g

DAIKON NOODLES

Yield: 2 servings   *Prep time:* 5 minutes   *Cook time:* 5 minutes

Daikon may be a new veggie for you. It is technically a radish but has an extremely mild flavor. If you have tried zucchini noodles and you were a bit disappointed by how wet the zucchini made the sauce, try daikon instead! It holds up great—even to the thickest, meatiest spaghetti sauce.

1 large daikon radish (about 2 pounds)

1 cup chicken or beef bone broth, homemade (page 344) or store-bought

SPECIAL EQUIPMENT:
Spiral slicer

1. Peel the daikon and cut off the ends. Using a spiral slicer, swirl it into long, thin noodlelike shapes.

2. Place the noodles and broth in a saucepan over medium-high heat. Cover and steam for 5 to 8 minutes, until the daikon is soft. Remove from the heat and drain the noodles. Serve with your favorite keto sauce or top with butter or coconut oil and a sprinkle of salt and serve as a side dish. Store in an airtight container in the refrigerator for up to 4 days.

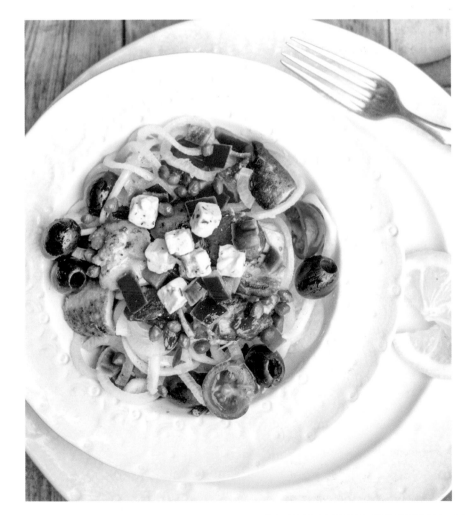

NUTRITIONAL INFO (per serving)

 CALORIES 179   FAT 13g   PROTEIN 11g   CARBS 10g   FIBER 0.1g

PURPLE CAULIFLOWER MASH

Yield: 4 servings   *Prep time:* 5 minutes   *Cook time:* 8 minutes

This Purple Cauliflower Mash tastes great with Broiled Salmon (page 318), as pictured.

2 cups chicken bone broth, homemade (page 344) or store-bought

Florets from 1 medium head purple or other color cauliflower, cut into bite-sized pieces

1 tablespoon dried chives, plus extra for garnish

1 clove garlic, minced

2 ounces cream cheese (¼ cup), softened

½ cup grated Parmesan cheese (about 1½ ounces)

Fine sea salt and ground black pepper

Butter, for serving

1. Pour the broth into a large saucepan. Use enough that you have about ½ inch of broth in the pan. Bring the broth to a boil, then add the cauliflower, chives, and garlic and cover the pan with a tight-fitting lid. Steam the cauliflower until tender, 6 to 8 minutes. Drain well. Pat it very dry between several layers of paper towels.

2. Place the cauliflower in a high-powered blender or food processor. Add the cheeses and puree until very smooth. Season to taste with salt and pepper. Transfer the mixture to a serving dish and garnish with pats of butter and chives.

3. Store in an airtight container in the refrigerator for up to 3 days. Reheat in a saucepan over medium heat for a few minutes or until warmed through.

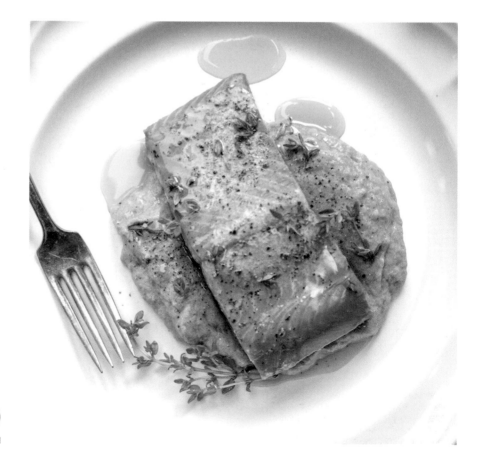

NUTRITIONAL INFO (per serving)

CALORIES	FAT	PROTEIN	CARBS	FIBER
178	12g	9g	9g	4g

BACON-WRAPPED
ASPARAGUS

Yield: 4 servings   *Prep time:* 5 minutes (not including time to make dressing)
Cook time: 10 to 20 minutes, depending on thickness of bacon and asparagus

24 spears asparagus (about 1 pound, depending thickness of asparagus)

2 tablespoons melted lard or coconut oil

½ teaspoon fine sea salt

¼ teaspoon ground black pepper

4 strips bacon

5 cloves garlic, minced

2 tablespoons chopped fresh chives, plus extra for garnish

½ cup Ranch Dressing (page 347)

1. Preheat the oven to 400°F. Trim the tough ends off the asparagus.

2. Coat the asparagus with the melted fat or oil. Season with the salt and pepper. Slice the bacon down the middle lengthwise, making 8 long, thin strips. Wrap 1 slice of bacon around 3 asparagus spears and secure the ends with a toothpick. Repeat with the remaining bacon strips and asparagus spears to make a total of 8 bundles.

3. Place on a rimmed baking sheet in one layer. Top the asparagus with the garlic and chives. Roast until the spears are slightly charred on the ends and the bacon is crispy, about 10 minutes for thin asparagus, 20 minutes for medium to thick spears.

4. Remove from the oven and garnish with additional chives. Serve with the dressing on the side. Best served fresh.

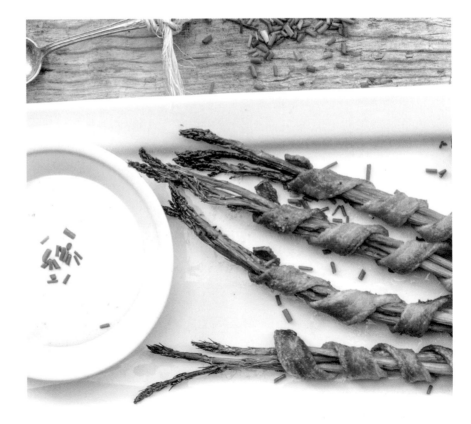

NUTRITIONAL INFO (per serving)

CALORIES 609 FAT 56g PROTEIN 14g CARBS 16g FIBER 6g

BLOODY MARY TOMATOES

Yield: 4 servings   *Prep time:* 4 minutes

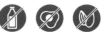

1 cup cherry tomatoes, cut in half

½ teaspoon celery salt

1 tablespoon hot sauce, such as Frank's RedHot (or more depending on how hot you prefer)

1 tablespoon avocado oil or extra-virgin olive oil

Place the sliced tomatoes on a serving platter. Sprinkle with the celery salt. Drizzle with the hot sauce and avocado oil. Store in an airtight container in the refrigerator for up to 4 days.

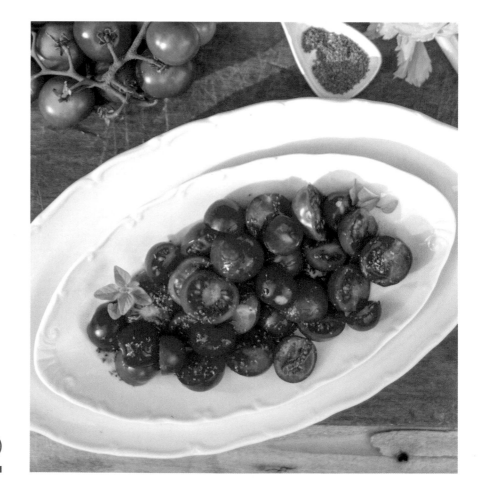

NUTRITIONAL INFO (per serving)

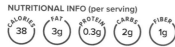

CALORIES	FAT	PROTEIN	CARBS	FIBER
38	3g	0.3g	2g	1g

FRIED ZUCCHINI BLOSSOMS

Yield: 4 servings   *Prep time:* 10 minutes   *Cook time:* 2 minutes

Coconut oil, for frying

4 ounces fresh (soft) goat cheese or cream cheese (½ cup)

1 teaspoon chopped fresh basil

8 zucchini blossoms

2 large eggs

Fine sea salt

Note:

I store a large mason jar of coconut oil for frying in the refrigerator and strain the used oil back into the jar through a fine-mesh strainer when I am finished frying. You can get about four uses out of the same batch of oil when you strain it and store it in the fridge.

1. Heat ½ inch of oil to 350°F in a large, deep cast-iron pan.

2. In a small bowl, mix together the goat cheese and basil. Clean the zucchini blossoms and fill each one with about 1½ teaspoons of the goat cheese mixture. Set aside.

3. Separate the eggs and whip the whites until soft peaks form. Lightly beat the egg yolks and add them to bowl with the whites; stir well to mix the yolks into the whites.

4. Dip the stuffed zucchini blossoms into the whipped egg mixture so they're covered on all sides.

5. Carefully place the dipped zucchini blossoms into the hot oil, working in batches if needed. Fry on all sides until golden brown, about 1 minute per side.

6. Remove to a paper towel to drain. Sprinkle with salt. Best served fresh.

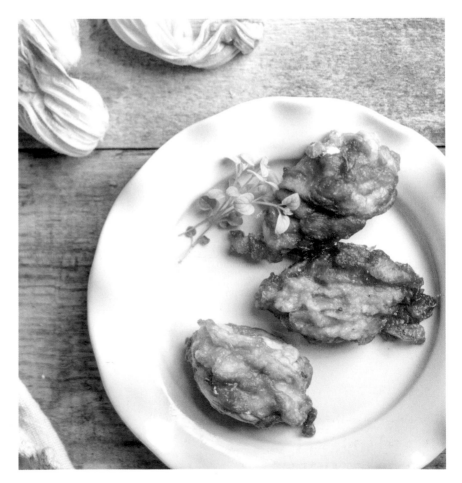

NUTRITIONAL INFO (per serving)

CALORIES 158 | FAT 12.2g | PROTEIN 11g | CARBS 1g | FIBER 0g

FAUXTATOES AU GRATIN

Yield: 8 servings   *Prep time:* 10 minutes   *Cook time:* 65 minutes

2 large daikon radishes (about 3 pounds)

Butter, for greasing the dish

1 teaspoon fine sea salt, divided

½ teaspoon ground black pepper, divided

4 ounces cream cheese (½ cup), softened, divided

2 cups grated Parmesan cheese (about 6 ounces), divided

1 cup shredded cheddar cheese (about 4 ounces), divided

1 cup heavy cream

Fresh thyme leaves, for garnish

2 strips bacon, fried until crispy and then crumbled, for garnish

1. Preheat the oven to 375°F.

2. Bring a large pot of water to a boil. Peel and slice the daikon. Add the daikon to the boiling water and boil for 15 minutes to soften. Drain.

3. Grease a 10 by 7½-inch baking dish with butter. Layer half the sliced daikon in the bottom of the baking dish. Sprinkle ½ teaspoon of the salt and ¼ teaspoon of the pepper on top. Spread half of the cream cheese on the daikon layer, then sprinkle the cream cheese with ½ cup of the Parmesan and ½ cup of the shredded cheddar. Top with the rest of the daikon, sprinkle with the remaining ½ teaspoon of salt and ¼ teaspoon of pepper, spread the remaining cream cheese on the layer of daikon, then top with the remaining 1½ cups of Parmesan and ½ cup of cheddar. Pour in the cream.

4. Bake for 50 minutes or until nice and golden brown on top. Let cool for 10 minutes before slicing and serving. Garnish with thyme leaves and crumbled bacon, if desired.

5. Store in an airtight container in the refrigerator for up to 4 days or in the freezer for up to a month. To reheat, place in a baking dish and heat in a preheated 375°F oven for 5 minutes or until heated through.

NUTRITIONAL INFO (per serving)

CALORIES	FAT	PROTEIN	CARBS	FIBER
303	28g	15g	6g	0.3g

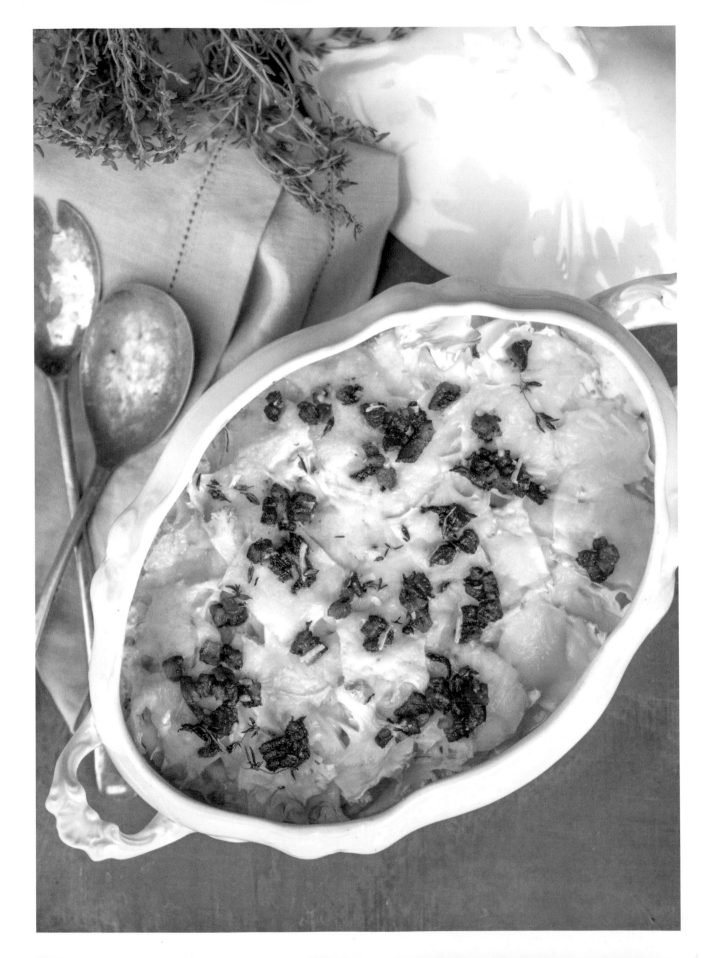

CAULIFLOWER PATTIES

Yield: 4 servings *Prep time:* 7 minutes *Cook time:* 30 minutes

2 (1-pound) bags frozen cauliflower

4 strips bacon, diced

½ cup diced onions

¾ cup blanched almond flour

4 ounces cream cheese (½ cup), softened

¾ cup shredded cheddar cheese (about 3 ounces)

2 large eggs

1 teaspoon fine sea salt

½ teaspoon ground black pepper

1. Bring a large pot of water to a boil. Add the cauliflower and cook for 8 minutes or until fork-tender.

2. While the cauliflower is cooking, cook the bacon in a large skillet over medium-high heat until it's crispy and the fat is rendered, about 4 minutes. Remove the bacon with a slotted spoon to a large mixing bowl, leaving the fat in the pan.

3. Add the onions to the skillet and cook over medium heat until the onions are translucent, about 4 minutes.

4. Add the cooked onions to the large mixing bowl with the bacon. Leave the bacon fat in the skillet for frying the patties.

5. Once the cauliflower is cooked until soft, drain the excess water and place the cauliflower on a cheesecloth to soak up any water still in the cauliflower. Squeeze tightly to remove any excess water and to mash the cauliflower a bit with the cloth.

6. When the excess water is out of the cauliflower, put the cauliflower in the large mixing bowl with the bacon and onion mixture and mash the cauliflower with a hand mixer on high speed. Add the almond flour, cream cheese, grated cheese, eggs, salt, and pepper and mix with a wooden spoon until well combined.

7. Using your hands, form the mixture into 3-inch balls, then flatten and shape them into small slider-sized patties, about ¾ inch thick.

8. Heat the skillet with the bacon fat to medium-high heat. Add the patties in batches and fry on both sides for about 3 minutes per side or until golden brown and cooked through.

9. Store in an airtight container in the refrigerator for up to 4 days or in the freezer for up to a month. To reheat, place in a greased skillet over medium-high heat for 5 minutes.

NUTRITIONAL INFO (per serving)

CALORIES 475 FAT 35g PROTEIN 24g CARBS 18g FIBER 8g

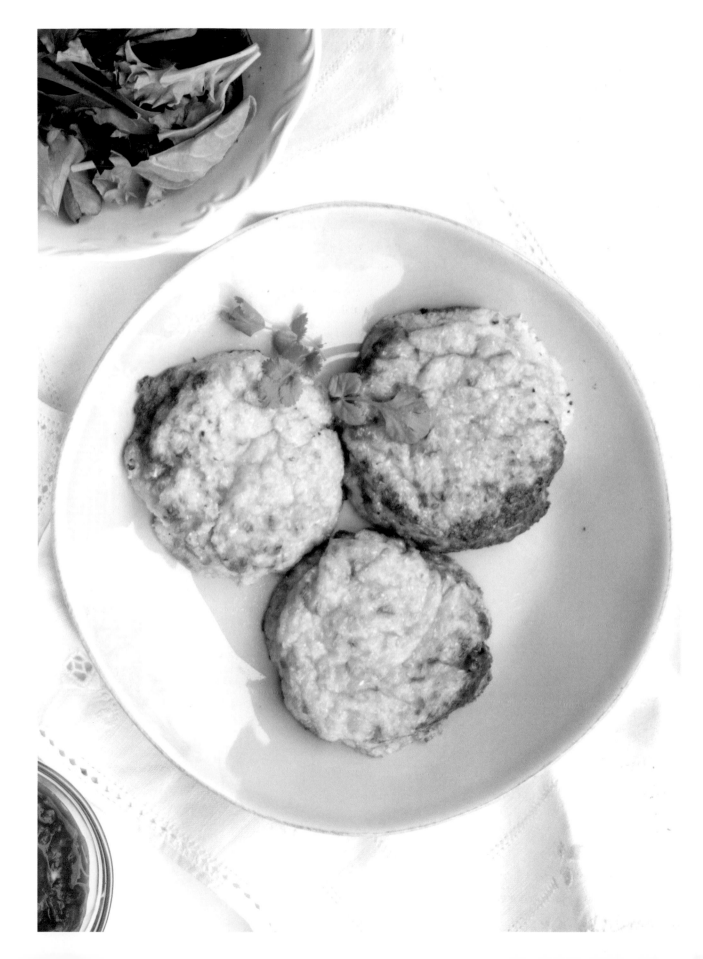

KIMCHI DEVILED EGGS

Yield: 2 dozen (2 halves per serving)   *Prep time:* 5 minutes   *Cook time:* 11 minutes

12 large eggs

4 strips bacon

½ cup mayonnaise, homemade (page 346) or store-bought

1 teaspoon hot sauce, such as Frank's RedHot, or more to taste

Fine sea salt

FOR GARNISH:

1½ cups chopped kimchi, homemade (page 296) or store-bought

Black sesame seeds (optional)

Korean red pepper flakes (see Note, page 296) (optional)

1. Hard-boil the eggs: Place the eggs in a saucepan and cover with cold water. Bring to a boil and immediately remove the pan from the heat. Cover and let the eggs cook in the hot water for 11 minutes.

2. While the eggs are cooking, cook the bacon in a large skillet over medium-high heat until it's crispy and the fat is rendered, about 4 minutes. Remove from the pan and, once cooled, crumble into very small pieces and set aside.

3. When the eggs have cooked for 11 minutes, remove the eggs from the hot water and rinse them under cold water until cooled. Peel the boiled eggs and cut them in half lengthwise. Remove the yolks and place into a small bowl. Mash the egg yolks with the mayonnaise, crumbled bacon, and kimchi. Stir in the hot sauce to desired heat. Season with salt to taste.

4. Fill the egg white halves with the yolk mixture and top each with about 1 tablespoon of the kimchi. Sprinkle with black sesame seeds and red pepper flakes, if using. Refrigerate until serving. Store in an airtight container in the fridge for up to 4 days.

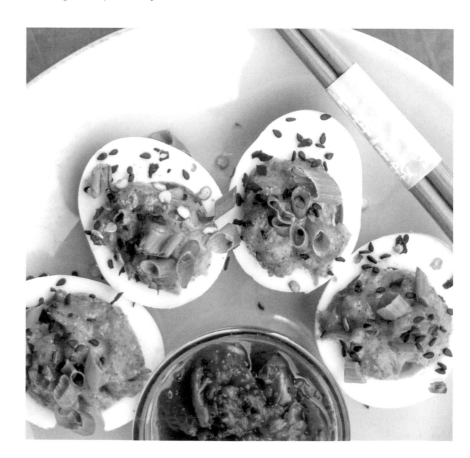

NUTRITIONAL INFO (per serving)

CALORIES	FAT	PROTEIN	CARBS	FIBER
158	14.2g	6.7g	0.7g	0g

HOT REUBEN DIP

Yield: 12 servings   *Prep time:* 5 minutes

2 (8-ounce) packages cream cheese, softened

½ pound corned beef, chopped

1 cup drained and chopped sauerkraut, homemade (page 294) or store-bought

½ cup shredded Swiss cheese (about 2 ounces)

2 tablespoons sauerkraut juice (from above)

Fine sea salt and ground black pepper

Serving suggestions:
Sliced bell peppers

Asparagus spears, trimmed

Thinly sliced corned beef (from the deli counter), for rolling

1. Place the softened cream cheese in a medium saucepan over medium heat. Stir to loosen the cream cheese.

2. Add the chopped corned beef, sauerkraut, Swiss cheese, and sauerkraut juice. Add the liquid from the sauerkraut to the mixture to thin the dip a little and stir until well combined. Taste and add salt and pepper to your liking.

3. Serve hot with sliced bell peppers, asparagus spears, and/or slices of deli corned beef rolled into logs for dipping or scooping the dip.

4. Store in an airtight container in the refrigerator for up to 4 days. To reheat, place in a medium saucepan over medium heat for 4 minutes or until heated through. Alternatively, this dip can be served cold, but it will be very thick.

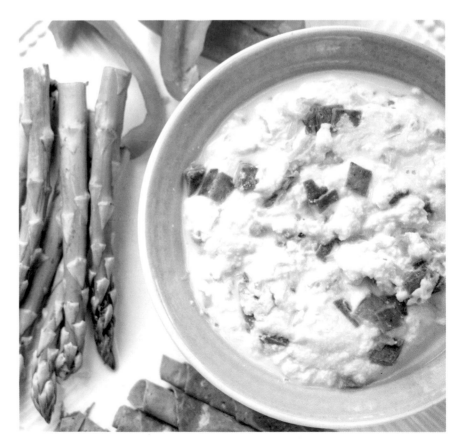

NUTRITIONAL INFO (per serving)

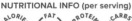

CALORIES	FAT	PROTEIN	CARBS	FIBER
175	14g	7g	1g	0g

GUACAMOLE

Yield: about 3 cups (½ cup per serving)   *Prep time:* 4 minutes

3 avocados, peeled, halved, and pitted

½ cup diced onions

2 cloves garlic, crushed to a paste

2 plum tomatoes, diced

3 to 4 tablespoons lime juice

3 tablespoons chopped fresh cilantro leaves

1 teaspoon fine sea salt

½ teaspoon ground cumin

1. Place the avocados in a large bowl and mash with a fork to the desired consistency.

2. Add the onions, garlic, tomatoes, 3 tablespoons of the lime juice, cilantro, salt, and cumin. Stir until well combined. Taste and add up to 1 tablespoon more lime juice, if desired.

3. Cover tightly and refrigerate for 1 hour for the best flavor, or serve immediately.

NUTRITIONAL INFO (per serving)

CALORIES (220)   FAT (20g)   PROTEIN (2.6g)   CARBS (11g)   FIBER (7.4g)

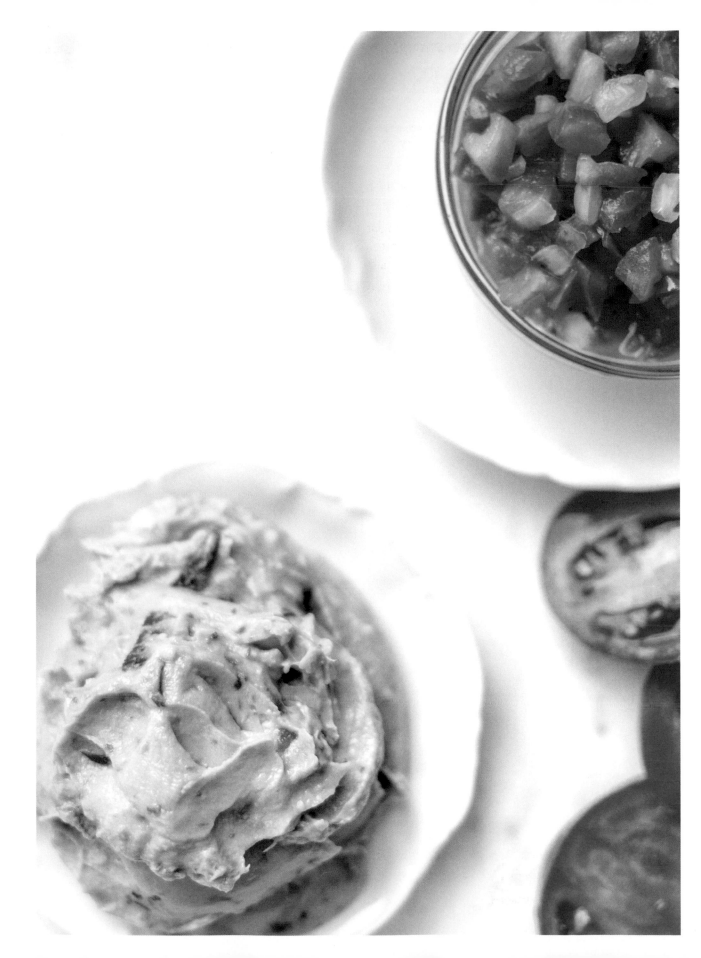

EASY CHICKEN FRIED RICE

Yield: 2 servings   *Prep time:* 5 minutes   *Cook time:* 14 minutes

3 strips bacon, diced

1 clove garlic, minced

¼ cup diced onions

2 boneless, skinless chicken thighs, cut into ¾-inch pieces

2 cups riced cauliflower florets (from about ½ small head cauliflower)

1 large egg, beaten

Sliced green onions, for garnish

1. In a large skillet over medium-high heat, cook the bacon until it's crispy and the fat is rendered, about 4 minutes. Using a slotted spoon, remove the bacon, but leave the drippings in the pan.

2. Add the garlic and onions to the skillet and sauté in the bacon drippings until the onions are translucent, about 2 minutes. Add the chicken and cook for 5 minutes or until it is cooked through and no longer pink in the center. Add the riced cauliflower and sauté for 4 minutes or until tender. Add the egg and sauté into the other ingredients for 1 minute or until the egg is cooked through.

3. Garnish with sliced green onions and serve.

4. Store in an airtight container in the refrigerator for up to 4 days or in the freezer for up to a month. To reheat, place in a skillet over medium-high heat for 3 minutes or until heated through.

NUTRITIONAL INFO (per serving)

CALORIES	FAT	PROTEIN	CARBS	FIBER
310	16g	30g	10g	2g

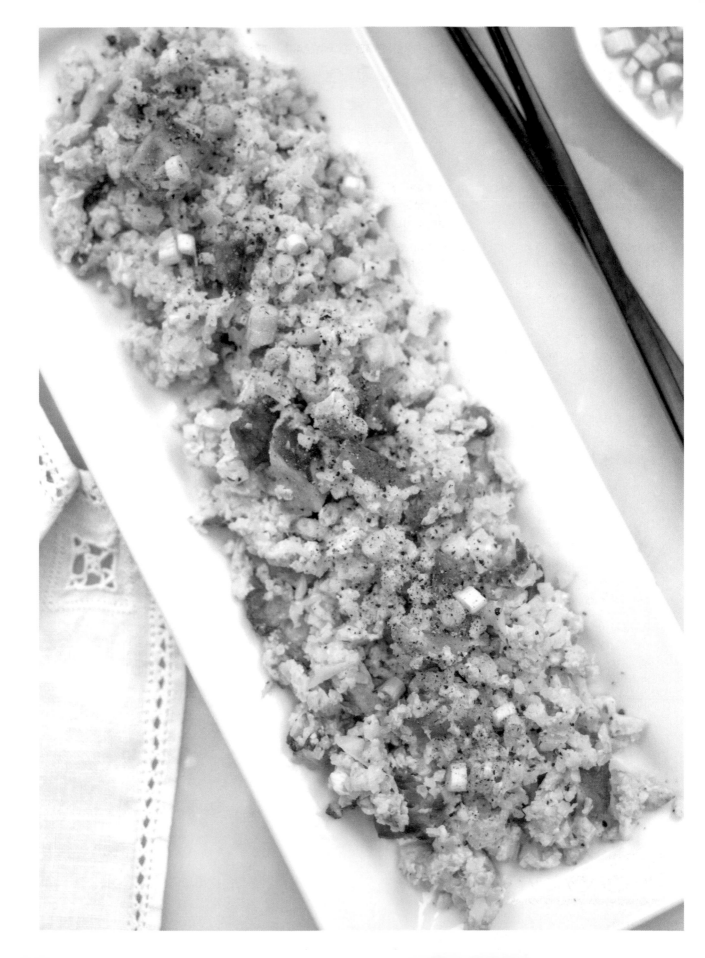

CHINESE CHICKEN AND BROCCOLI SOUP

Yield: 4 servings   *Prep time:* 10 minutes, plus time to marinate chicken   *Cook time:* 20 minutes

OPTION

1 pound boneless, skinless chicken thighs, cut into 1-inch pieces

¼ cup coconut aminos or wheat-free tamari

2 tablespoons unsalted butter or coconut oil

½ cup diced onions

3 cloves garlic, minced

1 tablespoon grated fresh ginger (optional)

¼ teaspoon fine sea salt

½ teaspoon ground black pepper

3 cups bite-sized fresh broccoli florets

3 cups chicken bone broth, homemade (page 344) or store-bought

1 tablespoon fish sauce

2 tablespoons Swerve confectioners'-style sweetener or equivalent amount of liquid or powdered sweetener (see page 271)

FOR GARNISH (OPTIONAL):
Red pepper flakes

Ground black pepper

1. Place the chicken in a medium bowl. Add the coconut aminos and toss to coat. Place in the refrigerator to marinate for at least 1 hour or overnight.

2. Heat the butter in a stockpot over medium-high heat. Add the onions, garlic, and ginger, if using. Toss to coat the onions with the butter, sprinkle with the salt and pepper, and cook for about 5 minutes, stirring occasionally. When the onions are tender, add the marinated chicken (discarding the marinating liquid) and sauté for 5 minutes or until the chicken in cooked through and no longer pink inside.

3. Add the broccoli and broth to the stockpot and bring to a simmer. Stir in the fish sauce and sweetener, then taste and adjust the saltiness or sweetness as desired. Simmer until the broccoli is soft, about 4 minutes. Serve hot and garnish with red pepper flakes and/or black pepper.

4. Store in an airtight container in the refrigerator for up to 4 days. To reheat, place in a saucepan over medium heat for 5 minutes or until heated through.

NUTRITIONAL INFO (per serving)

CALORIES	FAT	PROTEIN	CARBS	FIBER
294	15g	28g	11g	5g

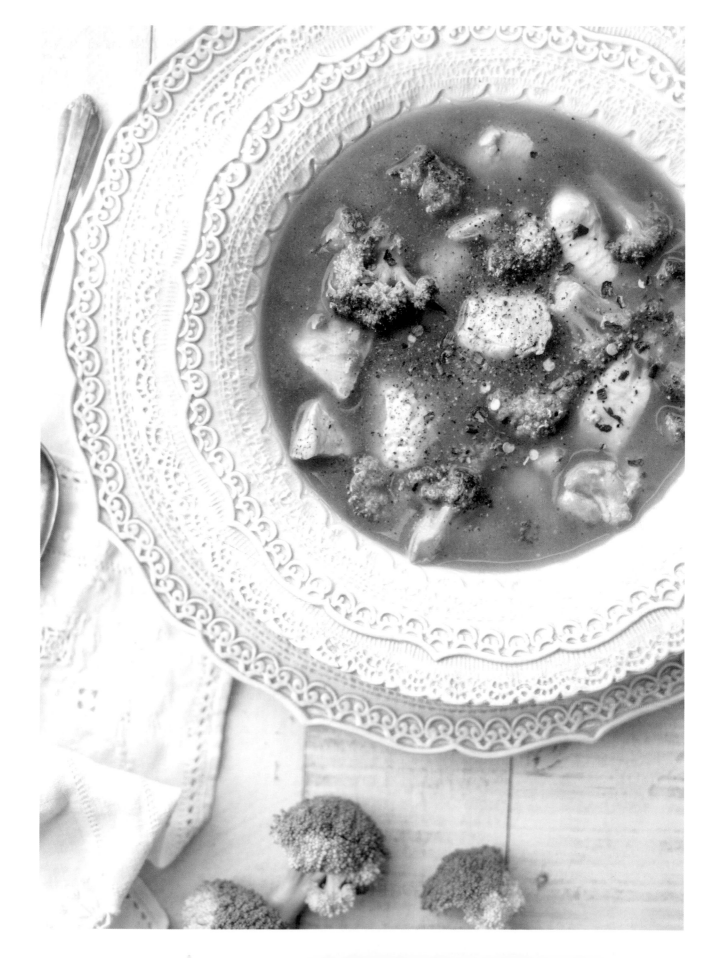

KIMCHI BURGERS

Yield: 4 servings   *Prep time:* 5 minutes   *Cook time:* 8 minutes

Burger tip: To keep burgers moist, salt only the outside of the meat. Salt removes water from meat and dissolves some of the meat protein, which causes the insoluble proteins to bind together, which is great for making sausages, when you want a springy, chewy texture. However, it's not great for creating tender, juicy burgers.

BURGERS:

1 tablespoon lard

1 pound ground beef

1½ teaspoons fine sea salt

1 teaspoon ground black pepper, divided

FOR SERVING:

8 lettuce leaves

½ cup kimchi, homemade (page 296) or store-bought

½ cup chopped red cabbage

1. Heat the lard in a cast-iron skillet over medium-high heat. Using your hands, form the ground beef into 4 patties, about 4 inches in diameter. Season the outsides with the salt and pepper. Fry the burgers for 3 minutes on each side for medium-done burgers or cook to your desired doneness (see the chart below).

2. Serve each burger on 2 lettuce leaves topped with 2 tablespoons of kimchi and 2 tablespoons of chopped red cabbage.

3. Store leftover burgers in an airtight container in the refrigerator for up to 4 days. Leftover mayo will keep in an airtight container in the refrigerator for up to 2 weeks. To reheat burgers, place in a skillet over medium-high heat for 3 minutes or until heated through.

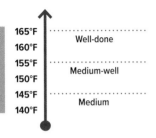

165°F
Well-done
160°F

155°F
Medium-well
150°F

145°F
Medium
140°F

NUTRITIONAL INFO (per serving)

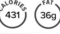   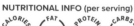

CALORIES (431)   FAT (36g)   PROTEIN (21g)   CARBS (4g)   FIBER (2g)

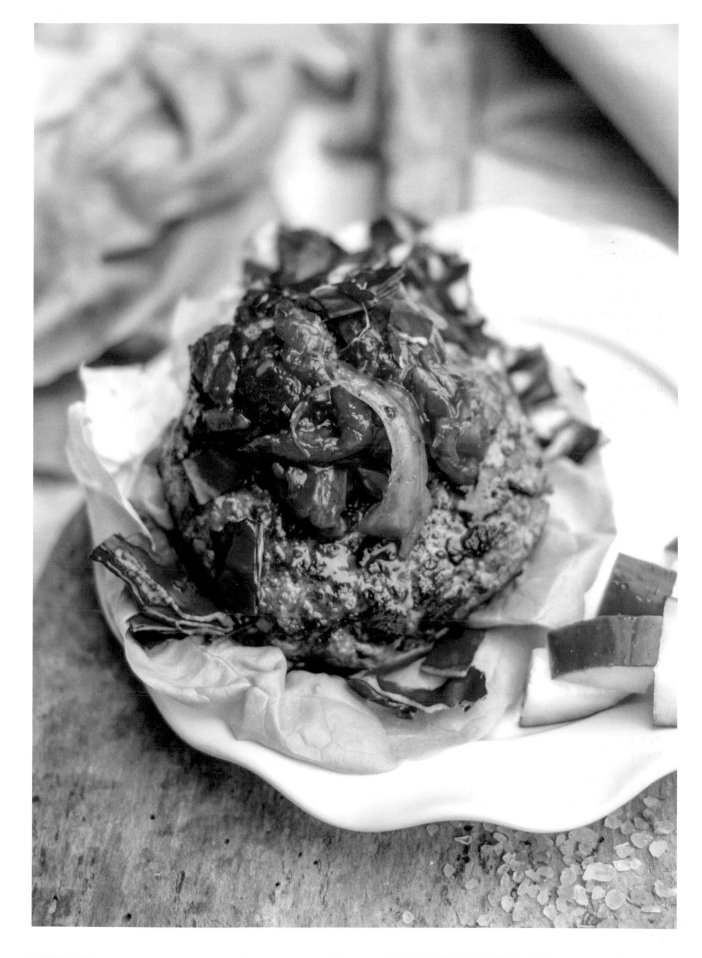

BROILED SALMON

Yield: 4 servings   *Prep time:* 4 minutes   *Cook time:* 8 minutes

OPTION

4 (4-ounce) wild-caught salmon fillets

1 teaspoon fine sea salt

¾ teaspoon ground black pepper

2 cups Purple Cauliflower Mash (page 300), for serving (optional; omit for dairy-free)

Extra-virgin olive oil, for drizzling (optional)

Fresh thyme leaves or other herb of choice, for garnish (optional)

1. Place an oven rack in the top position, about 4 inches below the broiler. Preheat the broiler to high.

2. Sprinkle the salmon with the salt and pepper, then place it on a broiler pan or rimmed baking sheet, skin side down.

3. Broil until the fish is opaque in the center and flakes easily with a fork, 8 to 10 minutes, depending on the salmon's thickness.

4. Serve on top of the Purple Cauliflower Mash and garnish with a drizzle of olive oil and with thyme, if desired.

5. Store in an airtight container in the refrigerator for up to 4 days. To reheat, place in a skillet over medium-high heat for 3 minutes or until heated through.

NUTRITIONAL INFO
(per serving, without cauliflower puree or garnishes)

CALORIES	FAT	PROTEIN	CARBS	FIBER
262	8g	44g	1g	0.3g

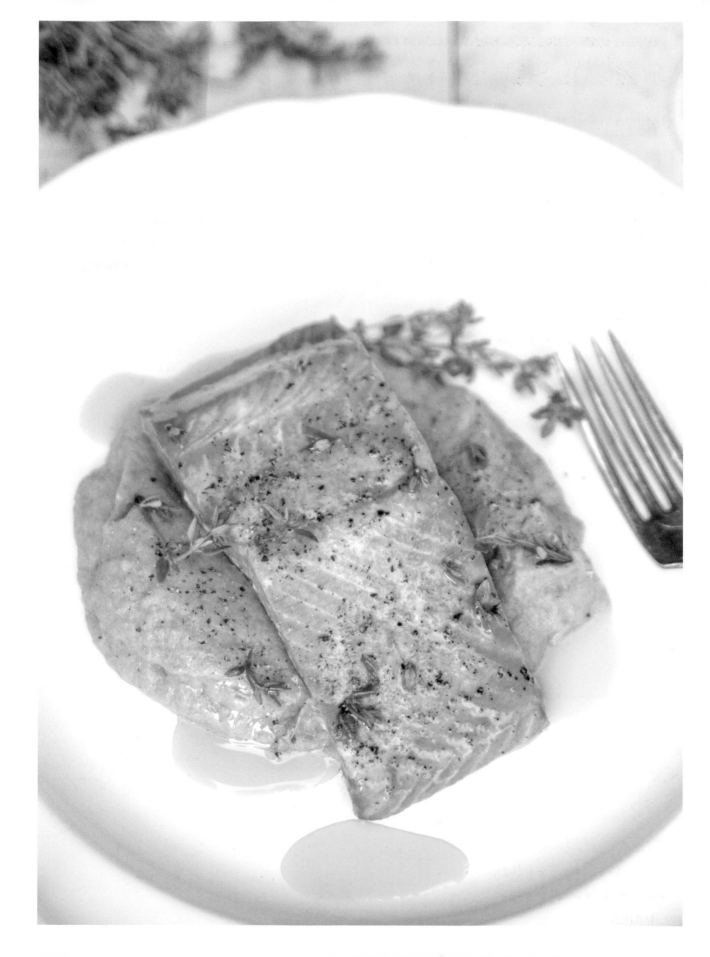

SPANAKOPITA

Yield: 4 servings   *Prep time:* 9 minutes   *Cook time:* 12 minutes

Coconut oil or lard, for greasing the pan

DOUGH:

1¾ cups shredded mozzarella cheese (about 7 ounces)

2 tablespoons cream cheese, softened

¾ cup blanched almond flour

1 large egg

⅛ teaspoon fine sea salt

FILLING:

1 tablespoon unsalted butter

4 cups fresh spinach

2 tablespoons jarred roasted, marinated red peppers, diced

1 tablespoon minced onions

1 teaspoon minced garlic

½ teaspoon fine sea salt

½ cup feta cheese crumbles (about 2 ounces), plus extra for garnish

Fresh parsley and/or oregano, for garnish

1. Preheat the oven to 400°F. Line a pizza stone or baking sheet (a pizza stone will create a crispier bottom crust) with parchment paper, then grease the paper with coconut oil or lard.

2. Make the dough: Place the mozzarella and cream cheese in a microwave-safe bowl and microwave for 1 to 2 minutes, or until the cheese is entirely melted. Stir well.

3. Add the almond flour, egg, and salt and combine well using a hand mixer. Use your hands and work it like a traditional dough, kneading for about 3 minutes. (Note: If the dough is too sticky, chill it in the refrigerator for at least 1 hour or overnight.)

4. Divide the dough into four equal portions. Put the dough on the greased parchment and pat each portion with your hands or use a rolling pin to make 4 squares, about 4½ inches.

5. Make the filling: Heat the butter in a skillet over medium heat. Add the spinach, red peppers, onions, garlic, and salt to the pan. Sauté for 4 minutes or until the spinach is wilted.

6. Place the filling mixture down the middle of each square of dough. Top with the feta cheese. Fold each square in half from corner to corner to make a triangle and press the edges together to seal. This dough is forgiving, so if you see a hole, just press it together with your fingers.

7. Place the pizza stone with the spanakopita in the oven and bake for 10 minutes or until the dough is golden brown and fully cooked. Remove from the oven. Garnish with feta and fresh parsley or oregano or both.

8. Store in an airtight container in the refrigerator for up to 4 days. To reheat, place on a baking sheet in a preheated 400°F oven for 3 minutes or until heated through.

NUTRITIONAL INFO (per serving)

CALORIES 260   FAT 21.5g   PROTEIN 9.7g   CARBS 7.2g   FIBER 3g

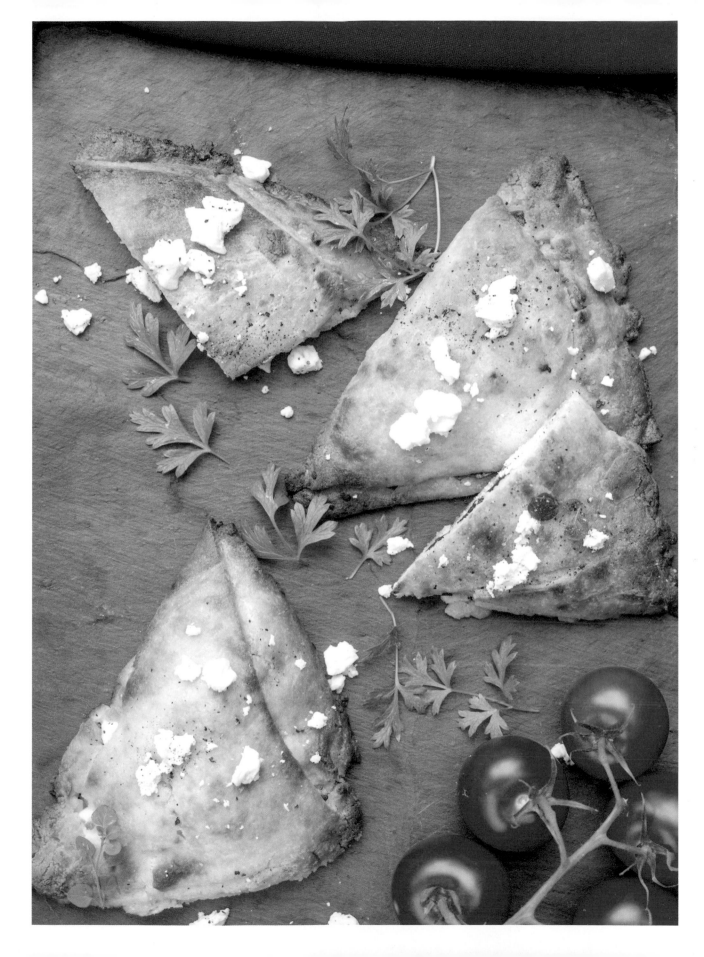

REUBEN SLIDERS

Yield: 8 sliders (2 per serving)   *Prep time:* 8 minutes (not including time to make dressing)
Cook time: 6 minutes

OPTION

Coconut oil or lard (if pan-frying burgers)

1 pound ground beef or pork

2½ teaspoons fine sea salt

1½ teaspoons ground black pepper

8 slices Swiss cheese (optional; omit for dairy-free)

8 butter lettuce leaves

½ cup sauerkraut, homemade (page 294) or store-bought, warmed

½ cup Thousand Island Dressing (page 349)

1. Heat a grill to medium-high heat. (Alternatively, heat about 1½ teaspoons of coconut oil or lard in a cast-iron skillet over medium-high heat.)

2. Using your hands, form the meat into 8 small patties that are about ½ inch thick. Season the outsides with the salt and pepper. Grill or pan-fry the burgers on both sides until they are medium done (if using beef, cook to a minimum of 145°F; if using pork, cook to a minimum of 160°F). Add slices of Swiss cheese, if using, and continue to heat until melted.

3. Remove the burgers from the grill or pan and place on butter lettuce leaves for wrapping.

4. Serve each burger with sauerkraut and Thousand Island dressing. These burgers are best served fresh because small burgers like these tend to become dry when reheated.

NUTRITIONAL INFO (per serving)

CALORIES 512 FAT 47g PROTEIN 20g CARBS 2g FIBER 0.4g

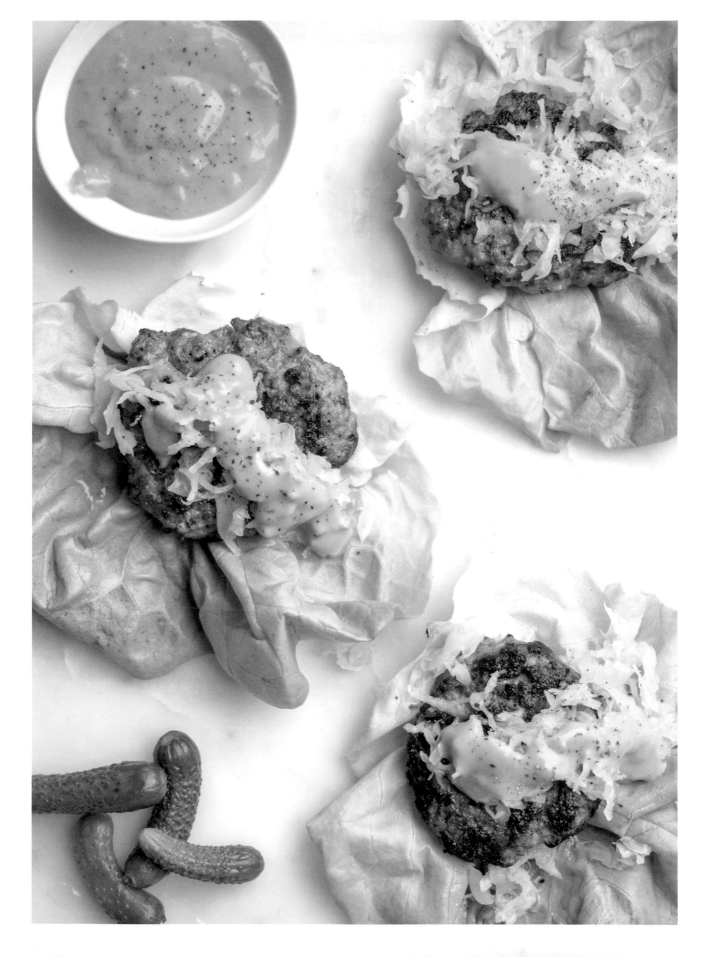

HEARTY CHICKEN ASPARAGUS
SALAD

Yield: 6 servings   *Prep time:* 10 minutes   *Cook time:* 20 minutes

I love to use leftover chicken for this recipe. If you don't have leftover chicken, feel free to pick up an organic rotisserie chicken on your way home!

1 tablespoon ghee or unsalted butter, plus more for greasing the dish

3 cups trimmed and ½-inch-sliced asparagus

1 tablespoon diced celery

1 tablespoon diced onions

1 clove garlic, crushed to a paste

3 cups diced roasted chicken

3 ounces cream cheese (⅓ cup), softened

2 tablespoons mayonnaise, homemade (page 346) or store-bought

½ teaspoon fine sea salt

¼ teaspoon ground black pepper

FOR GARNISH:

3 asparagus spears, trimmed and cut into 1-inch pieces (optional)

1 cup shredded sharp cheddar cheese (about 4 ounces) (optional)

⅓ cup chopped fresh dill or parsley

18 cherry tomatoes, halved

1. Melt the ghee or butter in a small skillet over medium-high heat. Add the asparagus, celery, and onions and sauté for 3 minutes, until the asparagus is starting to soften and the onions are translucent. Add the garlic and sauté for another minute. Transfer the asparagus mixture to a medium mixing bowl. Add the chicken, cream cheese, mayonnaise, salt, and pepper to the bowl and mix well to combine.

2. Divide the salad among serving bowls and sprinkle with the asparagus pieces and cheese, if using. Garnish with dill or parsley and cherry tomato halves.

3. Store in an airtight container in the refrigerator for up to 4 days.

NUTRITIONAL INFO (per serving)

CALORIES 314   FAT 21g   PROTEIN 26g   CARBS 4g   FIBER 1g

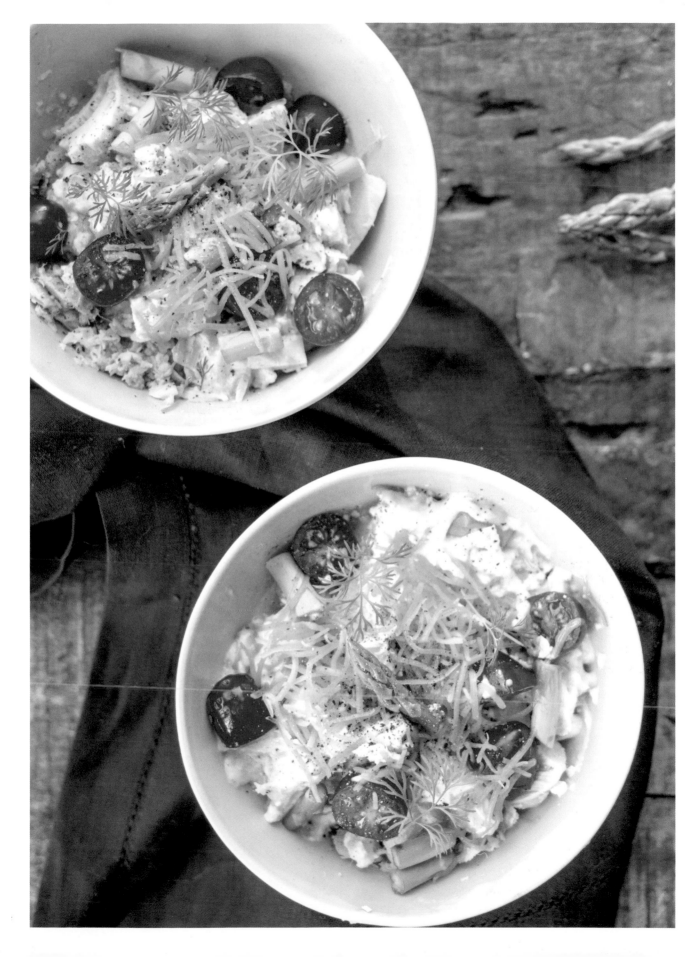

MEXICAN TENDERLOIN

Yield: 4 servings
Prep time: 10 minutes, plus time to marinate meat (not including time to make seasoning or guacamole)
Cook time: 15 minutes

4 cloves garlic, minced

1 tablespoon lime juice

1 tablespoons MCT oil or avocado oil

4 teaspoons Taco Seasoning (page 350)

1 pound beef or venison tenderloin

1 tablespoon lard

2 teaspoons fine sea salt

FOR SERVING:
4 cups arugula

2 limes, quartered and sliced

Salsa

Guacamole (page 310)

1. Combine the garlic, lime juice, oil, and taco seasoning in a baking dish. Add the tenderloin and roll it in the seasoning mixture to coat. Cover and refrigerate for at least 30 minutes or overnight.

2. Preheat the oven to 450°F.

3. Heat the lard in a large cast-iron skillet over medium-high heat. Season the loin on all sides with the salt, then place the loin in the hot skillet. Sear on all sides for about 2 minutes per side, or until a nice crust forms.

4. Use an oven mitt to transfer the skillet to the hot oven. Cook the loin for 7 to 8 minutes, until medium done.

5. Remove the loin from the oven and allow to rest on a cutting board for 10 minutes before slicing. Set the sliced tenderloin on a bed of arugula and serve with lime quarters, salsa, and guacamole. Store in an airtight container in the refrigerator for up to 4 days. To reheat, place in a skillet over medium-high heat for 3 minutes or until heated through.

NUTRITIONAL INFO (per serving)

CALORIES 253 | FAT 11g | PROTEIN 34g | CARBS 1g | FIBER 0g

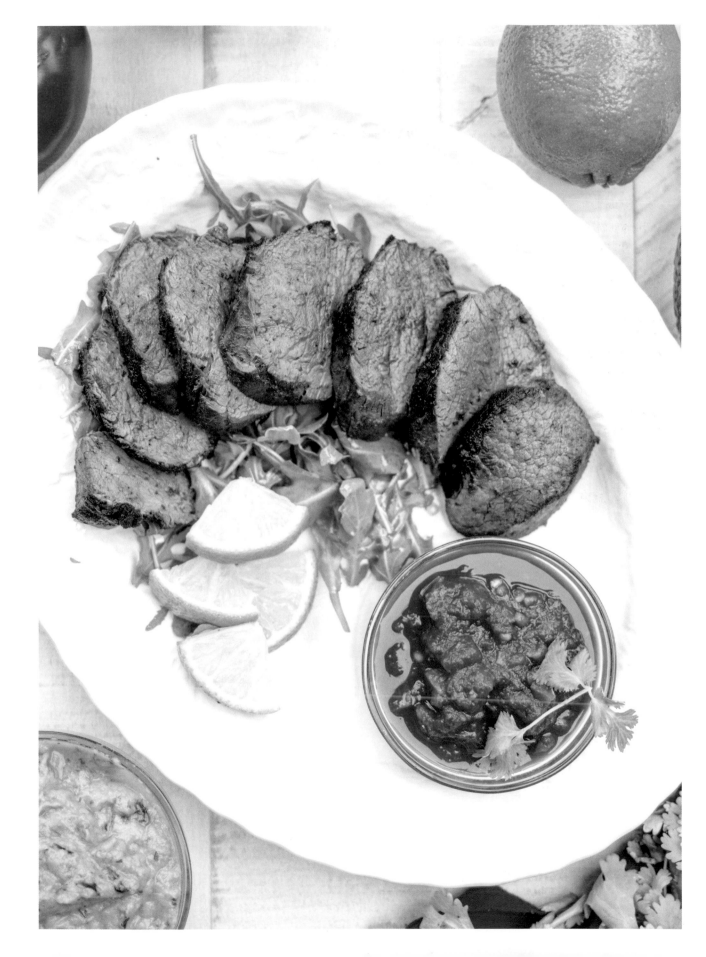

ONE-POT
PIZZA-RONI

Yield: 8 servings   *Prep time:* 10 minutes   *Cook time:* 15 minutes

3 cups peeled and ½-inch cubed eggplant

1 teaspoon fine sea salt

2 tablespoons unsalted butter

½ yellow onion, diced

½ green bell pepper, diced

1 teaspoon minced garlic

1½ pounds bulk Italian sausage

2 cups pizza sauce

½ cup shredded mozzarella cheese (about 2 ounces)

½ cup grated Parmesan cheese (about 1½ ounces)

Red pepper flakes, for garnish (optional)

1. Place the eggplant in a colander over a sink. Sprinkle with the salt and allow to sit for 5 minutes while you sauté the onion.

2. Heat the butter in a large skillet over medium-high heat. Add the onion and sauté for 3 minutes or until soft. Add the green pepper and garlic and sauté for another minute. Add the Italian sausage and salted eggplant and cook, while crumbling the sausage, until the meat is cooked through, about 5 minutes.

3. Stir in the pizza sauce. Cook over medium-low heat, uncovered, for 5 minutes. Top with the cheeses and red pepper flakes, if using, and serve.

4. Store in an airtight container in the refrigerator for up to 4 days. To reheat, place in a skillet over medium heat for 3 minutes or until heated through.

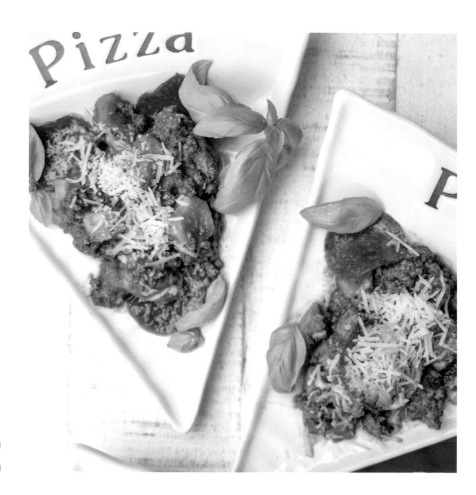

NUTRITIONAL INFO (per serving)

CALORIES	FAT	PROTEIN	CARBS	FIBER
329	25g	19g	6g	2g

EASY
COBB-STUFFED AVOCADOS

Yield: 12 servings   *Prep time:* 8 minutes (not including time to make dressing)   *Cook time:* 18 minutes

2 strips bacon, diced

2 (5-ounce) cans chicken meat, drained

3 tablespoons mayonnaise, homemade (page 346) or store-bought

1 teaspoon prepared yellow mustard

Fine sea salt (optional)

6 Hass avocados, halved and pitted

12 tablespoons shredded sharp cheddar cheese (about 3 ounces)

12 tablespoons Ranch Dressing (page 347)

1. Preheat the oven to 375°F.

2. Cook the diced bacon in a skillet over medium-high heat or until crispy and the fat is rendered, about 4 minutes. Remove from the pan and set aside.

3. In a medium bowl, stir the chicken, mayonnaise, and mustard together until well combined. Taste and adjust the seasoning to your liking, adding a touch of salt if needed.

4. Place the avocado halves in a baking dish and carefully fill each half with the chicken salad.

5. Top each avocado half with 1 tablespoon of cheese and some diced bacon. Bake for 10 to 12 minutes, until the cheese is melted. Remove from the oven and drizzle each avocado half with 1 tablespoon of the dressing. Serve warm.

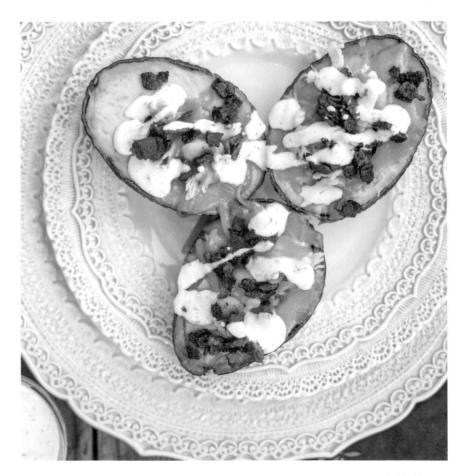

NUTRITIONAL INFO (per serving)

 CALORIES 311   FAT 29g   PROTEIN 8g   CARBS 10g   FIBER 7g

MAPLE BACON APPLE CAKE

Yield: 12 servings   *Prep time:* 18 minutes, plus time to freeze the cakes   *Cook time:* 20 minutes

Use the following tips to make it easier to assemble the cake:

- *Use 6-inch springform pans if you have them. It's easier to release the cake layers from springform pans than regular pans.*

- *Freeze the cake before frosting. If you try to frost a warm or room-temperature cake, the cake will crumble, and you will have frosting full of cake pieces.*

- *If the cake breaks as you slice it into layers, don't worry. The frosting is like an amazing duct tape that holds it all together.*

- *Use room-temperature frosting. If the frosting is too cool, it will be difficult to spread. If you make the frosting the day before, remove it from the refrigerator and allow it to come to room temperature before using. (I actually set my chilled frosting in the toaster oven on the warm setting for 3 minutes to warm it so it was nice and spreadable.)*

CAKE:
Coconut oil spray, for greasing the pan

6 large eggs, separated

1 cup Swerve confectioners'-style sweetener or equivalent amount of liquid or powdered sweetener (see page 271)

⅓ cup unsweetened cashew milk or almond milk, homemade (page 345) or store-bought

1 teaspoon apple extract or maple extract

1 cup blanched almond flour

1½ teaspoons baking powder

FROSTING:
1½ cups (3 sticks) unsalted butter, softened

1½ cups Swerve confectioners'-style sweetener or equivalent amount of liquid or powdered sweetener (see page 271)

12 ounces cream cheese or mascarpone cheese (1½ cups)

1 teaspoon maple extract

2 to 4 tablespoons unsweetened almond milk, homemade (page 345) or store-bought

FOR GARNISH:
4 strips bacon, fried until crispy and then crumbled

1. Preheat the oven to 350°F. Grease the bottoms of two 6-inch springform pans or two 6-inch round cake pans with coconut oil spray.

2. Using a hand mixer, beat the egg yolks with the sweetener on high speed until light in color. Add the milk and extract and stir to combine well. Then add the almond flour and baking powder and combine well with the hand mixer.

3. In a small bowl, beat the egg whites until stiff peaks form. Fold the whites into the yolk mixture.

4. Pour the batter into the prepared pans. Bake for 20 to 25 minutes or until a cake tester or toothpick inserted in the middle comes out clean. Remove the cakes from the oven and allow to cool to room temperature, then set the cakes (still in the pans) in the freezer until semi-frozen, about 2 hours. Loosen the edges with a knife before removing the cakes from the pans.

5. Make the frosting: Place the butter, sweetener, cream cheese, and extract in small bowl. Using a hand mixer, beat on medium speed to combine well, then, with the mixer running, gradually add enough milk for desired spreading consistency.

6. To assemble, use a long serrated knife to cut each semi-frozen cake layer in half horizontally by using a gentle sawing motion. (Remember, if the cake breaks, the frosting will hold it together.) Put 1 layer, cut side up, on a cake stand or large plate and spread with about ¾ cup of the frosting. Stack the remaining cake layers, spreading about ¾ cup of frosting on each layer and ending with top cake layer cut side down. Frost the top and sides of the cake. Garnish with crumbled bacon and serve.

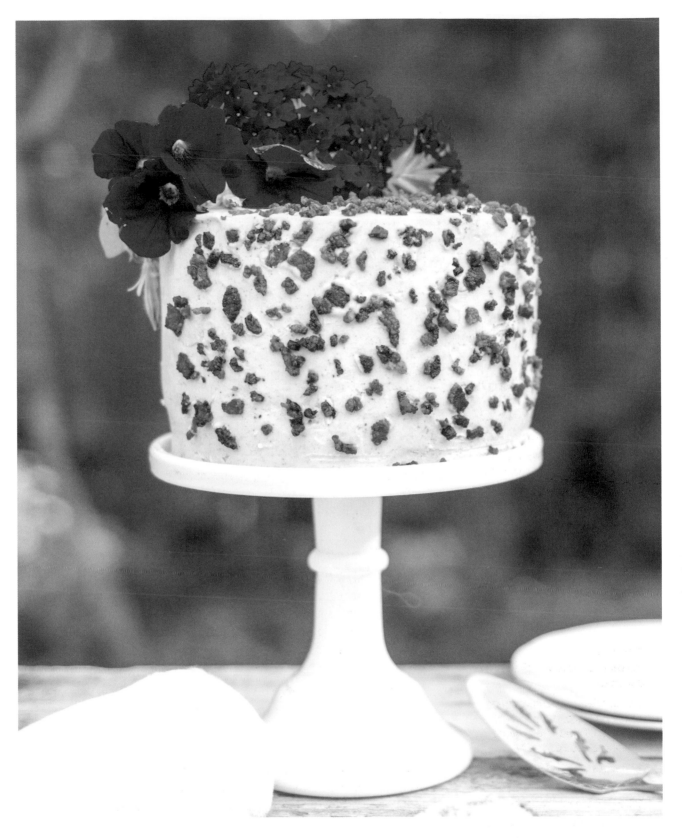

NUTRITIONAL INFO (per serving)

CALORIES 427   FAT 43g   PROTEIN 8g   CARBS 3.5g   FIBER 1.1g

7. Store in an airtight container in the refrigerator for up to 5 days or in the freezer for up to a month.

CHOCOLATE
ALMOND BÛCHE DE NOËL

Yield: 10 servings   *Prep time:* 1 hour, plus 4 hours to chill

This is such an elegant-looking dessert. You don't have to be an artist to make it—all you need is a special Bûche de Noël mold. If you don't have one, you can always make the cake in loaf pan, though I have to admit the special mold is what makes this look so classy.

ALMOND CHEESECAKE LAYER

½ cup unsweetened almond milk, homemade (page 345) or store-bought

1 teaspoon grass-fed powdered gelatin

1 (8-ounce) package cream cheese, softened

1 cup creamy almond butter (unsweetened and salted)

¾ cup Swerve confectioners'-style sweetener or equivalent amount of liquid or powdered sweetener (see page 271)

½ cup heavy cream

CHOCOLATE MOUSSE LAYER

¼ cup hot unsweetened almond milk, homemade (page 345) or store-bought

1 teaspoon grass-fed powdered gelatin

½ cup Swerve confectioners'-style sweetener or equivalent amount of liquid or powdered sweetener (see page 271)

3 large egg yolks

3 ounces unsweetened baking chocolate, finely chopped

1 cup heavy cream

CHOCOLATE SAUCE

¾ cup heavy cream

2 ounces unsweetened chocolate, finely chopped

⅓ cup Swerve confectioners'-style sweetener or equivalent amount of liquid or powdered sweetener (see page 271)

Seeds scraped from 1 vanilla bean (about 6 inches long), or 1 teaspoon vanilla extract

Crushed toasted nuts of choice, for garnish

SPECIAL EQUIPMENT:
Silicone Bûche de Noël mold, about 10 by 3½ inches (optional)

1. Have on hand a silicone Bûche de Noël mold or a 9 by 5-inch loaf pan. If using a loaf pan, line it with parchment paper, leaving some paper overhanging.

2. Make the cheesecake layer: Place the almond milk in a medium saucepan and use a whisk to stir in the gelatin. Heat over medium-high heat until the gelatin dissolves, about 2 minutes. (Or heat in the microwave for 10 seconds or until liquefied). Add the cream cheese, almond butter, sweetener, and cream and mix well with an electric mixer. Pour the batter into the silicone Bûche de Noël pan or lined loaf pan. Carefully set the mold in the freezer; allow the layer to freeze until frozen solid, about 2 hours.

3. Make chocolate mousse layer: Place the almond milk a saucepan and whisk in the powdered gelatin. Let soften for a minute. Then heat the mixture over medium heat until hot. Slowly whisk in the sweetener and egg yolks. Cook over medium heat, stirring constantly, for 5 minutes or until the mixture thickens and coats the back of a spoon. Add the chopped chocolate and stir until the chocolate is totally melted, about 3 more minutes. Place in the refrigerator to cool slightly.

4. When the chocolate custard is no longer hot but still slightly warm, whip the cream until stiff peaks form and gradually fold the whipped cream into the chocolate custard until combined. Smooth the chocolate mousse over the cheesecake layer in the pan and smooth the top. Cover and freeze until frozen solid, at least 3 hours or overnight.

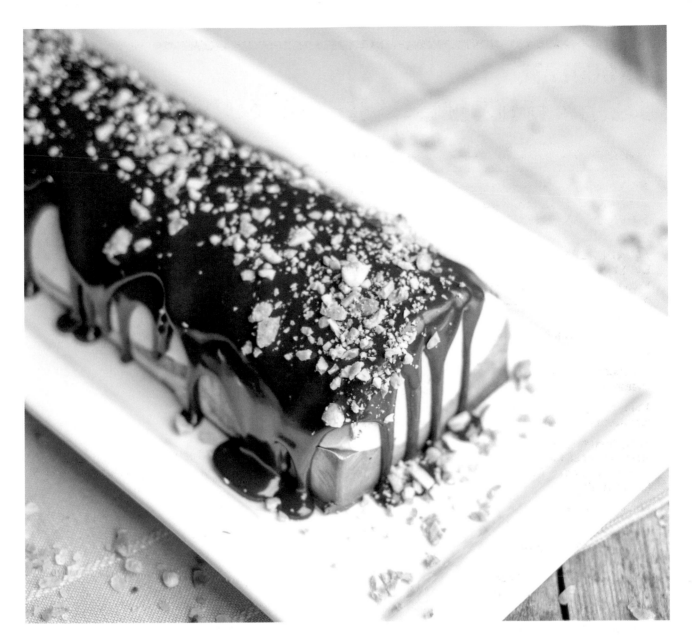

Serving Tip:

Slice when slightly frozen (before dinner) and allow to warm at room temperature until soft but still chilled.

5. To unmold, place the Bûche de Noël pan over a wire rack. Gently peel the sides of the mold away from the mousse. Press the top of the mold gently with your hands until the mousse releases. Place the Bûche de Noël on a serving platter and store in the refrigerator while you prepare the sauce.

6. Make the sauce: Place the cream, chopped chocolate, and sweetener in a double boiler or in a heat-safe bowl over a pan of simmering water. Heat on low, while stirring, just until the chocolate melts. Remove from the heat and stir in the vanilla bean seeds.

7. Remove the Bûche de Noël from the refrigerator and pour the chocolate sauce over the top. Garnish with the nuts, cover loosely, and refrigerate until ready to serve.

8. Store in the refrigerator for up to 4 days or the freezer for up to 2 weeks.

NUTRITIONAL INFO (per serving)

CALORIES 450 | FAT 41g | PROTEIN 11g | CARBS 11g | FIBER 4g

CHOCOLATE RASPBERRY
ICE POPS

Yield: 4 servings   *Prep time:* 4 minutes, plus 4 hours to set

OPTION

1 cup unsweetened almond milk, homemade (page 345) or store-bought

2 teaspoons Swerve confectioners'-style sweetener or equivalent amount of liquid or powdered sweetener (see page 271)

3 tablespoons unsweetened cocoa powder (see Note)

2 ounces cream cheese (¼ cup) (or coconut cream if dairy-free)

2 teaspoons raspberry extract

½ teaspoon fine sea salt

SPECIAL EQUIPMENT:
4 (3-ounce) ice pop molds

Note:

Three tablespoons of cocoa powder will create pops with a milk chocolate flavor. If you would like dark chocolate pops, increase the amount of cocoa powder to 5 tablespoons.

1. Place all of the ingredients in a blender and blend until smooth.

2. Pour into four 3-ounce ice pop molds. Place in the freezer until set, about 4 hours.

3. Store in the freezer for up to a month.

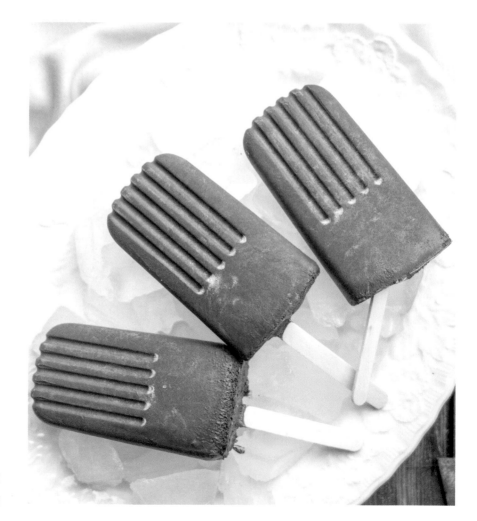

NUTRITIONAL INFO (per serving)

CALORIES	FAT	PROTEIN	CARBS	FIBER
73	6g	2g	2g	1g

STRAWBERRY CHEESECAKE
ICE POPS

Yield: 4 servings   *Prep time:* 5 minutes

One thing that I always have stocked in my freezer are keto ice pops, and this new strawberry cheesecake ice pop is my kids' favorite one yet! In the summer I am all about easy recipes. Ice pops are something that even my boys can make, and they are so tasty on a hot summer day.

4 ounces cream cheese (½ cup)

½ cup unsweetened almond milk, homemade (page 345) or store-bought

¼ cup Swerve confectioners'-style sweetener or equivalent amount of powdered or liquid sweetener (see page 271)

2 teaspoons strawberry extract

Pinch of fine sea salt

4 ounces fresh strawberries, hulled

SPECIAL EQUIPMENT:
4 (3-ounce) ice pop molds

1. Place all of the ingredients in a blender and puree until smooth. Taste and adjust the sweetness to your liking.

2. Pour the mixture into four 3-ounce ice pop molds. Place in the freezer for at least 4 hours before serving.

3. Store in an airtight container in the freezer for up to a month.

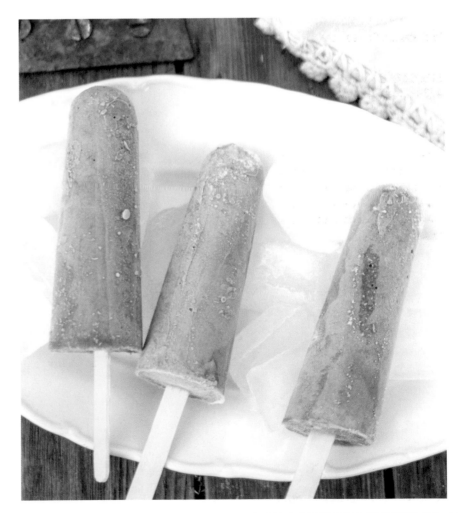

NUTRITIONAL INFO (per serving)

     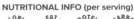

CALORIES	FAT	PROTEIN	CARBS	FIBER
112	10g	2.4g	3.5g	1g

ALMOND JOYFUL FAT BOMBS

Yield: 16 servings   **Prep time:** 5 minutes, plus 20 minutes to set

½ cup coconut oil, melted

½ cup unsweetened cocoa powder

¼ cup creamy almond butter (unsweetened and salted)

¼ cup coconut flour

1 teaspoon coconut-flavored liquid stevia

1. Line a 6-inch square baking dish with parchment paper, leaving some overhanging for easy removal.

2. Place the melted coconut oil in a medium bowl. Stir in the cocoa powder. Add the almond butter and mix until smooth. Add the coconut flour and stevia. Taste and adjust the sweetness to your liking.

3. Pour the mixture into the prepared baking dish. Freeze for at least 20 minutes or until set. Remove the chilled fat bombs from the dish using the parchment paper. Cut into 16 squares.

4. Store in an airtight container in the refrigerator for up to 5 days or in the freezer for up to a month.

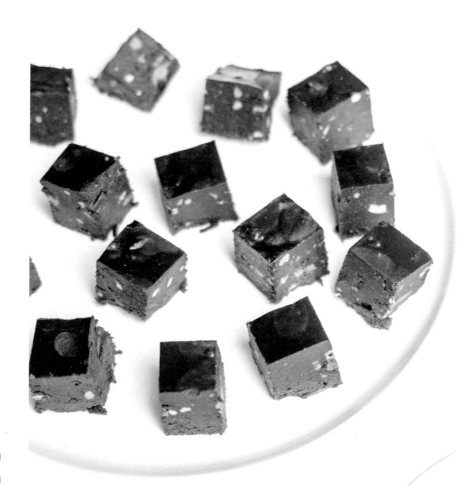

NUTRITIONAL INFO (per serving)

CALORIES	FAT	PROTEIN	CARBS	FIBER
100	10g	2g	3g	2g

ALMOND BRITTLE

Yield: 12 servings *Prep time:* 5 minutes, plus 15 minutes to chill *Cook time:* 5 minutes

¼ cup (½ stick) unsalted butter

1 cup Swerve confectioners'-style sweetener or equivalent amount of powdered erythritol (see page 271)

Seeds scraped from 1 vanilla bean (about 6 inches long), or
1 teaspoon vanilla extract

1 cup raw almonds, chopped

1. Line an 8-inch square baking dish with parchment paper, leaving some overhanging for easy removal.

2. In a medium saucepan, simmer the butter until it froths and brown flecks appear. Whisk in the sweetener and vanilla bean seeds (discard the pod) and continue to heat for about 5 minutes, until well combined. Remove from the heat and stir in the almonds. Pour into the prepared pan and let cool to room temperature, then place in the refrigerator to set, about 15 minutes.

3. Remove the cooled brittle from the refrigerator. Break into pieces for serving.

4. Store in an airtight container in the refrigerator for up to 2 weeks.

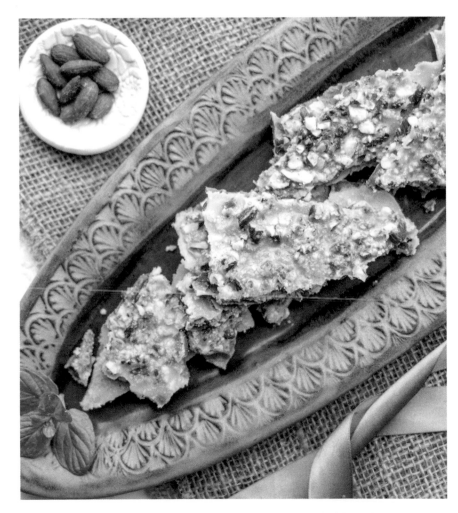

NUTRITIONAL INFO (per serving)

 CALORIES 88 FAT 8g   PROTEIN 2g   CARBS 2g   FIBER 1g

CHOCOLATE ALMOND
WHOOPIE PIES

Yield: 6 servings   *Prep time:* 9 minutes   *Cook time:* 12 minutes

CAKES:

1¼ cups blanched almond flour

¼ cup unsweetened cocoa powder

½ teaspoon baking soda

¼ teaspoon fine sea salt

⅓ cup Swerve confectioners'-style sweetener or equivalent amount of liquid or powdered sweetener (see page 271)

¼ cup (½ stick) unsalted butter or coconut oil, softened, plus extra for greasing the pans

3 large eggs

1 teaspoon almond extract

FILLING:

¾ cup (1½ sticks) unsalted butter, softened

6 ounces cream cheese (¾ cup), softened

¾ cup Swerve confectioners'-style sweetener or equivalent amount of liquid or powdered sweetener (see page 271)

2 tablespoons unsweetened cocoa powder

1 tablespoon heavy cream

1 teaspoon almond extract

ALMOND CHOCOLATE SAUCE:

¼ cup heavy cream

2 tablespoons Swerve confectioners'-style sweetener or equivalent amount of liquid or powdered sweetener (see page 271)

½ ounce unsweetened chocolate, finely chopped

½ teaspoon almond extract

Fresh raspberries, for garnish

SPECIAL EQUIPMENT:

12-well whoopie pie pan or muffin top pan

1. Preheat the oven to 325°F. Grease a 12-well whoopie pie or muffin top pan with butter or coconut oil.

2. Make the cakes: In a mixing bowl, whisk together the almond flour, cocoa powder, baking soda, and salt until blended. In a separate bowl, beat the sweetener, butter, eggs, and extract with a hand mixer until smooth. Stir the wet ingredients into the flour mixture.

3. Spoon the batter into the prepared pan, filling each well about two-thirds full. Bake for 12 minutes or until a toothpick inserted in the center of a cake comes out clean. Allow to cool in the pan.

4. Meanwhile, make the filling: Using the hand mixer, cream the butter, cream cheese, and sweetener in a medium bowl. Add the cocoa powder and stir well. Add the cream to thin the filling a little, then add the extract and stir to combine. Set the filling aside.

5. To make the chocolate sauce, place the cream, sweetener, and chopped chocolate in a double boiler or in a heat-safe bowl set over a pan of simmering water. Heat on low, stirring, just until the chocolate is melted. Remove from the heat and stir in the extract. Taste and add more sweetener, if desired.

6. To assemble, place one cake flat side up on a plate. Place 2 tablespoons of the filling on the cake, then top with another cake. Repeat with the rest of the cakes and filling. Drizzle the chocolate over the filled whoopie pies. Garnish with fresh raspberries.

7. Store in an airtight container in the refrigerator for up to 4 days.

NUTRITIONAL INFO (per serving)

 CALORIES 615
 FAT 60g
 PROTEIN 12g
 CARBS 9g
 FIBER 4g

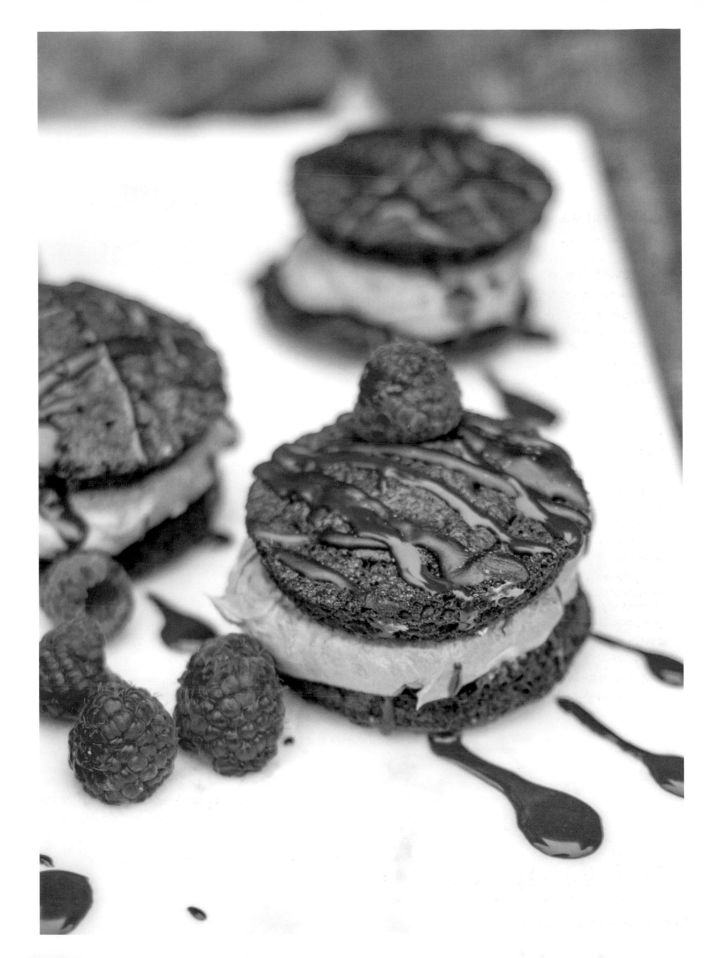

KETO EGGNOG

Yield: 4 servings (¾ cup per serving)   *Prep time:* 5 minutes, plus time to chill   *Cook time:* 10 minutes

4 large eggs, separated

¼ cup Swerve confectioners'-style sweetener or equivalent amount of liquid or powdered sweetener (see page 271)

2 cups unsweetened almond milk, homemade (page 345) or store-bought

1 teaspoon ground nutmeg, plus more for garnish

1 teaspoon rum extract

Note:

The egg whites used in this recipe are not cooked. If you're concerned about salmonella, you may use pasteurized eggs to make this recipe. Though salmonella is rare—only about 1 in 20,000 eggs are infected—young children, pregnant women, the elderly, and people with compromised immune systems should probably avoid raw eggs just in case. Interestingly, some studies show that the occurrence of salmonella is higher in factory-farmed eggs than in pastured eggs.

1. In a medium mixing bowl, beat the egg yolks with a hand mixer until they lighten in color. With the mixer running, gradually add the sweetener until combined, then set the egg yolk mixture aside.

2. In a medium saucepan over high heat, bring the milk and nutmeg just to a boil, stirring occasionally. Remove from the heat and gradually stir the hot milk mixture into the egg yolk mixture. Then return everything to the pan and cook over moderate heat, stirring constantly, until the mixture reaches 160°F (it will have thickened and will coat the back of a spoon). Remove from the heat and stir in the extract. Pour the custard into a clean mixing bowl, then set it in a larger bowl of ice water. Once it's cooled to room temperature, put the bowl of custard in the refrigerator to chill completely.

3. In another medium mixing bowl, beat the egg whites with the hand mixer until stiff peaks form. Fold the beaten whites into the chilled custard. Divide among four 4-ounce cups or glasses, garnish with nutmeg, if desired, and serve.

4. Store in an airtight container in the refrigerator for up to 3 days.

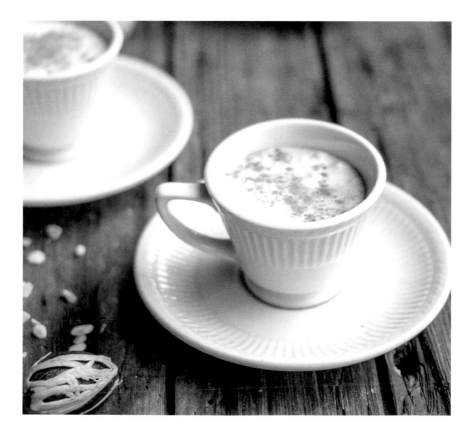

NUTRITIONAL INFO (per serving)

CALORIES	FAT	PROTEIN	CARBS	FIBER
82	5g	6g	1g	0.2g

EGGNOG LATTE

Yield: 1 serving   *Prep time:* 5 minutes (not including time to make eggnog)   *Cook time:* 3 minutes

⅔ cup Keto Eggnog (opposite)

⅓ cup unsweetened almond milk, homemade (page 345) or store-bought

2 tablespoons Swerve confectioners'-style sweetener or equivalent amount of liquid or powdered sweetener (see page 271)

2 shots decaffeinated espresso, hot, or ½ cup freshly brewed decaffeinated coffee

Pinch of ground nutmeg

Melted ghee, for garnish

1. Pour the eggnog, milk, and sweetener into a saucepan. Heat on high for a few minutes, until the mixture starts to bubble. Remove from the heat. Using an immersion blender, froth the mixture until doubled in size with air bubbles.

2. Pour the hot espresso into an 8-ounce mug. Holding back the foam with a spoon, carefully pour the milk mixture into the coffee. Do not stir. Gently spoon the foam over the top. Sprinkle with nutmeg and drizzle with melted ghee, if desired. Best served fresh.

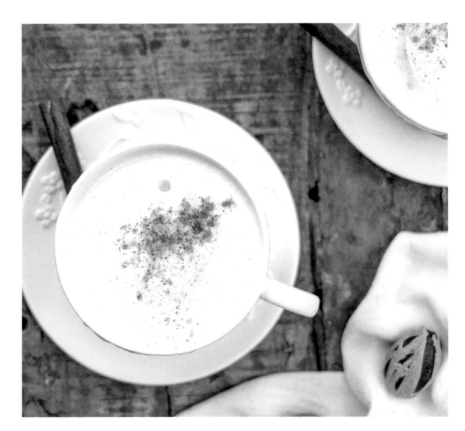

NUTRITIONAL INFO (per serving)

 CALORIES 68   FAT 5g   PROTEIN 4g   CARBS 2g FIBER 1g

KOMBUCHA

Yield: 1 liter (1 cup per serving)   *Prep time:* 10 minutes, plus up to 10 days to ferment

Whether kombucha is keto-friendly or not is a source of debate in the keto community. I choose not to consume it because of the sugar used to make it, but Jimmy and Christine believe it is fine in moderation, especially given its benefits to gut health. They asked me to come up with a healthy, low-sugar version for you.

When making fermented foods or beverages, it's essential to give the healthy bacteria every chance of surviving by starting off with clean equipment. Here are some tips:

- *Make sure the containers are sterile and very clean.*
- *Use filtered water; chlorine will damage the fermentation process.*
- *Use glass containers. Metal will react with the acid.*

1 liter filtered water

¼ cup organic sugar

2 organic black tea bags

½ cup unflavored kombucha (from a previous batch or a store-bought one)

1 kombucha culture (also known as a SCOBY)

1. Bring the water to a boil in a large stockpot over high heat. Add the sugar and stir until it dissolves. Remove from the heat and add the tea bags. Allow to steep and cool to room temperature before adding the SCOBY. (Too much heat would kill it.)

2. Once the tea has cooled, pour it into a sterile 2-quart glass jar. Add the premade kombucha and SCOBY. Cover the jar with cheesecloth and use a rubber band to secure it. Place in a warm area (around 75°F to 85°F) and allow to ferment for 8 to 10 days, until the kombucha is bubbly and tangy to the taste. The longer you ferment it, the tangier it will taste.

3. Pour the kombucha into glass bottles and store covered in the refrigerator until ready to consume. The kombucha will keep for up to 2 months.

NUTRITIONAL INFO (per serving)

 CALORIES 32   FAT 0g   PROTEIN 0g   CARBS 8g   FIBER 0g

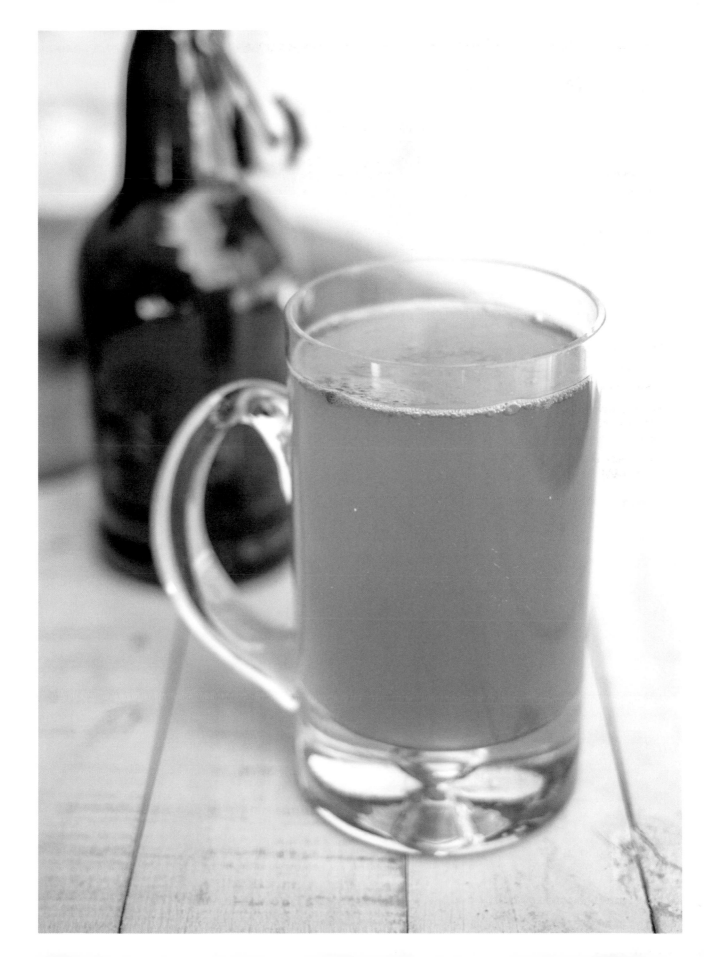

BEEF, CHICKEN, OR FISH
BONE BROTH

Yield: 4 quarts (1 cup per serving)   *Prep time:* 10 minutes   *Cook time:* 1 to 3 days

4 quarts cold water (reverse-osmosis water or filtered water is best)

4 large beef bones (about 4 pounds), or leftover bones and skin from 1 pastured chicken (ideally with the feet, too), or 4 pounds fish bones and heads

1 medium onion, chopped

2 stalks celery, sliced ¼ inch thick

2 tablespoons coconut vinegar or apple cider vinegar

2 tablespoons fresh rosemary leaves or other herb of choice

2 teaspoons minced garlic

2 teaspoons fine sea salt

1 teaspoon fresh thyme leaves, or ¼ heaping teaspoon dried thyme leaves

1. Place all of the ingredients in a 6-quart slow cooker. Set the heat to high, then, after 1 hour, turn the heat to low. Simmer for a minimum of 1 day and up to 3 days. The longer the broth cooks, the more nutrients and minerals will be extracted from the bones!

2. When the broth is done, pour it through a strainer and discard the solids, but do not skim the fat off the top. The fat makes this broth even more keto-friendly.

3. Store in the refrigerator for up to 5 days or in the freezer for up to several months.

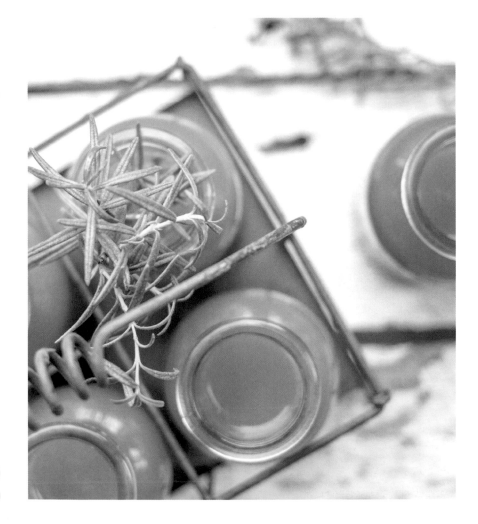

NUTRITIONAL INFO (per serving)

CALORIES 21 | FAT 1g | PROTEIN 2g | CARBS 1g | FIBER 0.2g

ALMOND MILK

Yield: 1 quart (½ cup per serving)   *Prep time:* 2 minutes, plus 8 hours to soak nuts

1½ cups raw almonds, soaked in water overnight

4 cups reverse-osmosis or filtered water

1. Drain the soaked nuts, then place them in a high-powdered blender or food processor with the 4 cups of reverse-osmosis or filtered water. Puree until the milk has a smooth, somewhat thick texture, about the consistency of a smoothie.

2. Strain in a colander lined with cheesecloth or in a fine-mesh strainer to remove the almond pulp. Discard the pulp. Store the milk in an airtight container in the refrigerator for up to 1 week.

Variation: Vanilla Almond Milk.

Add the seeds scraped from 1 vanilla bean (about 6 inches long) or 1 teaspoon vanilla extract to the blender in Step 1 when you add the 4 cups of reverse-osmosis or filtered water.

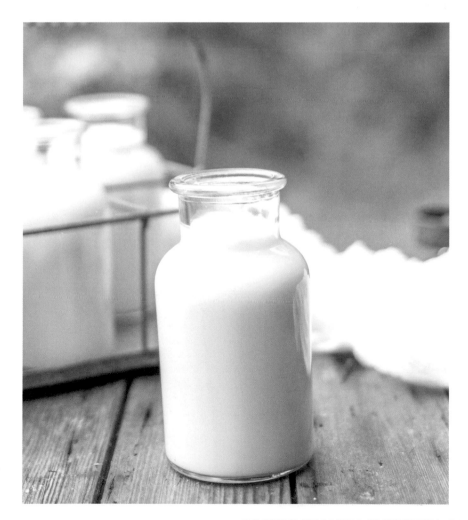

NUTRITIONAL INFO (per serving)

 CALORIES 55   FAT 5g   PROTEIN 1.2g   CARBS 1.6g   FIBER 1g

EASY MAYO

Yield: 1½ cups (about 1 tablespoon per serving)   *Prep time:* 5 minutes

Homemade mayonnaise has a milder and more neutral flavor than store-bought mayo—plus, it's so much healthier! You can personalize this basic mayo to your taste by adding finely chopped or roasted garlic or your favorite herb.

2 large egg yolks

2 teaspoons lemon juice

1 cup MCT oil or other neutral-flavored oil, such as macadamia nut or avocado oil

1 tablespoon Dijon mustard

½ teaspoon fine sea salt

Place the ingredients in the order listed in a wide-mouth, pint-sized mason jar or similar-sized container. Place an immersion blender at the bottom of the jar. Turn the blender on and very slowly move the blender to the top. Be patient! It should take you about a minute to reach the top. Moving the blender slowly is key to getting the mayonnaise to emulsify. Voilà! Simple mayo! Store in the refrigerator for up to 5 days.

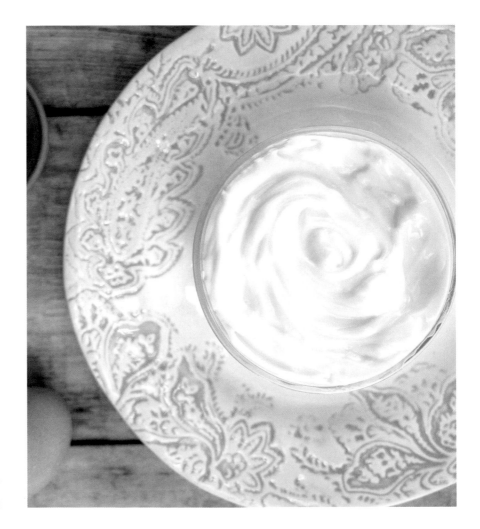

NUTRITIONAL INFO (per serving)

CALORIES	FAT	PROTEIN	CARBS	FIBER
92	10g	0.3g	0.1g	0g

RANCH DRESSING

Yield: 1½ cups (2 tablespoons per serving)   *Prep time:* 5 minutes, plus 2 hours to chill

1 (8-ounce) package cream cheese, softened

½ cup chicken or beef bone broth, homemade (page 344) or store-bought

½ teaspoon dried chives

½ teaspoon dried dill weed

½ teaspoon dried parsley

¼ teaspoon garlic powder

¼ teaspoon onion powder

⅛ teaspoon fine sea salt

⅛ teaspoon ground black pepper

In a blender or large bowl, mix together all of the ingredients. Transfer to a mason jar, cover, and refrigerate for 2 hours before serving. (It will thicken as it rests.) Store in the refrigerator for up to 2 weeks.

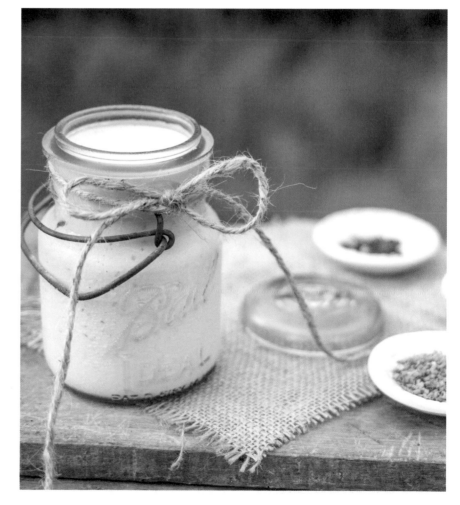

NUTRITIONAL INFO (per serving)

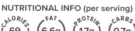

CALORIES	FAT	PROTEIN	CARBS	FIBER
69	6.6g	1.7g	0.7g	0g

THE BEST BLUE CHEESE
DRESSING

Yield: 2 cups (2 tablespoons per serving)   *Prep time:* 4 minutes

2 cups blue cheese crumbles (about 8 ounces), plus more if desired for a chunky texture

¼ cup sour cream

¼ cup beef bone broth, homemade (page 344) or store-bought

¼ cup red wine vinegar or coconut vinegar

1 tablespoon avocado oil or MCT oil

1 clove garlic, minced

Place the ingredients in a food processor and blend until smooth. Stir in chunks of extra blue cheese, if desired, for a chunky-style dressing. Store in an airtight container in the refrigerator for up to 5 days.

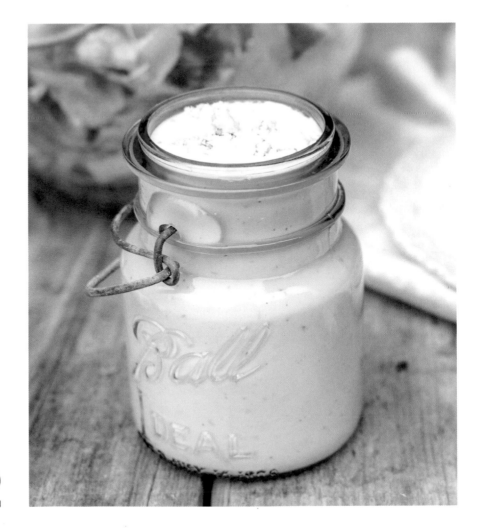

NUTRITIONAL INFO (per serving)

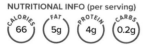

CALORIES 66 | FAT 5g | PROTEIN 4g | CARBS 0.2g | FIBER 0g

THOUSAND ISLAND
DRESSING

Yield: 1¼ cups (2 tablespoons per serving)   *Prep time:* 4 minutes

¾ cup mayonnaise, homemade (page 346) or store-bought

¼ cup chopped dill pickles

¼ cup tomato sauce (preferably from a glass jar)

2 tablespoons Swerve confectioners'-style sweetener or equivalent amount of liquid or powdered sweetener (see page 271)

⅛ teaspoon fine sea salt

⅛ teaspoon fish sauce

Place all of the ingredients in a jar and shake well. Store in an airtight container in the refrigerator for up to 2 weeks.

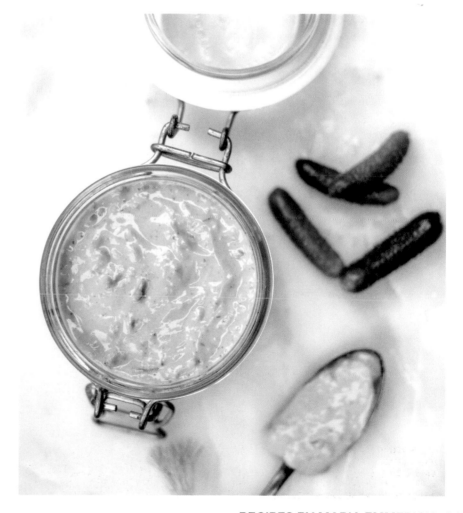

NUTRITIONAL INFO (per serving)

CALORIES	FAT	PROTEIN	CARBS	FIBER
307	36g	0.2g	1g	0g

TACO SEASONING

Yield: ½ cup (1 tablespoon per serving)   *Prep time:* 2 minutes

This seasoning tastes great on Mexican Tenderloin (page 326), but it also is a great seasoning to have on hand to make seasoned ground beef for a simple taco night supper. I use this whole batch of seasoning for 1 pound of ground beef.

2 tablespoons chili powder

1 tablespoon ground cumin

2 teaspoons fine sea salt

2 teaspoons ground black pepper

1 teaspoon paprika

1 teaspoon ground coriander

½ teaspoon garlic powder

½ teaspoon onion powder

½ teaspoon ground dried oregano

½ teaspoon red pepper flakes

In a bowl, mix together all of the ingredients until well combined. Store in an airtight container away from heat and light for up to 2 months.

NUTRITIONAL INFO (per serving)

CALORIES 16 FAT 0.6g PROTEIN 0.5g CARBS 2.2g FIBER 1.1g

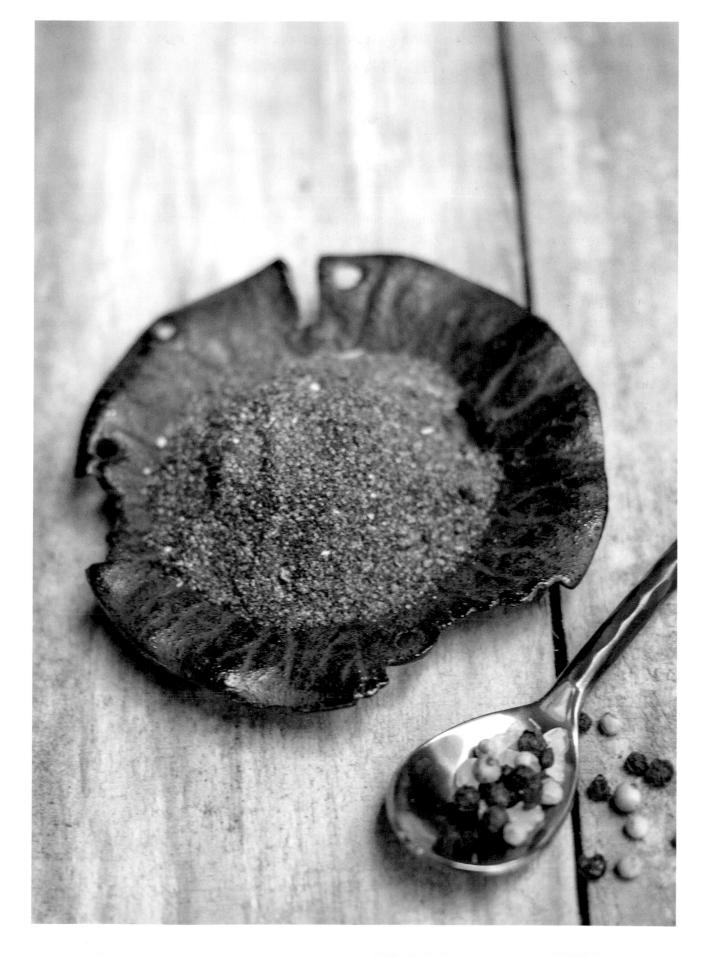

ACKNOWLEDGMENTS

FROM CHRISTINE MOORE

If you had asked me when I was a child if I thought I would write a book and get it published, I probably would have laughed at you. Well, that very opportunity has happened, and I'm very proud of this book you're holding. I've heard people talk about the book-writing process and how hard it can be, but I never really understood that until I tried writing a book. Needless to say, I now get it! But I'm so happy to have had this amazing opportunity.

There are several people I want to thank for helping to make this book possible.

To Jimmy Moore, my husband, best friend, and coauthor: I couldn't have done this book without you. You have always been there encouraging me and loving me every day. I can't tell you how many times I wanted to quit the Nutritional Therapy Practitioner program because it was difficult at times, and life had a way of throwing curve balls at us, especially during that time. I was overwhelmed several times, but you kept telling me to keep going and that I could do it—and I did. You did the same as we were writing the book, and I am so grateful to you for that. Thank you for loving me and putting up with my quirkiness and love of *Star Trek*, LEGOs, Precious Moments figurines, and rocks. I love you so much!

To my parents, John and Elizabeth Woodward, who have always encouraged me, even from a very young age, not to give up on anything: You taught me that even though I had some physical limitations with my eyesight, I was no different than all the other children. You sacrificed so much time, energy, and money due to my premature birth and challenges that came along with that. Thank you for always being there for me and loving me! I am so blessed to have you as my parents! I love you both so much!

To my brother, John Woodard, Jr., and sister, Jennifer Stephan: You both mean so much to me. You always look out for me and are there for me any time I need to talk. It was interesting growing up with the both of you because you guys could definitely antagonize me at times. Of course, I know I did the same thing to you. That's what siblings do. I could not have asked for a better brother and sister! I love you both so very much!

To my NTA tribe: Thank you for being a wonderful family! Thank you to my wonderful and patient instructors, Christie Banners and Brook Reyns, and my group leaders. You made going through the NTP program so fun!! Thank you to my classmates of the 2017 Herndon class for being such wonderful people! WE DID IT!! Woo-hoo!! And last but not least, thank you to Gray Graham for your friendship and leadership. Because you followed through with your vision of starting the NTA, many lives will change for the better!

To my team at Victory Belt Publishing: Thank you for giving me this opportunity to write this book. Thank you for all the hard work you did behind the scenes to make this book the best it could be! I fully believe that this book is going to make a huge difference in people's lives because the information in this book is not regularly talked about in the general health community. I will always be grateful to you!

And last but not least, to my Lord God Almighty: Thank you for blessing me with the gifts and talents to do what I do. I know that whenever I get discouraged, I can talk to you about things. You have always been there for me giving me the strength to keep going, even when times get tough. Thank you for loving me!

FROM JIMMY MOORE

I've been a word nerd since I was a little kid (I was the spelling bee champ and poetry contest winner growing up), and I knew I'd be an author someday. But because I was the fat kid my entire childhood, the fact I've written six books on the subject of health with a major publisher (and written eight books overall) is simply unbelievable and even miraculous. God definitely has a sense of humor. The honor and privilege of writing books that have changed people's lives for the better is the lasting legacy that will follow me the rest of my life. And now I'm getting to do it again—with my wife Christine this time!

Christine, I am so proud of you for putting in the work and effort to become a Nutritional Therapy Practitioner. After hearing me jibber-jabber on and on about nutritional health concepts over the years, now turnabout is fair play (prostaglandin, duodenum, chyme, oh my!). You'll never forget this very first book of what I'm sure will be many more in the years to come. Cherish every moment of this accomplishment that you will always have. You go, girl!

There are so many people in the ketogenic and health communities that I consider genuine friends, and I'm so grateful for all the work we are doing together to promote this way of eating to the masses: Maria Emmerich, Dr. Jason Fung, Suzanne Ryan, Dr. Will Cole, Danny Vega, Dr. John Limansky, Brian Williamson, Shawn Mynar, Meg Doll, Daniele Della Valle, Dr. Eric Westman, Dr. Ken Berry, Megha Barot and Matt Gaedke, Vanessa Spina, Drew Manning, Robert Sikes and Crystal Love, Mike Mutzel, Jessica Tye, Trent Holbert—and far too many others for me to list here! I'm so honored to walk alongside some of the best and brightest minds in the world of healthy living.

Erich at Victory Belt Publishing, what can I say? You took a chance on this health podcaster in 2012 when you gave me my first book contract, and here we are all these years later pumping out book after book. I'm so grateful for your belief in me and continued support of all the ideas that pop in my head for book ideas. You're rocking the health community by pumping out the best books on this subject on the planet! Thanks so very much for letting me be a part of this wild and crazy ride with you guys. I appreciate all that Lance, Dena, Charlotte, and the team did to make this book magical.

Finally, to the reader, get ready—this book is about to blow you away! Other than my seminal book *Keto Clarity,* this is the hardest I've worked on a book, and the payoff is one of the best books I've ever written. Soak it all in, take back control of your health, and then get healthy. One real food bite at a time!

REAL FOOD SOURCES OF MINERALS AND VITAMINS

BORON
Tomatoes, hazelnuts, almonds, Brazil nuts, walnuts, raw cashews, celery, olives, broccoli, onions

CALCIUM
Full fat dairy (milk, cheese, yogurt), collard greens, turnip greens, spinach, dandelion greens, kale, beet greens, arugula, lamb, rhubarb, okra, salmon, perch, rainbow trout, sardines, cabbage, sauerkraut, anchovies, caviar, bone broth, garlic, broccoli rabe

CHLORIDE
Sea salt, seaweed, tomatoes, lettuce, celery, olives

CHROMIUM
Oysters, liver, seafood, cheese, chicken, broccoli, free range eggs, grass-fed beef

COBALT
Fish, nuts, spinach, cabbage, broccoli, meat, liver, milk, oysters, clams, cocoa, chocolate, coffee, scallops

COPPER
Beef liver, chicken liver, Brazil nuts, cashews, almonds, sunflower seeds, dark chocolate, asparagus, kale, mushrooms, turnip greens, sauerkraut, cabbage, lobster, oysters, squid, clam, shrimp, crab, coconut, garlic

GERMANIUM
Broccoli, celery, garlic, shiitake mushrooms, milk, onions, rhubarb, sauerkraut, aloe vera, comfrey, ginseng, suma root

IODINE
Seaweed, kombu, dulce, kelp, arame, wakame, hiziki, nori, haddock, cod, shrimp, herring, oysters, scallops, clams, lobster, crab, mackerel, mussels, sardines, salmon, tuna, yogurt, strawberries, cheese (raw cheddar)

IRON
Liver, amaranth, ground beef, seaweed, chard, collard greens, mustard greens, spinach, beet greens, dandelion greens, Jerusalem artichokes, leeks, oysters, clams, sardines, halibut, haddock, perch, caviar, salmon, tuna, octopus, sardines, shrimp, chicken, turkey, pumpkin seeds, sesame seeds, squash seeds, sunflower seeds, pecans, walnuts, pistachios, roasted almonds, roasted cashews, coconut, broccoli, sauerkraut, cabbage, asparagus

LITHIUM
Seaweed, some mineral waters (such as Pellegrino and Lithia Spring Water), mustard greens, kelp, sardines, raw or roasted pistachios, mushrooms, summer squashes, okra, cucumbers, cabbage, cauliflower

MAGNESIUM
Almonds, cashews, dark chocolate, avocados, seeds, some fatty fish (salmon, mackerel, halibut, pollack, sardines, tuna, bass, cod), caviar, conch, snails, crabs, oysters, shrimp, kale, spinach, collard greens, turnip greens, mustard greens, cabbage, sauerkraut, coconut, ginger

MANGANESE
Pecans, hazelnuts, Swiss chard, mustard greens, kale, spinach, beet greens, turnip greens, cabbage, sauerkraut, broccoli, coconut, garlic, endive, mollusks, clams, blackberries, raspberries, strawberries, coconut milk, oysters

PHOSPHORUS
Pumpkin seeds, squash seeds, Romano cheese, salmon, scallops, Brazil nuts, pork, beef, veal, yogurt

POTASSIUM

Avocado, cantaloupe, parsnips, sardines, yogurt, tomato paste, spinach, beet greens, dandelion greens, Swiss chard, arugula, kale, mustard greens, watercress, bass, halibut, salmon, sardines, snapper, trout, tuna, garlic, ginger, acorn squash, Jerusalem artichokes, broccoli, Brussels sprouts, cauliflower, kohlrabi, squash, pork, chicken

RUBIDIUM

Asparagus, coffee, black tea, poultry, fish, mineral water

Sources of rubidium have not been researched intensively. Some fruits and vegetables have been shown to contain rubidium, and it may also be found in some water sources.

SELENIUM

Brazil nuts, yellowfin tuna, halibut, sardines, anchovies, caviar, oysters, lobster, tuna, swordfish, bass, squid, cod, tuna, haddock, snapper, catfish, clams, eel, mackerel, salmon, whitefish, shrimp, tilapia, grass-fed beef, liver (beef, chicken), turkey, kidney (beef, lamb, pork), chicken, bison, lamb, pork, turkey, Swiss chard, sunflower seeds, free range eggs, spinach

SILICON

Bell peppers, kale, spinach, asparagus, Jerusalem artichokes, parsley, sunflower seeds

SODIUM

Sea salt, sausage, sardines, bacon, ham, salted nuts, cabbage, sauerkraut, bouillon cubes, salami, beef jerky, olives, pickles, ham

SULFUR (METHYLSULFONYLMETHANE OR MSM)

Garlic, eggs, cabbage, kale, cauliflower, asparagus, mustard greens, Brussels sprouts, onions, tomatoes, broccoli, avocado, bok choy, turnips, turnip greens, nuts

VANADIUM

Mushrooms, shellfish, black pepper, parsley, dill weed, kelp, wine

ZINC

Oysters, lobster, crab, anchovies, clams, mollusks, grass-fed beef, turkey, chicken, chicken liver and heart, lamb, pork liver, cheese, Swiss chard, spinach, pumpkin seeds, cocoa powder, cashews, kifir, yogurt, mushrooms, coconut, garlic

VITAMINS AND ACCESSORY NUTRIENTS

ALLICIN

Garlic

ARGININE

Almonds, turkey, pork loin, pumpkin seeds, spirulina, dairy products

BETAINE

Beets (especially the tops and the greens), spinach, veal, turkey breast, beef

CHOLINE

Egg yolks, liver, meat, poultry, fish, dairy foods, spinach, beets

COENZYME Q10

Organ meats (liver, kidney, heart), beef, sardines, mackerel, broccoli, spinach, cauliflower

FIBER SUPPLEMENTS

Psyllium seed husk and pectins (found in all plant cell walls and in the outer skin and rind of fruits and vegetables), lignans (flaxseeds and flaxseed oil)

Lignans have anticancer, antibacterial, antifungal, and antiviral properties.

FLAVONOIDS
Berries, green tea, onions, parsley, red wine

GLANDULAR PRODUCTS
Organ meats

Toxins conjugate in the organs of animals. Make sure your organ meats come from sources that are free of hormones and antibiotics and aren't subjected to inferior feeding methods.

GLUCOSAMINE
Shrimp, lobster, crawfish, crab

The foods listed have trace amounts of glucosamine. Larger amounts of glucosamine have to come from supplementation.

INOSITOL
Nuts, seeds, beef, liver, and leafy greens

INULIN
Jerusalem artichokes, ground chicory root, dandelion root, asparagus, leeks, onions, garlic

LIPOIC ACID
Liver, heart, kidneys from beef or chicken, broccoli, spinach, red meat, Brussels sprouts, tomatoes, beets, brewer's yeast

MELATONIN
Ginger, tomatoes, radishes, red wine

You can eat foods that have tryptophan in them because tryptophan helps to induce serotonin production, which is needed for melatonin production. Some foods that contain tryptophan include dairy products (except cheese), nuts, seafood, turkey, chicken, eggs, sesame seeds, and sunflower seeds

PHOSPHATIDYLSERINE
Bovine brain, mackerel, chicken heart, herring, tuna, chicken, chicken liver, veal, beef, turkey, Atlantic cod, anchovies, sardines, trout, sheep's milk, cow's milk (raw), soy lecithin

PROBIOTICS
Kombucha, cultured yogurt, tempeh, sauerkraut, miso, kimchi, kefir, tempeh, miso, natto

If you have gut health issues, slowly introduce fermented foods to your diet. Adding too much too quickly can cause issues like gas and bloating.

S-ADENOSYLMETHIONINE (SAME)
Chicken, fish, milk (raw), red meat, eggs

VITAMIN A
Liver, fish, egg yolks, butter, parsley, kale, chili peppers, dandelion root, collard greens, blueberries, whitefish, cabbage, sauerkraut, cod liver oil

VITAMIN B1 (THIAMINE)
Pork, beef, liver, heart, kidneys, dandelion root, eggs, sunflower seeds, Brazil nuts, pecans

VITAMIN B2 (RIBOFLAVIN)
Eggs, meat, milk, poultry, fish, liver, lamb, full-fat plain yogurt (unsweetened and raw), mushrooms, spinach, almonds, and sun-dried tomatoes

VITAMIN B3 (NIACIN)
Beef, beef liver, veal, lamb, pork, poultry, eggs, tuna, salmon, halibut, sardines in spring water, haddock, Atlantic herring, cod, shrimp, goat cheese, turkey, shiitake mushrooms, enoki mushrooms, portobella mushrooms

VITAMIN B5 (PANTOTHENIC ACID)
Meat, liver, fish, raw milk, salmon, sunflower seeds, avocados, sun-dried tomatoes, broccoli, mushrooms

VITAMIN B6 (PYRIDOXINE)
Meat, organ meats, poultry, salmon, tuna, eggs, kombucha, strawberries, pistachios, avocados, spinach, chestnuts, halibut, sunflower seeds, walnuts

VITAMIN B7 (BIOTIN)

Liver, egg yolks, strawberries, almonds, cauliflower, mushrooms, spinach, milk, cheese, butter

VITAMIN B9 (FOLATE/FOLIC ACID)

Beets, strawberries, broccoli, spinach, avocados, collard greens, turnip greens, okra, Brussels sprouts, asparagus, egg yolks, liver

VITAMIN B12 (CYANOCOBALAMIN)

Meat, poultry, fish, eggs, milk, liver, sardines, herring, salmon, tuna, halibut, cheese

VITAMIN C

Fennel, radishes, strawberries, blueberries, red peppers, kale, Brussels sprouts, broccoli, cabbage, sauerkraut, green bell peppers

VITAMIN D

Sardines, salmon, mackerel, tuna, cod liver oil, eggs, milk, cheese, mushrooms, caviar

VITAMIN E

Cod liver oil, sunflower seeds, pecans, walnuts, hazelnuts, almonds, Swiss chard, mustard greens, spinach, turnip greens, kale, pine nuts, avocados, broccoli, parsley, olives

VITAMIN K

Organ meats, full-fat cheeses, grass-fed butter and cream, animal fats, egg yolks, turnip greens, broccoli, cabbage, lettuce, sauerkraut, pickles, asparagus

VITAMIN U (ENZYME METHYLMETHIONINE)

Cabbage and cabbage juice, almonds, sauerkraut, celery, parsley, onions, beets, asparagus, tomatoes, spinach, turnips

RESOURCES

We've included links to each product's website, but you also can find many of these items through other online sources, such as Amazon.com.

BEAUTY PRODUCTS

Kelly Miskovic's beauty products: www.beautycounter.com/kellymiskovic

Kim McCreary's beauty products: http://theripenedavocado.com/beautycounter.html

BONE BROTH

Ali Anderson's Abundant Broth: www.abundantbroth.com

Bare Bones Broth: www.barebonesbroth.com

FERMENTED FOODS

Bubbies: bubbies.com/pantry

Firefly Kitchens fermented foods: www.fireflykitchens.com

GT's Living Foods: www.gtslivingfoods.com/

MISCELLANEOUS

Heart to Heart Farm Share Program: www.Heart2HeartFarms.com

Real Good Food Co. pizzas and enchiladas: www.realgoodfoods.com

NUTS AND NUT BUTTERS

Justin's: http://justins.com/

Love You Foods: www.dropanfbomb.com/pages/jimmy-loves-fbomb

Pili Hunters: www.eatpilinuts.com

OILS, SALAD DRESSINGS, AND CONDIMENTS

AlternaSweets: www.alternasweets.com

Kasandrinos: www.kasandrinos.com

Nutiva: www.nutiva.com

Perfect Keto: shop.perfectketo.com

Primal Kitchen: www.primalkitchen.com

Pure Indian Foods (ghee): www.pureindianfoods.com

SUPPLEMENTS AND KETO ACCESSORIES

Adapt Your Life Keto Bar: www.adaptyourlife.com

Best Ketone Test: www.bestketonetest.com

Jigsaw Electrolyte Supreme (powder): www.jigsawhealth.com

Just Thrive: http://thriveprobiotic.com/

Keto Living: www.ketoliving.com

KetoVitals High Dose Electrolytes (capsules): www.keto-vitals.myshopify.com/products/keto-vitals-30-day-supply

Perfect Keto (collagen powder): shop.perfectketo.com

WEBSITES

Darryl Edwards: www.primalplay.com

Diet Doctor: www.dietdoctor.com

Jimmy Moore: livinlavidalowcarb.com

Maria Emmerich: mariamindbodyhealth.com

Matt & Megha from Keto Connect: www.ketoconnect.net

Nutritional Therapy Association: www.nutritionaltherapy.com

Sharon Merriman, CHHC: www.healingfoods.us

Smiley Gut Hacker: www.smileyguthacker.com/

Trent Holbert: www.trentholbertfitness.com/

The Weston A. Price Foundation: www.westonaprice.org

BOOKS

The Big Fat Surprise: Why Butter, Meat and Cheese Belong in a Healthy Diet by Nina Teicholz

Cholesterol Clarity: What the HDL Is Wrong with My Numbers by Jimmy Moore and Dr. Eric C. Westman, MD

Eat Rich Live Long: Use the Power of Low-Carb and Keto for Weight Loss and Great Health by Ivor Cummins and Jeffry Gerber, MD

Fresh and Fermented: 85 Delicious Ways to Make Fermented Carrots, Kraut, and Kimchi Part of Every Meal by Julie O'Brien and Richard J. Climenhage

Keto: The Complete Guide to Success on the Ketogenic Diet, Including Simplified Science and No-Cook Meal Plans by Maria Emmerich and Craig Emmerich

Keto Clarity: Your Definitive Guide to the Benefits of a Low-Carb, High-Fat Diet by Jimmy Moore and Dr. Eric C. Westman, MD

Keto Comfort Foods: Family Favorite Recipes Made Low-Carb and Healthy by Maria Emmerich

The Keto Cure: A Low-Carb, High-Fat Dietary Solution to Heal Your Body and Optimize Your Health by Jimmy Moore and Adam S. Nally, DO, with recipes by Maria Emmerich

Keto Essentials: 150 Ketogenic Recipes to Revitalize, Heal, and Shed Weight by Vanessa Spina

Keto Made Easy: 100+ Easy Keto Dishes Made Fast to Fit Your Life by Megha Barot and Matt Gaedke

Keto Restaurant Favorites: More Than 175 Tasty Classic Recipes Made Fast, Fresh, and Healthy by Maria Emmerich

The Ketogenic Cookbook: Nutritious Low-Carb, High-Fat Paleo Meals to Heal Your Body by Jimmy Moore and Maria Emmerich

Nourishing Traditions: The Cookbook That Challenges Politically Correct Nutrition and Diet Dictocrats by Sally Fallon with Mary G. Enig, PhD

Quick and Easy Ketogenic Cooking: Meal Plans and Time-Saving Paleo Recipes to Inspire Health and Shed Weight by Maria Emmerich

Simply Keto: A Practical Approach to Health & Weight Loss, with 100+ Easy Low-Carb Recipes by Suzanne Ryan

Why We Get Fat And What To Do About It by Gary Taubes

Your Body's Many Cries for Water by F. Batmanghelidj, MD

NUTRITIONAL THERAPY PRACTITIONERS

The following nutritional therapy practitioners offer ketogenic diets as an option. If you don't see a Nutritional Therapy Practitioner or Nutritional Therapy Consultant on this list who's close to you, go to www.nutritionaltherapy.com/provider-search/ to find a provider in your area.

ALI ANDERSON
Johns Island, South Carolina
www.ali-anderson.com

LAUREN ARONSTAM
Body and Soul Sustenance
Coral Springs, FL
www.bodyandsoulsustenance.com

TRACI BABINI
24 Carrot Nutrition
New Holland, Pennsylvania
www.24carrotnutritiontherapy.com

DAWN COUGHLIN
Nourishing Streams LLC
Strasburg, Virginia
www.nourishingstreams.com

TAYLOR DEITRICK
Arrow Nutritional Therapy
Harrisburg, Pennsylvania
www.arrownutritionaltherapy.com/

KATIE DILLON
Empowered Nutrition
Melbourne, Australia
www.empowerednutrition.com.au

MANDIE DUKE
Howell, Michigan
www.facebook.com/againstthegrainwithmandie/

KATRINA FOE
Personalized Pilates
Scottsdale, Arizona
www.PersonalizedPilates.com/nutritionaltherapy

JAIME LUBICH HARTMAN
Alexandria, Virginia
http://gutsybynature.com

APRIL LUEDER
Bourbonnais, Illinois
www.facebook.com/AprilLuederFitness/

KIM MCCREARY
Alexandria, Virginia
www.theripenedavocado.com

SHARON MERRIMAN, CCHC, AADP
Healing Foods
Mystic, Connecticut
http://healingfoods.us

CHRISTINE MOORE
Spartanburg, South Carolina
www.rebootingyournutrition.com

SHAWN MYNAR
Shawn Mynar Holistic Health
Boulder, Colorado
www.shawnmynar.com

KATIE NEWMAN
White Bear Lake, Minnesota
www.katienewman.com

CHRISTINA RICE
www.christinaricewellness.com

CAROLE ST. LAURENT
Food Heal Thrive
Greenwood Holistic Nutrition
Greenwood, South Carolina
www.foodhealthrive.com

SARA UZZLE
Naturally Nourished
Knoxville, Tennessee
www.getnaturallynourished.com

DAWN VAN WERT
Tampa, Florida
www.facebook.com/146801545972545/
posts/176564646329568/

SERINA VASSAR
Wise Bear Functional Nutrition
Chalfont, Pennsylvania
www.wisebearfn.com

JINA WELTER
3 Nourishing Bowls
Ashburn, Virginia
www.3nourishingbowls.com

LEAH WILLIAMSON
Brisbane Paleo Group
Brisbane, Australia
www.nourishingconversations.com
brisbanepaleo.com.au

EVENTS

KetoCon: www.ketocon.org/

KetoFest: ketofest.com

Low Carb USA: www.lowcarbusa.org

Low Carb Cruise and Keto 101 Cruise: www.
lowcarbcruiseinfo.com

Nutritional Therapy Association Annual Conference: www.
nutritionaltherapy.com/annual-conference

GLOSSARY

acetoacetate: A ketone body formed in the liver when fatty acids are broken down; measured in the urine.

acetone: A colorless liquid ketone made by oxidizing isopropanol; measured in the breath.

achlorhydria: A more serious form of **hypochlorhydria**, which is low or no hydrochloric acid production in the stomach.

acidic: Having the properties of an acid, or containing acid; having a pH lower than 7. An acidic substance has more hydrogen (H+) than hydroxide (OH-) in it.

adrenal fatigue: A condition or state (due to chronic stress or infections) in which the adrenal glands are exhausted and can no longer produce adequate amounts of hormones, primarily **cortisol**. Traditional medicine often doesn't diagnose adrenal fatigue; you have to see a practitioner in alternative medicine. Also known as hypoadrenia.

adrenaline: A hormone secreted by the adrenal glands, especially in conditions of stress, which increases rates of blood circulation, rate of breathing, and **carbohydrate** metabolism and prepares muscles for exertion. Also known as **epinephrine**.

advanced glycation end products (AGEs): Proteins or lipids that become glycated as a result of exposure to sugars. They can be a factor in aging and in the development or worsening of many degenerative diseases, such as **diabetes**, **atherosclerosis**, chronic kidney disease, and Alzheimer's disease.

alkaline: Having the properties of an alkali, or containing alkali; having a pH greater than 7. This substance will have more hydroxide (OH-) than hydrogen (H+) in it.

allergy: A damaging immune response by the body to a substance, especially pollen, fur, a particular (protein-based) food, or dust, to which it has become hypersensitive.

alpha cells: Cells of the pancreas that produce the hormone **glucagon** to help regulate blood sugar levels, especially between meals, when blood sugar gets too low. Alpha cells turn stored sugar (**glycogen**) into **glucose**.

amines: Derivatives from ammonia in which one or more hydrogen atoms have been replaced with an alkyl or aryl group.

amino acids: The building blocks of **protein** that play important roles in almost all biological processes. There are twenty-two amino acids, and twenty are considered essential amino acids. All amino acids combine to make **peptide** chains.

atherosclerosis: A disease of the arteries characterized by plaques of fatty material being deposited on their inner walls.

autoimmune: Description for a disease in which the antibodies of the immune system attack healthy tissue and organs in the body. An autoimmune disease can manifest in many conditions like Hashimoto's thyroiditis, Graves' disease, rheumatoid arthritis, psoriasis, lupus, multiple sclerosis, **type 1 diabetes**, myasthenia gravis, and many others.

beta cells: Cells in the pancreas that produce the hormone **insulin**, which shuttles **glucose** into the muscles and liver for storage to be used as fuel at a later point.

beta-hydroxybutyrate: A ketone body or salt of 3-hydroxybutyric acid involved in fatty acid metabolism; measured in the blood.

betaine: A methyl donor created by choline in combination with the **amino acid** glycine. Betaine aids the liver in its functions, helps with **detoxification**, and supports cellular functions.

bioindividuality: The concept that each person has unique needs regarding **nutrition**, differences in anatomy, a particular way the metabolism functions, and so much more. Consequently, there's no one-size-fits-all diet; whereas a particular diet will work for one person, it might not necessarily work for the next person.

bolus: Food that has been chewed and is ready to be swallowed.

bone remodeling (or bone metabolism): A process that occurs throughout one's life in which mature bone tissue is removed from the skeleton and new bone tissue is formed.

carbohydrates: Organic compounds that exist in foods and living tissues. They include sugars, starch, and cellulose. Carbohydrates can typically be broken down and used as energy in the body.

cellular respiration: A chemical process that generates most of the energy in the cell and supplies the molecules needed to make the metabolic reactions (see **metabolism**) of an organism run. Note: The main carrier of energy in metabolism is adenosine triphosphate or ATP.

cholecystokinin: A hormone secreted by cells in the duodenum to stimulate the gall bladder to release bile to help break down the **fat** we consume.

chyme: A substance that consists of gastric juices and partially digested food that passes from the stomach to the small intestine.

coenzyme: A nonprotein molecule, mostly derived from **vitamins**, that binds with a **protein** to facilitate enzyme reactions in the body.

cofactor: A substance (metal ions or **coenzymes**) that's essential for the activity of an **enzyme**.

colonic: A procedure in which the colon is irrigated for therapeutic benefit.

complete protein: A **protein** that contains all the essential **amino acids** (amino acids that can't be produced by the body) in quantities necessary for the dietary needs of humans. Animal products are our only source of complete proteins. Also known as a whole protein.

cortisol: A hormone released by the adrenal cortex when blood sugar levels are not being sufficiently supported by glucagon. It also aids in the process known as **gluconeogenesis**. See also **hydrocortisone**.

deficiency: A lack or shortage.

detoxification: The process of removing toxic substances from the body.

diabetes: See **type 1 diabetes** and **type 2 diabetes**.

digestion: The process of breaking down food by mechanical and enzymatic action into substances like amino acids, fatty acids, and glucose that can be used by the body.

disaccharide: A sugar that contains two **monosaccharides**.

eicosanoids: Compounds derived from fatty acids (like arachidonic acid) and involved in cellular activity. Examples of eicosanoids are **prostaglandins**, **leukotrienes**, and **thromboxanes**.

electrolytes: Minerals like calcium, potassium, chloride, sodium, and magnesium that carry electrical charges that help with cell membrane stability and the contraction and relaxation of muscles. Cells would not be able to communicate with each other without electrolytes.

enema: A procedure in which liquid or gas is injected into the bowel via the rectum, typically for the purpose of emptying and cleansing the bowel, but it also can be used to administer drugs or permit X-ray imaging.

enzyme: A substance that works in conjunction with other substances (such as vitamins) in the body to speed up reactions and aid in digestion and metabolism.

epigenetics: The study of how genes express themselves due to external factors like diet, stress, exercise, smoking, consumption of alcohol, place of residence, and many more.

epinephrine: A hormone secreted by the adrenal glands, especially in conditions of stress. Epinephrine increases blood circulation, rate of breathing, and the metabolism of **carbohydrates**. It also prepares the muscles for exertion. Also known as **adrenaline**.

essential fatty acids (EFAs): Fatty acids that humans and other animals must ingest because the body can't make them but that are required for good health. Those **fats** that aren't considered essential are referred to as nonessential fatty acids.

essential nutrient: A **nutrient** required for normal body functioning that cannot be made by the body. Examples of essential nutrients are **vitamins**, dietary minerals, **essential fatty acids**, and essential **amino acids**.

fasting hypoglycemia: See **nonreactive hypoglycemia**.

fat: A major, long-lasting source of fuel for the body, which provides 9 calories per gram (twice as much as **protein** and **carbohydrates**, which provide 4 calories per gram). Fat comes in several forms such as saturated fats, monounsaturated fats, and polyunsaturated fats.

fermentation: The chemical breakdown of a substance by bacteria, yeasts, or other microorganisms.

gastrin: A **protein** hormone that stimulates secretion of gastric acid (HCl) by the parietal cells of the stomach to aid in the contractions of smooth muscles in the stomach.

genetics: The study of heredity and the variation of inherited characteristics.

glucagon: A hormone formed by the **alpha cells** in the pancreas to promote the breakdown of **glycogen** to **glucose** in the liver.

gluconeogenesis: A process that occurs in the liver for the purpose of breaking down some of the protein and fat a person eats and converting it to glucose to be used as energy for the body.

glucose: A simple sugar that is an important energy source in living organisms and is a component of many **carbohydrates**. Glucose provides a quick source of energy for the body but is not as long lasting as fat.

glycation: The bonding of a sugar molecule to a **protein** or lipid molecule without enzymatic regulation, which turns the proteins into "sticky proteins" that can't be used by the body. The speed at which glycation takes place is increased by a diet high in refined **carbohydrates**. As the glycation process continues, the proteins begin to harden.

glycogen: A form of sugar stored in the muscles and liver that can be converted back to glucose through a process known as **glycogenolysis**.

glycogenesis: The formation of **glycogen** from sugar.

glycogenolysis: The breakdown of glycogen to turn it back into glucose so the body can use it as fuel.

health: As defined by The World Health Assembly, health is "A dynamic state of complete physical, mental, spiritual, and social well-being and not merely the absence of disease or infirmity."[1]

hormone: Product of the endocrine system; a regulatory substance that's transported by blood and other tissue fluids to help stimulate cells or tissues to action. Examples of hormones are **insulin**, **melanin**, thyroxin, dopamine, calcitonin, and ghrelin.

hydrocortisone: A **steroid hormone** produced by the adrenal cortex and used in medicine to treat inflammation due to various factors or conditions such as chronic injury, eczema, or rheumatism. Hydrocortisone also helps with the regulation of blood sugar when it's not sufficiently supported by glucagon, and it aids in the process of gluconeogenesis. Another word for **cortisol**.

hydrogenated oil: Oil that has undergone a chemical process in which hydrogen is added to liquid oil to turn it into a solid. Hydrogenated oils are completely saturated with hydrogen, and partially hydrogenated oils are not completely saturated with hydrogen. Some of the unsaturated **fat** in the partially hydrogenated oil turns into **trans fatty acids**, and they may be the worst type of fat you can consume. Also can be called partially hydrogenated oil.

hydrogenation: To treat with hydrogen. Organic compounds become more "saturated" through the process of hydrogenation, meaning that liquid oil fats are turned into oils that are semi-solid or solid fats.

hyperglycemia: An excess of glucose in the bloodstream that's often associated with diabetes mellitus (**type 2 diabetes**). This occurs when fasting blood sugar levels reach 130 mg/dL and higher.

hyperthyroidism: Overactivity of the thyroid gland that can result in a rapid heartbeat and an increased rate of metabolism.

hypoadrenia: See **adrenal fatigue**.

hypochlorhydria: A condition in which the production of hydrochloric acid in gastric secretions of the stomach and other digestive organs is absent or low. Symptoms include fingernails that chip or break easily, undigested or partially digested food in stools, a sense of excessive fullness after meals, and heartburn or acid reflux. The more serious form of hypochlorhydria is known as **achlorhydria**.

hypothyroidism: Abnormally low activity of the thyroid gland, resulting in retardation of growth and mental development in children and adults.

insulin: A hormone produced in the pancreas by the **beta cells** that regulates the amount of glucose in the blood. Insulin takes excess glucose and puts it in the muscles, fat cells, and liver cells to be stored as fuel for the body.

insulin resistance (IR): A pathological condition in which cells fail to respond normally to insulin. When the body produces insulin under conditions of insulin resistance, the cells are resistant to the insulin and are unable to use it as effectively, which leads to high blood sugar.

ketogenesis: The production of **ketone bodies** during the metabolism of fats.

ketogenic: Relating to or causing **ketogenesis**.

ketone or ketone body: An organic compound and alternative source of fuel for the body when the body is primarily burning **fat** rather than **glucose**. The simplest ketone body is **acetone**. Other forms are **beta-hydroxybutyrate** and **acetoacetate**.

ketosis: A state in which the body is burning **fat** for fuel rather than glucose and therefore has higher levels of ketones. Ketosis often is a result of consuming a diet low in **carbohydrates**.

kombucha: A beverage produced by fermenting sweet tea with a culture of yeast and bacteria known as a SCOBY (symbiotic culture of bacteria and yeast).

leaky gut: A condition in which the lining of the small intestine becomes more permeable, which results in undigested food particles, toxic waste products, and bacteria entering the rest of the body. Leaky gut often leads to autoimmune conditions. Also known as increased intestinal permeability.

leukotrienes: Compounds in the immune system that are released by mast cells and help mediate inflammation.

lipolysis: The breakdown of fats and other lipids by hydrolysis to release fatty acids.

lipotropic factors: Substances produced naturally in the body that promote the flow of fat and bile through the liver to help keep it from getting congested with fat.

macromineral: Major minerals that the body requires in amounts of 100 milligrams or more per day through diet or supplementation. These macrominerals are calcium, phosphorus (phosphates), magnesium, sulfur, sodium, chloride, and potassium.

macronutrient: A substance required in larger amounts than **micronutrients** for living organisms to grow and develop. Examples of food macronutrients are **fat**, **protein**, and **carbohydrates**, and examples of chemical macronutrients are potassium, magnesium, and calcium.

melanin: A dark brown to black pigment in the hair, skin, and iris of the eye in people and animals. When skin is exposed to sunlight, this pigment is what makes the skin tan or get darker.

metabolic syndrome: Syndrome of several different conditions that occur together, which increases the risk of cardiovascular disease and diabetes. These conditions can include high blood pressure, high blood sugar, excess fat around the waist, and high triglyceride levels.

metabolism: Processes that happen in the body, either physical or chemical, that are necessary for life. In some processes, food is broken down to make energy.

microbe: A microorganism, especially a bacterium, that causes disease or fermentation. Having good microbes in the gut can help with the production of vitamins B1 (thiamine), B2 (riboflavin), B12 (cobalamin), and K2 in the intestines.

microbiome: The microorganisms living in a particular environment (including the body or a part of the body).

microbiota: The microorganisms of a particular site, habitat, or geological period.

microminerals: Minerals that are present at low levels in the body. We need to obtain small amounts of these minerals from dietary sources or supplementation. Also known as trace minerals. Microminerals include chromium, cobalt, copper, fluorine, iodine, iron, manganese, molybdenum, selenium, and zinc.

micronutrient: A chemical element or substance required in trace amounts for the normal growth and development of living organisms. They consist of **vitamins** and **minerals**.

mineral: An inorganic substance needed by the human body for good health. They include **macrominerals** and **microminerals**.

monosaccharide: The simplest form of sugar, which cannot be broken down further.

native microbes: Microbes that enter our bodies through environmental sources like air, soil, and the water supply. They have antifungal, anti-parasitic, and antiviral properties.

neurotransmitters: Chemical messengers that can cross the synapse (the gap between neurons) to send information to the next neuron.

neutral: A substance that's neither **acidic** nor **alkaline** and has a pH of about 7. This substance has a balance of hydrogen (H+) and hydroxide (OH-).

nonreactive hypoglycemia: Condition that happens mainly in type 1 or type 2 diabetics when their blood sugar drops below 60 mg/dL for any reason. Causes could be stress, an illness (especially affecting the liver, heart, or kidneys), pregnancy, or medications. Also known as fasting hypoglycemia.

nutrients: The chemical substances contained in food that are necessary to sustain life. Nutrients have many important functions in the body, including providing energy (also known as calories), helping to form the body's structure, and working with **enzymes** and **hormones** to complete bodily processes.

nutrition: A science that focuses on the interactions between living organisms and their food, including the processes used in consuming the food and the ability to use the **nutrients** in food.

oligosaccharide: A **carbohydrate** whose molecules are composed of a relatively small number of **monosaccharide** units.

osteoblast activity: A process that builds bone.

osteoclast activity: A process that breaks down bone.

parasympathetic nervous system: Part of the nervous system that controls processes when the body is in a relaxed state.

partially hydrogenated oil: See **hydrogenated oil**.

peptide: A compound consisting of two or more **amino acids** linked in a chain.

pH scale: A measurement system for indicating the acidity or alkalinity of a solution. A pH of 0 is pure acidity, 7 is **neutral**, and 14 is pure alkalinity. The more **acidic** a solution, the more hydrogen (H+) it contains; the more **alkaline** a solution, the more hydroxide (OH-) it contains. pH stands for the power of hydrogen.

phospholipid: A lipid containing a phosphate group in its molecule that helps form cell membranes and control what goes in and out of each cell.

polysaccharide: A **carbohydrate**, like cellulose, starch, or glycogen, whose molecules consist of a number of sugar molecules bonded together.

prebiotic: An undigestible food ingredient that promotes the growth of beneficial microorganisms in the intestines.

probiotic: A substance that encourages the growth of microorganisms. Most probiotics, like those in the intestines, have beneficial properties.

prostaglandin: Fatty acid compounds with varying hormonelike effects, one of which is to help regulate inflammation. There are three groups: prostaglandin 1 or PG1, which are derived from omega-6 fatty acids and are anti-inflammatory in nature; prostaglandin 2 or PG2, which are derived from saturated fats and are inflammatory in nature; and prostaglandin 3 or PG3, which are derived from omega-3 fatty acids and are anti-inflammatory in nature.

proteins: Long chains of **amino acids** that are essential for all living organisms for building structures including things like muscle, hair, and collagen. Proteins also play important roles in forming **enzymes** and antibodies.

purgatives: In **nutrition**, a laxative.

reactive hypoglycemia: A condition when blood sugar levels drop below baseline after eating. This occurs when blood sugars are 60 mg/dL and lower or 90 mg/dL with symptoms such as fatigue, trouble sleeping, mood disorders, infertility, and weight gain.

secretin: A hormone released into the bloodstream by the duodenum in response to acidity that stimulates the pancreas to release pancreatic juices and bicarbonate.

sensitivity: Occurs when a person has difficulty digesting a particular food. This can lead to symptoms such as intestinal gas, abdominal pain, or diarrhea. A food sensitivity is sometimes confused with or mislabeled as a food **allergy**.

steroid hormones: Members of a class of chemical compounds known as steroids. They are secreted by three glands: the adrenal glands (adrenal cortex), testes, and ovaries. When a woman is pregnant, the placenta also can release these hormones. All steroid hormones are derived from cholesterol.

sympathetic nervous system: Part of the autonomic nervous system that prepares your body for physical activity and controls the body for fight-or-flight mode.

thromboxane: A hormone that helps with blood clotting and the constriction of blood vessels.

thyroid hormones: Chemical substances made by the thyroid gland that are released into the bloodstream. The thyroid gland needs iodine to make thyroid hormones. The two most important thyroid hormones are thyroxine (T4) and triiodothyronine (T3).

toxin: Any substance that is harmful to the body. Toxins can come from environmental factors like water pollution or air pollution, household cleaners, and many other sources. Toxins also can come from internal sources like harmful microorganisms in the body that cause disease.

trans fatty acid: An unsaturated fatty acid that results from the hydrogenation process, like those found in margarines and manufactured cooking oils. Consuming this type of fatty acid can increase the risk of **atherosclerosis**.

transient microbes: Microbes that enter the body through dietary sources. They do their work, then leave through the stool. They work alongside native microbes.

type 1 diabetes: An **autoimmune** disease that is often the result of the immune system attacking the pancreas. The beta cells of the pancreas can no longer produce **insulin**. Also known as juvenile diabetes or insulin-dependent diabetes.

type 2 diabetes: A long-term metabolic disorder that is characterized by high blood sugar, **insulin resistance**, and the reduced ability of the beta cells of the pancreas to produce adequate amounts of **insulin** to control blood sugar levels. Also known as diabetes mellitus type 2.

vitamins: Organic compounds that are necessary for life. They are required in smaller quantities in the body than **macronutrients** like **fat**, **protein**, and **carbohydrates**.

REFERENCES

INTRODUCTION

[1] "Vitamin D Deficiency," reviewed by Christine Mikstas, RD, LD, last modified on May 16, 2018, accessed June 1, 2018, www.webmd.com/diet/guide/vitamin-d-deficiency.

CHAPTER 1

[1] Beth Hoffman, "Behind the Brands: Food Justice and the 'Big 10' Food and Beverage Companies," Behind the Brands website, February 26, 2013, accessed June 4, 2018, www.behindthebrands.org/images/media/Download-files/bp166-behind-brands-260213-en.pdf, www.forbes.com/sites/bethhoffman/2013/02/26/who-owns-your-favorite-food-brands.

[2] Craig Elmets, "How Much Sunlight Is Equivalent to Vitamin D Supplementation?" *Journal of American Academy of Dermatology* 62, no. 6 (2010): 935, www.jwatch.org/jd201006040000002/2010/06/04/how-much-sunlight-equivalent-vitamin-d.

CHAPTER 2

[1] Param Dedhia, "Integrative Approaches to Health and Performance," presentation from Live Nourished: The Nutritional Therapy Association Conference 2018, Vancouver, WA, March 2018, www.nutritionaltherapyconference.com/wp-content/uploads/2018/03/1-Dedia.pdf.

[2] Ritamarie Loscalzo, "Nutrigenomics in Action: Using the Power of Food to Optimize Gene Expression," presentation from Live Nourished: The Nutritional Therapy Association Conference 2018, Vancouver, WA, March 2018, www.nutritionaltherapyconference.com/wp-content/uploads/2018/03/3-Loscalzo-1.pdf.

[3] Merriam-Webster Online, s.v. "nutrition," accessed June 4, 2018, www.merriam-webster.com/dictionary/nutrition.

[4] Keesha Ewers, "From Sabotage to Success in Business, Love and Health: The Psychology of Nourishment," presentation from Live Nourished: The Nutritional Therapy Association Conference 2018, Vancouver, WA, March 2018, www.nutritionaltherapyconference.com/wp-content/uploads/2018/03/2-Ewars-1.pdf.

CHAPTER 3

[1] Weston A. Price, *Nutrition and Physical Degeneration,* Eighth Edition (Lemon Grove, California: Price-Pottenger Nutrition Foundation, 2009).

[2] Francis Pottenger, *Pottenger's Cats: A Study in Nutrition,* Second Edition (Lemon Grove, CA: Price-Pottenger Nutrition Foundation, 1995).

[3] Sarah Pope, "Proper Preparation of Grains and Legumes," video on The Weston A. Price Foundation website, September 19, 2011, www.westonaprice.org/proper-preparation-of-grains-and-legumes-video-by-sarah-pope/.

[4] Darryl Edwards, Primal Play website, www.primalplay.com.

[5] Anthony Wayne and Lawrence Newell, "The Hidden Hazards of Microwave Cooking," accessed July 26, 2018, https://pdfs.semantic-scholar.org/53a1/d37f97fb2115db9fbe449793fd6897235cc5.pdf.

[6] "Are Microwave Ovens a Source of Danger?" *The Journal of Natural Science* 1, no. 2, offprint (2002): 2–12, www.naturalscience.org/wp-content/uploads/2015/01/wfns_special-report_microwave_02-02_english.pdf.

[7] Amy Morin, "Scientifically Proven Benefits of Gratitude," *Psychology Today* website, April 3, 2015, accessed July 16, 2018, www.psychologytoday.com/us/blog/what-mentally-strong-people-dont-do/201504/7-scientifically-proven-benefits-gratitude.

[8] Keesha Ewers, "From Sabotage to Success in Business, Love and Health: The Psychology of Nourishment," presentation from Live Nourished: The Nutritional Therapy Association Conference 2018, Vancouver, WA, March 2018, www.nutritionaltherapyconference.com/wp-content/uploads/2018/03/2-Ewers-1.pdf.

CHAPTER 4

[1] Param Dedhia, "Integrative Approaches to Health and Performance," presentation from Live Nourished: The Nutritional Therapy Association Conference 2018, Vancouver, WA, March 2018, www.nutritionaltherapyconference.com/wp-content/uploads/2018/03/1-Dedia.pdf.

[2] John Yudkin, *Pure, White, and Deadly: How Sugar Is Killing Us and What We Can Do to Stop It* (New York: Penguin Group, 2012).

[3] Cristin Kearns, Laura Schmidt, and Stanton Glantz, "Sugar Industry and Coronary Heart Disease Research: A Historical Analysis of Internal Industry Documents," *JAMA Internal Medicine* 176, no. 11 (2016): 1680–85, https://jamanetwork.com/journals/jamainternalmedicine/article-abstract/2548255.

[4] Anahad O'Connor, "How the Sugar Industry Shifted Blame to Fat," *New York Times,* September 12, 2016, accessed July 20, 2018, www.nytimes.com/2016/09/13/well/eat/how-the-sugar-industry-shifted-blame-to-fat.html.

[5] "Food Pyramid," Viral Rang website, November 24, 2016, accessed July 20, 2018, https://viralrang.com/food-pyramid/.

[6] MyPlate, last updated May 11, 2017, accessed June 7, 2018, https://choosemyplate-prod.azureedge.net/sites/default/files/myplate/myplate_green1.jpg.

[7] Nina Teicholz, *The Big Fat Surprise: Why Butter, Meat & Cheese Belong in a Healthy Diet* (New York: Simon & Schuster, Inc., 2014).

[8] Cheryl Fryar, Margaret Carroll, and Cynthia Ogden, "Prevalence of Overweight, Obesity, and Extreme Obesity Among Adults: United States, Trends 1960–1962 Through 2009–2010," U.S. Centers for Disease Control and Prevention website, National Center for Health Statistics, accessed June 12, 2018, www.cdc.gov/nchs/data/hestat/obesity_adult_09_10/obesity_adult_09_10.htm.

[9] Daisy Whitbread, "Top 10 Foods Highest in Saturated Fat," My Food Data website, accessed June 8, 2018, www.myfooddata.com/articles/foods-highest-in-saturated-fat.php.

[10] "Facts About Monounsaturated Fats," MedlinePlus website, updated April 24, 2016, accessed June 8, 2018, https://medlineplus.gov/ency/patientinstructions/000785.htm.

11 "Facts About Polyunsaturated Fats," MedlinePlus website, updated April 24, 2016, accessed June 8, 2018, https://medlineplus.gov/ency/patientinstructions/000747.htm.

12 Elizabeth Brown, "Foods High in Linoleic Acid," SFGate website, updated June 30, 2017, accessed June 8, 2018, http://healthyeating.sfgate.com/foods-high-linoleic-acid-9573.html.

13 "15 Omega-3 Foods Your Body Needs Now," Dr. Axe website, accessed June 8, 2018, https://draxe.com/omega-3-foods/.

14 Clay McKnight, "Why Is Hydrogenated Oil Bad for You?" LIVESTRONG website, October 3, 2017, accessed June 8, 2018, www.livestrong.com/article/272066-why-is-hydrogenated-oil-bad-for-you/.

15 Jimmy Moore and Eric Westman, *Cholesterol Clarity: What the HDL Is Wrong with My Numbers?* (Las Vegas, NV: Victory Belt Publishing, 2013).

CHAPTER 5

1 Maia Appleby, "List of the 22 Known Amino Acids," The Nest website, accessed June 8, 2018, https://woman.thenest.com/list-22-known-amino-acids-10296.html.

2 Sally Fallon and Mary Enig, *Nourishing Traditions: The Cookbook That Challenges Politically Correct Nutrition and Diet Dictocrats* (Washington, DC: NewTrends Publishing, 2001).

CHAPTER 6

1 "Types of Sugar," IvyRose Holistic website, accessed June 11, 2018, www.ivyroses.com/HumanBiology/Nutrition//Types-of-Sugar.php.

CHAPTER 7

1 Madlen Davies, "The Hiker Who Died from Drinking TOO MUCH Water: Excess Fluid and Lack of Food Caused Her Brain to Fatally Swell," DailyMail.com, October 5, 2015, accessed June 11, 2018, www.dailymail.co.uk/health/article-3260684/The-hiker-died-drinking-water-Excess-fluid-lack-food-caused-brain-fatally-swell.html.

2 Lianna Roth Hursh, "9 Signs You're Drinking Too Much Water," *Reader's Digest* online, accessed June 11, 2018, www.rd.com/health/wellness/drinking-too-much-water/.

3 Fereydoon Batmanghelidj, *Your Body's Many Cries for Water* (Falls Church, VA: Global Health Solutions, Inc., 2008).

CHAPTER 8

1 "The pH Scale," Talk2Bio website, accessed June 14, 2018, http://talk2bio.com/the-ph-scale/.

2 Monica Reinagel, "How Birth Control Pills Affect Your Nutritional Needs," *Scientific American* website, September 23, 2015, accessed June 14, 2018, www.scientificamerican.com/article/how-birth-control-pills-affect-your-nutritional-needs/.

3 M. Palmery, A. Saraceno, A. Vaiarelli, and G. Carlomagno, "Oral Contraceptives and Changes in Nutritional Requirements," *European Review for Medical and Pharmacological Sciences* 17, no. 13 (2013): 1804–13, www.ncbi.nlm.nih.gov/m/pubmed/23852908/.

4 James DiNicolantonio, *The Salt Fix: Why the Experts Got It All Wrong and How Eating More Might Save Your Life* (New York: Harmony Books, 2017).

CHAPTER 9

1 Julius Goepp, "Vitamin K's Delicate Balancing Act," Life Extension website, April 2006, accessed June 19, 2018, www.lifeextension.com/Magazine/2006/4/report_vitamink/Page-01.

2 Sally Fallon and Mary Enig, *Nourishing Traditions: The Cookbook That Challenges Politically Correct Nutrition and Diet Dictocrats* (Washington, DC: NewTrends Publishing, 2001).

3 Teodoro Bottiglieri, "S-Adenosyl-L-Methionine (SAMe): From the Bench to the Bedside—Molecular Basis of a Pleiotrophic Molecule," *The American Journal of Clinical Nutrition* 75, no. 5 (2002): 1151S–57S, https://academic.oup.com/ajcn/article/76/5/1151S/4824259.

4 Ritamarie Loscalzo, "Nutrigenomics in Action: Using the Power of Food to Optimize Gene Expression," presentation from Live Nourished: The Nutritional Therapy Association Conference 2018, Vancouver, WA, March 2018, www.nutritionaltherapyconference.com/wp-content/uploads/2018/03/3-Loscalzo-1.pdf.

CHAPTER 10

1 Jennifer Russo, "List of Good Bacteria," LIVESTRONG website, August 14, 2017, accessed June 21, 2018, www.livestrong.com/article/26093-list-good-bacteria/.

2 Jonathan Wright and Lane Lenard, *Why Stomach Acid Is Good for You* (Lanham, MD: M. Evans, 2001).

3 George Goodheart, "The Acid-Alkaline Balance and Patient Management," *Digest of Chiropractic Economics,* September/October 1962, accessed on July 26, 2018, www.seleneriverpress.com/historical/acid-alkaline-balance-and-patient-management/.

CHAPTER 11

1 Michael Pollan, *The Omnivore's Dilemma: A Natural History of Four Meals* (London: Bloomsbury Publishing, PLC, 2006).

2 Adam Nally and Jimmy Moore, *The Keto Cure: A Low-Carb, High-Fat Dietary Solution to Heal Your Body and Optimize Your Health* (Las Vegas, NV: Victory Belt Publishing, 2018).

3 Natasha Campbell-McBride, *Put Your Heart in Your Mouth* (White River Junction, VT: Medinform Publishing, 2016).

4 U.S. Centers for Disease Control, "New CDC Report: More Than 100 Million Americans Have Diabetes or Prediabetes," CDC press release, July 18, 2017, www.cdc.gov/media/releases/2017/p0718-diabetes-report.html.

5 World Health Organization, *Global Report on Diabetes* (Geneva, Switzerland: World Health Organization, 2016).

CHAPTER 12

1 James Wilson, *Adrenal Fatigue: The 21st Century Syndrome* (Petaluma, CA: Smart Publications, 2001).

2 "Food Intolerance Fact Sheet," Food Intolerance Network website, updated August 2006, accessed June 26, 2018, https://fedup.com.au/factsheets/additive-and-natural-chemical-factsheets/amines.

3 "Peptides & Proteins," Michigan State University Department of Chemistry website, William Reusch faculty page, updated May 5, 2013, accessed June 26, 2018, www2.chemistry.msu.edu/faculty/reusch/virttxtjml/protein2.htm.

4 "Medical Definition of Prostaglandin," MedicineNet.com website, updated May 13, 2016, accessed June 26, 2018, www.medicinenet.com/script/main/art.asp?articlekey=16461.

5 "Medical Definition of Thromboxane," MedicineNet.com website, updated May 13, 2016, accessed June 26, 2018, www.medicinenet.com/script/main/art.asp?articlekey=32482.

6 J. N. Sharma and L. A. Mohammed, "The Role of Leukotrienes in the Pathophysiology of Inflammatory Disorders: Is There a Case for Revisiting Leukotrienes as Therapeutic Targets?" *Inflammopharmacology* 14, no. 1–2 (2006): 10–16, www.ncbi.nlm.nih.gov/pubmed/16835707.

CHAPTER 13

1 Jason Fung and Jimmy Moore, *The Complete Guide to Fasting: Heal Your Body Through Intermittent, Alternate-Day, and Extended Fasting* (Las Vegas, NV: Victory Belt Publishing, 2016).

2 Nithya Shrikant, "Top 10 Health Benefits of Diaphoretic Herbs," Instah website, March 19, 2017, accessed June 28, 2018, www.instah.com/herbs/health-benefits-of-diaphoretic-herbs/.

3 "About Oil Pulling," Innovative Medicine website, accessed June 28, 2018, https://innovativemedicine.com/solutions/oil-pulling/.

GLOSSARY

1 Param Dedhia, "Integrative Approaches to Health and Performance," presentation from Live Nourished: The Nutritional Therapy Association Conference 2018, Vancouver, WA, March 2018, www.nutritionaltherapyconference.com/wp-content/uploads/2018/03/1-Dedia.pdf.

RECIPE INDEX

BREAKFAST

276 Strawberries and Cream Smoothie

277 Pumpkin Smoothie

278 Pecan Pie Waffles

280 Baked Eggs with Corned Beef and Sauerkraut Hash

282 Spring Dutch Baby

284 No-Bake Mini Breakfast Cheesecakes

286 Glazed Cinnamon Fritters

287 Breakfast Cobbler

288 Denver Omelet

SALADS & SIDES

   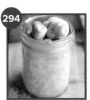 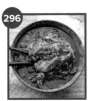

290 Roast Beef Salad Kabobs

291 Cobb Salad Stacks

292 Greek Cucumber Salad

294 Sauerkraut

296 Kimchi

298 Quick Asian Fermented Cucumbers

299 Daikon Noodles

     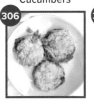

300 Purple Cauliflower Mash

301 Bacon-Wrapped Asparagus

302 Bloody Mary Tomatoes

303 Fried Zucchini Blossoms

304 Fauxtatoes au Gratin

306 Cauliflower Patties

308 Kimchi Deviled Eggs

309 Hot Reuben Dip

310 Guacamole

MAINS

 312
Easy Chicken
Fried Rice

 314
Chinese Chicken
and Broccoli Soup

 316
Kimchi Burgers

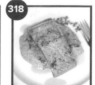 318
Broiled Salmon

 320
Spanakopita

 322
Reuben Sliders

 324
Hearty Chicken
Asparagus Salad

 326
Mexican
Tenderloin

 328
One-Pot
Pizza-Roni

 329
Easy
Cobb-Stuffed
Avocados

DESSERTS & DRINKS

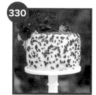 330
Maple Bacon
Apple Cake

 332
Chocolate
Almond
Bûche de Noël

 334
Chocolate
Raspberry Ice
Pops

 335
Strawberry
Cheesecake
Ice Pops

 336
Almond Joyful
Fat Bombs

 337
Almond Brittle

 338
Chocolate
Almond
Whoopie Pies

 340
Keto Eggnog

 341
Eggnog Latte

 342
Kombucha

BASICS

 344
Beef, Chicken, or
Fish Bone Broth

 345
Almond Milk

 346
Easy Mayo

 347
Ranch Dressing

 348
The Best Blue
Cheese Dressing

 349
Thousand Island
Dressing

 350
Taco Seasoning

ALLERGEN INDEX

RECIPES	PAGE	DAIRY-FREE	EGG-FREE	NUT-FREE
Strawberries and Cream Smoothie	276		✓	
Pumpkin Smoothie	277		✓	
Pecan Pie Waffles	278	✓		
Baked Eggs with Corned Beef and Sauerkraut Hash	280			✓
Spring Dutch Baby	282			O
No-Bake Mini Breakfast Cheesecakes	284		✓	
Glazed Cinnamon Fritters	286	✓		O
Breakfast Cobbler	287			
Denver Omelet	288			✓
Roast Beef Salad Kabobs	290			✓
Cobb Salad Stacks	291			✓
Greek Cucumber Salad	292	O	✓	✓
Sauerkraut	294	✓	✓	✓
Kimchi	296	✓	✓	✓
Quick Asian Fermented Cucumbers	298	✓	✓	✓
Daikon Noodles	299	✓	✓	✓
Purple Cauliflower Mash	300		✓	✓
Bacon-Wrapped Asparagus	301		✓	✓
Bloody Mary Tomatoes	302	✓	✓	✓
Fried Zucchini Blossoms	303			✓
Fauxtatoes au Gratin	304		✓	✓
Cauliflower Patties	306			
Kimchi Deviled Eggs	308	✓		✓
Hot Reuben Dip	309		✓	✓
Guacamole	310	✓	✓	✓
Easy Chicken Fried Rice	312	✓		
Chinese Chicken and Broccoli Soup	314	O	✓	✓
Kimchi Burgers	316	✓		✓
Broiled Salmon	318	O	✓	✓
Spanakopita	320			
Reuben Sliders	322	O		✓
Hearty Chicken Asparagus Salad	324			✓
Mexican Tenderloin	326	✓	✓	✓
One-Pot Pizza-Roni	328		✓	✓
Easy Cobb-Stuffed Avocados	329			✓
Maple Bacon Apple Cake	330			
Chocolate Almond Bûche de Noël	332			
Chocolate Raspberry Ice Pops	334	O	✓	
Strawberry Cheesecake Ice Pops	335		✓	
Almond Joyful Fat Bombs	336	✓	✓	
Almond Brittle	337		✓	
Chocolate Almond Whoopie Pies	338			
Keto Eggnog	340	✓		
Eggnog Latte	341	✓		
Kombucha	342	✓	✓	✓
Beef, Chicken, or Fish Bone Broth	344	✓	✓	✓
Almond Milk	345	✓	✓	
Easy Mayo	346	✓		✓
Ranch Dressing	347		✓	✓
The Best Blue Cheese Dressing	348		✓	✓
Thousand Island Dressing	349	✓		✓
Taco Seasoning	350	✓	✓	✓

GENERAL INDEX

hormone replacement therapy (HRT), 147
hormones
  bioidentical, 147
  blood sugar and imbalances in, 217
  fat-soluble, 240–242
  produced by endocrine system, 240–242
  water-soluble, 240–242
hot and cold towel therapy, 261
Hot Reuben Dip recipe, 309
HRT (hormone replacement therapy), 147
human growth hormone (HGH), 100, 234
hunger control, fats and, 78–79
hydration, 129–130, 259
hydrochloric acid (HCL), 142, 186, 187, 191–192
hydrogenated oils/foods, 62, 88–89, 363
hydrogenation, 60, 88–89
hyperactivity, 148
hypercalciuria, 101
hyperchloremia, 149
hyperglycemia, blood sugar and, 219
hyperthyroidism, 237, 363
hypochlorhydria, 154
  causes of, 201–203
  signs of, 204
hypoglycemia, 153, 218–219
hyponatremia, 120
hypothalamus, 234, 239
hypothyroidism, 150, 236–237, 363

I

ICSH (interstitial cell-stimulating hormone), 235
IGF-1 hormone, 101
immune function
  accessory nutrients and, 178
  blood sugar and, 223–224
  fats and, 81
  minerals and, 138
  water and, 124
  zinc and, 154
immunoglobulins, 100
impaired growth, 151
infection, 149, 177
inflammation, fats and, 81, 83
ingestion, in digestion, 185
inositol
  deficiencies in, 173
  food sources for, 357

insect repellent, 163
insoluble fiber, 197
insomnia, 148
insulin, 214–215, 363
insulin resistance (IR), 26–27, 106–107, 214, 219, 363
intermedin, 235
interstitial cell-stimulating hormone (ICSH), 235
inulin, 109, 161, 172, 357
iodine, 44, 139, 141, 144, 150, 236–237, 239, 355
iron, 44, 141, 144, 150, 355
irregular breathing, 151
irritability, 151
Islamic traditions for detoxification, 253
isoleucine, 44, 99
Italian sausage
  One-Pot Pizza-Roni, 328

J

Jerusalem artichokes, for digestion, 205
jet lag, 177
Jewish traditions for detoxification, 252
joint pain, 177

K

kale
  for blood sugar regulation, 226
  for digestion, 205
kefir, 114, 206
Keto (Emmerich and Emmerich), 359
keto, reasons for, 32–36
Keto Clarity (Moore and Westman), 8, 26, 32, 36, 359
Keto Comfort Foods (Emmerich), 359
Keto Connect (website), 359
Keto Eggnog recipe, 340
  Eggnog Latte, 341
Keto Essentials: 150 Ketogenic Recipes to Revitalize, Heal, and Shed Weight (Spina), 359
keto flu, 135, 136
Keto Living (website), 93, 163
Keto Made Easy (Barot and Gaedke), 359
Keto Restaurant Favorites (Emmerich), 359
Keto Talk with Jimmy Moore & Dr. Will Cole (podcast), 8
Keto Vitals (website), 121, 136
ketoacidosis, vs. nutritional ketosis, 128
The Ketogenic Cookbook (Moore and Emmerich), 8, 26, 359
The KetoHacking MD Podcast, 8, 221